T0198204

Practice Management

Editor

PETER WEINSTEIN

VETERINARY CLINICS
OF NORTH AMERICA:
SMALL ANIMAL PRACTICE

www.vetsmall.theclinics.com

March 2024 • Volume 54 • Number 2

ELSEVIER

1600 John F. Kennedy Boulevard ● Suite 1800 ● Philadelphia, Pennsylvania, 19103-2899

http://www.vetsmall.theclinics.com

VETERINARY CLINICS OF NORTH AMERICA: SMALL ANIMAL PRACTICE Volume 54, Number 2
March 2024 ISSN 0195-5616, ISBN-13: 978-0-443-13145-5

Editor: Stacy Eastman

Developmental Editor: Varun Gopal

Veterinary Clinics of North America: Small Animal Practice (ISSN 0195-5616) is published bimonthly by Elsevier Inc., 360 Park Avenue South, New York, NY 10010-1710. Months of issue are January, March, May, July, September, and November. Business and Editorial Offices: 1600 John F. Kennedy Blvd., Ste. 1800, Philadelphia, PA 19103-2899. Customer Service Office: 3251 Riverport Lane, Maryland Heights, MO 63043. Periodicals postage paid at New York, NY and additional mailing offices. Subscription prices are $391.00 per year (domestic individuals), $100.00 per year (domestic students/residents), $503.00 per year (Canadian individuals), $544.00 per year (international individuals), $100.00 per year (Canadian students/residents), and $220.00 per year (international students/residents). For institutional access pricing please contact Customer Service via the contact information below. To receive student/resident rate, orders must be accompanied by name of affiliated institution, date of term, and the *signature* of program/residency coordinator on institution letterhead. Orders will be billed at individual rate until proof of status is received. Foreign air speed delivery is included in all *Clinics* subscription prices. All prices are subject to change without notice. **POSTMASTER:** Send address changes to *Veterinary Clinics of North America: Small Animal Practice*, Elsevier Health Sciences Division, Subscription Customer Service, 3251 Riverport Lane, Maryland Heights, MO 63043. Customer Service (orders, claims, online, change of address): Elsevier Periodicals Customer Service, Elsevier Health Sciences Division Subscription **Customer Service 3251 Riverport Lane Maryland Heights, MO 63043. Tel: 1-800-654-2452 (U.S. and Canada); 314-447-8871 (outside U.S. and Canada). Fax: 314-447-8029. E-mail: journalscustomerservice-usa@elsevier.com (for print support); journalsonlinesupport-usa@elsevier.com (for online support).**

Reprints. For copies of 100 or more of articles in this publication, please contact the Commercial Reprints Department, Elsevier Inc., 360 Park Avenue South, New York, NY 10010-1710. Tel.: 212-633-3874; Fax: 212-633-3820; E-mail: reprints@elsevier.com.

Veterinary Clinics of North America: Small Animal Practice is also published in Japanese by Inter Zoo Publishing Co., Ltd., Aoyama Crystal-Bldg 5F, 3-5-12 Kitaaoyama, Minato-ku, Tokyo 107-0061, Japan.

Veterinary Clinics of North America: Small Animal Practice is covered in *Current Contents/Agriculture, Biology and Environmental Sciences, Science Citation Index, ASCA, MEDLINE/PubMed (Index Medicus), Excerpta Medica,* and *BIOSIS.*

Contributors

EDITOR

PETER WEINSTEIN, DVM, MBA
President, PAW Consulting, Simple Solutions 4 Vets, Inc, Irvine, California, USA

AUTHORS

LOWELL ACKERMAN, DVM, MBA, MPA, CVA, MRCVS
Diplomate, American College of Veterinary Dermatology (Emeritus); Global Veterinary
Consultant, Author and Lecturer, Westborough, Massachusetts, USA

JULES BENSON, BVSc, MRCVS
Chief Veterinary Officer, Nationwide Mutual Insurance Company, Nationwide Insurance
(Pet), Columbus, Ohio, USA

ROBIN BROGDON, MA
Owner/CEO BluePrints Veterinary Marketing Group, Huntington Beach, California, USA

ADAM CHRISTMAN, DVM, MBA
Chief Veterinary Officer, dvm360 & Fetch Conferences

RICHARD M. DEBOWES, DVM, MS
Diplomate, American College of Veterinary Surgeons; Professor of Surgery, Clinical
Communication, Leadership and Practice Management, Washington State College of
Veterinary Medicine, Pullman, Washington, USA

CAITLIN DEWILDE, DVM
Founder, The Social DVM, LLC, St Louis, Missouri, USA

KAREN E. FELSTED, CPA, MS, DVM, CVPM, CVA
President, PantheraT Veterinary Management Consulting, Richardson, Texas, USA

JENNI GEORGE, BA, CVPM
Co-Owner and Hospital Administrator, Deerfield Veterinary Clinic, Co-Host of
The Veterinary Survival Show Podcast, Deerfield, New Hampshire, USA

LESLIE A. MAMALIS, CVA (Emeritus)
Senior Consultant, Summit Veterinary Advisors, Lakewood, Colorado, USA

NATALIE MARKS, DVM, CVJ
President, MarksDVMConsulting, Chicago, Illinois, USA

DAN MARKWALDER, DVM
Chief Veterinary Officer, Mission Veterinary Partners

DAVE NICOL, BVMS Cert Mgmt MRCVS, CEO
VetX International, MD of Roundwood Vets Ltd, Founder Roundwood Pet Hospice,
Brighton, London, United Kingdom

MONICA DIXON PERRY, BS, CVPM
Director of Veterinary Consulting Services, Burzenski & Co, PC, Mariner's Point, East Haven, Connecticut, USA; Raleigh, North Carolina, USA

HEATHER PRENDERGAST, RVT, CVPM, SPHR
Chief Executive Officer, Synergie Consulting, Las Cruces, New Mexico, USA

MATTHEW SALOIS, PhD
President, Veterinary Management Groups, Johns Creek, Georgia, USA

JEFFREY R. SANFORD, MBA
Director of Financial Literacy and Practice Outreach, University of Georgia College of Veterinary Medicine, Office of Academic Affairs, Athens, Georgia, USA

EMILY M. TINCHER, DVM
Sr. Director of Pet Health, Nationwide Mutual Insurance Company, Nationwide Insurance (Pet), Columbus, Ohio, USA

PETER WEINSTEIN, DVM, MBA
President, PAW Consulting, Simple Solutions 4 Vets, Inc, Irvine, California, USA

Contents

Preface: Veterinary Practice Management   xi

Peter Weinstein

The Economics of Small Animal Veterinary Practice   207

Matthew Salois

> Recent economic cycles and unique factors like the COVID-19 pandemic have all affected small animal veterinary practice, changing both demand and supply-side factors. One-time events exacerbated cyclical macro-economic factors, increasing the highs and worsening the lows. Behind the perceived labor shortage, the mental health concerns, and the challenges of staff turnover in the profession's daily work to meet client expectations and provide the best possible medical care lurks a productivity problem. The good news is that veterinary practices can take steps to improve productivity and resilience in the face of these challenging trends.

The Future of Small Animal Veterinary Practice   223

Lowell Ackerman

> The future may be difficult or even impossible to predict with any accuracy, but appreciating the likely path forward for small animal veterinary practices is possible with some defensible assumptions. With advancements in technology, a growing appreciation of the human–animal bond, and changing societal norms, the role of small animal veterinary teams will become even more important in the years to come. Although there may be challenges, there will also be new opportunities and a greater need for qualified professionals and paraprofessionals in this field, who can deliver services that clients want and pets need.

Cost of Care, Access to Care, and Payment Options in Veterinary Practice   235

Jules Benson and Emily M. Tincher

> Accessing veterinary care is increasingly challenging for US pet families. Although there are many contributing factors, the cost of care presents the greatest challenge. This article explores the ways in which payment options, a spectrum of care approach, and the stratification of care might improve access to care.

The True Benefits of Veterinary Practice Ownership   251

Dan Markwalder

> Many believe that the era of independent veterinary practice ownership is over but evidence suggests that now is a great time to be a practice owner. Corporate consolidation is becoming more prevalent but this presence in the industry provides benefits for independent owners. For those willing to

learn and develop the necessary business skills, practice ownership has numerous advantages, and individuals who decide they want to own their own practice have several routes they can take to reach their goal. The future of veterinary medicine has never been brighter, and now is a wonderful time to invest in yourself.

The Progressive Veterinary Practice   265

Natalie Marks

Veterinary practices must be forward-thinking to effectively serve today's pet owners and move into the future. The progressive practice considers every aspect of a pet owner's journey, from searching for a veterinarian to paying their invoice, and seeks ways to improve their experience. Many tools and methods can be used to reach these goals, while also improving efficiency and veterinary team well-being. Digital tools and artificial intelligence in particular provide significant advances that allow veterinary practices to better serve and build relationships with their clients and patients.

Leadership in Veterinary Practice   277

Dave Nicol

Veterinary practice ownership has long been a financially rewarding option. High time it was an emotionally rewarding one for all concerned, too. This is the gift that strong leaders bestow on those lucky enough to work on their team. If more of us developed these skills, the course of veterinary medicine would change inevitably for the good.

Building a Veterinary Practice Team   293

Monica Dixon Perry

Building a successful veterinary team is foundational and a driving force to having an all-around accomplished veterinary practice, one that provides quality customer service and medical care while being financially healthy and creating an environment for team members to thrive and be happy, highly productive employees. This article focuses on new and innovative approaches to cultivating a practice personality and culture that is employee centered. This article provides a road map to assist in implementing and achieving the next big steps needed to have an employee-focused business. Taking care of employees, unlike ever before, is desperately needed in veterinary practices.

Culture: Building Happier, Healthier Teams and Practices in Veterinary Medicine   307

Jenni George

A positive culture is important to team retention and a successful business. Building a culture is not a fast process, but it is worth the hard work and time. Building up and supporting leaders is necessary to building a good team and a great culture. Team leadership must be courageous and open to communication as it is key to a successful and positive culture. The practice must be a psychologically safe workplace that encourages the team to learn from mistakes and take risks. The team needs to be involved in building and maintaining a great culture.

Optimal Veterinary Team Utilization Leads to Team Retention   317

Heather Prendergast

> Retaining and attracting talent in VetMed has become an increasingly difficult challenge and applies to all roles in the veterinary practice. Culture, leadership, training and development, and full role utilization are key factors in retaining current talent, as well as attracting future team members. These elements must work synergistically together to create an environment that team members do not want to leave while also being able to deliver exceptional patient care (fulfilling each team member's sense of purpose).

Practice (In)Efficiency in Veterinary Medicine: Moving from Chaos to Control   337

Peter Weinstein

> The veterinary profession has long struggled with inefficiency. The challenges of the pandemic and the increase in case load have truly highlighted how significant the in-efficiencies were. By working on more efficient use of the physical plants where veterinary care is delivered; more efficient use of the inventory that is sold; more efficient use of the people that deliver service and care; and more efficient use of systems, processes, and checklists, the veterinary profession can improve its efficiency, its profitability, and even the enjoyment of working in the profession.

The Magic of Customer Service in Veterinary Practice   355

Adam Christman

> Disney sets the bar very high when it comes to customer service and employee engagement. There are many parallels that align with the ways in which we deliver client service in veterinary medicine. This article will share the quality standards that can be easily implemented into every day practice for veterinary professionals. Learning the customer psychographic will empower the veterinary team to exceed client expectations.

Traditional Marketing Is Not Dead in Veterinary Practice   369

Robin Brogdon

> Contrary to popular belief, not only is traditional marketing alive and well but also it is making a comeback. The right marketing mix typically includes a variety of both traditional and digital tactics. By understanding your practice's key differentiators and ideal client, you can target just the right combination of messages to thrive.

Social Media and Digital Marketing for Veterinary Practices   381

Caitlin DeWilde

> This comprehensive article on digital marketing in veterinary medicine guides practice members through the process of developing an effective online presence. Focusing on strategic planning, it explores the importance of understanding the purpose and target audience when implementing a multimodal digital marketing strategy. Specific platforms, like Facebook, Instagram, and others, are examined, alongside email marketing, texting, online review platforms, Web sites, and search engine

optimization. Paid digital advertising, content creation, tracking metrics, and streamlining marketing efforts for efficiency are discussed. This article equips veterinary practices with the necessary knowledge and tools to navigate the digital landscape and optimize marketing endeavors.

Veterinary Practice Profitability: You Have to Measure It to Manage It   395

Karen E. Felsted

There are many actions a practice can take to improve its profitability but the management team must first know what the profitability of the practice actually is. Fortunately, there are multiple resources available to practice owners and managers to get this information. Understanding not only the profitability of the practice but the kinds of factors that lead to this state is critical. Until the practice has an idea of the root causes of the problem, it is difficult to determine what the correct solution is. Fortunately, there are also many resources available to help a practice change and improve.

Building Value for Veterinary Practice Sale   409

Leslie A. Mamalis

This article provides an overview of the factors that lead to veterinary practice value. People do not enter veterinary medicine with the primary goals of owning and operating a small business. However, those who spend their careers in private practice may start or purchase a veterinary practice. To maximize value, the business must be profitable and carry as little risk to a potential buyer as possible. This article discusses the adjustments a professional valuation analyst is likely to make to calculate profits, the elements that measure risk, and how to mitigate that risk to increase value.

Top Veterinary Practice Issues that Negatively Affect Culture, Retention, and Performance   423

Jeffrey R. Sanford and Richard M. DeBowes

With over 70 years of experience and having consulted with nearly 2000 veterinary hospitals in the United States and abroad, this top 10 list has been consistent through the years with some different approaches since the pandemic. Beyond consulting and advising, we teach practice management for veterinary students at Washington State University (Rick) and University of Georgia (Jeff). As a part of the 4th year curriculum, we conduct on-site evaluations for practices where the veterinary students observe appointments, interpret practice and financial data, and make recommendations for improvement to the owners. From these reports, often over 100 pages long and from debrief meetings with owners, we offer the following as our list of the TOP 10challenges we see in practices today. For each issue, we identify the issue, describe common findings, and then suggest some changes that practices can institute to either treat or avoid these issues for their practices.

VETERINARY CLINICS OF NORTH AMERICA: SMALL ANIMAL PRACTICE

FORTHCOMING ISSUES

May 2024
Small Animal Oncology
Craig A. Clifford and Philip J. Bergman, *Editors*

July 2024
Small Animal Endoscopy
Boel A. Fransson, *Editor*

September 2024
Diversity, Equity, and Inclusion in Veterinary Medicine, Part I
Christina V. Tran, *Editor*

RECENT ISSUES

January 2024
Canine and Feline Behavior
Carlo Siracusa, *Editor*

November 2023
Advancements in Companion Animal Cardiology
Joshua A. Stern, *Editor*

September 2023
Small Animal Theriogenology
Bruce W. Christensen, *Editor*

Preface

Veterinary Practice Management

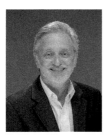

Peter Weinstein, DVM, MBA
Editor

I considered asking ChatGPT to write this preface, but I was afraid they would identify ideas we hadn't even addressed.

For the first time in over 17 years (2006), *Veterinary Clinics of North America: Small Animal Practice* is hosting an issue on Practice Management. As fast as veterinary health care is morphing, so is the business of small animal clinical medicine. The American Pet Products Manufacturers Association (APPMA) reported that spending on veterinary care and services in 2005 was $9.4B[1]; the American Pet Products Association (APPA) reported that in 2022 it was $35.9B.[2]

Rather than looking back at the way things were or the topics covered in the past, the authors were asked to focus on the current needs and future trends of the business of veterinary medicine. The business-scape of the profession reflects global changes in where animals fit into people's lives. It also reflects a philosophic change as our health care field moves more toward a service industry that provides health care. The changes and disruption that the profession is enduring demand a greater and greater need to understand the business of veterinary medicine.

Each of the authors shares their unique background and their own perspective on the various topics that they cover. Trying to cover ALL the issues that are happening is impossible in this issue. In addition, from the time that the articles were commissioned to the time that they are published allows for new tools, new technologies, and new concerns.

On behalf of the entire veterinary profession, I want to extend my appreciation to the contributors. They have worked tirelessly and stressfully to create useful, practical resources for current and future business owners and managers.

Vet Clin Small Anim 54 (2024) xi–xii
https://doi.org/10.1016/j.cvsm.2023.11.001
0195-5616/24/© 2023 Published by Elsevier Inc.

vetsmall.theclinics.com

Finally, to quote Michael E. Gerber in *The E-Myth Revisited* (1995), when it comes to your business, it is time to "work on it, not just in it." With great expectations, I think this tome will be front and center as you work on your business.

Peter Weinstein, DVM, MBA
PAW Consulting
Simple Solutions 4 Vets, Inc
3972 Barranca Parkway
Suite J-137
Irvine, CA 92606, USA

E-mail address:
peterweinsteindvmmba@gmail.com

REFERENCES

1. AVMA. Spending on Pets Projected to Hit All-Time High. Available at: https://www. avma.org/javma-news/2006-08-01/spending-pets-projected-hit-all-time-high. Accessed June 5, 2023.
2. Industry Trends and Stats. Available at: https://www.americanpetproducts.org/ press_industrytrends.asp. Accessed June 5, 2023.

The Economics of Small Animal Veterinary Practice

Matthew Salois, PhD

KEYWORDS

- Veterinary practice • Practice productivity • Veterinary labor • Productivity

KEY POINTS

- Recent disruptions in the veterinary market are a result of supply and demand side, cyclical and one-time factors.
- The short-term pent-up demand for veterinary care from the pandemic is decreasing, returning the profession to more familiar levels of growth.
- Decreased labor force participation by veterinarians and staff, the impact of inflation, and staff burnout and turnover can all decrease practice performance, but practice owners can take steps to manage these challenges.
- Increasing veterinary practice productivity provides a triple win, by improving staff retention, relieving hiring pressure, and reducing the cost of care.

INTRODUCTION

Insiders have long considered small animal veterinary practice to be insulated from larger economic forces. Some have even gone so far as to call small animal practice "recession proof."[1] The last few years have shown us how wrong that view can be.

This article discusses how recent economic cycles and unique factors like the COVID-19 pandemic affect small animal veterinary practice. It examines the impact on the demand for veterinary care and veterinary labor and supply-side factors such as labor productivity and labor force participation. It also suggests responses to improve the veterinary practice's resilience in the face of these challenging trends.

DEMAND FOR VETERINARY CARE

The disruption of the COVID years led to unprecedented swings in consumer spending. Consider real personal consumption expenditure per capita or the amount that people actually spend on their personal needs. Although year-on-year growth in this expenditure is usually 2% to 4%, in early 2020 it crashed to −15%, then rebounded in mid-2021 to more than 25%, delivering a tremendous economic shock (**Fig. 1**).[2]

Veterinary Management Groups, 6455 East Johns Crossing, Johns Creek, GA 30097, USA
E-mail address: matt@myvmg.com

Vet Clin Small Anim 54 (2024) 207–221
https://doi.org/10.1016/j.cvsm.2023.10.001
0195-5616/24/© 2023 Elsevier Inc. All rights reserved.

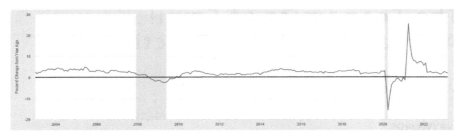

Fig. 1. Real personal consumption expenditures, January 2003 to March 2023. Blue line indicates real personal consumption expenditures. Shaded areas indicate US recessions. (*From* U.S. Bureau of Economic Analysis; fred.stlouisfed.org)

Veterinary revenues mimicked this pattern. After a precipitous drop in early 2020, year-on-year growth in practice revenue began increasing, from 8%, to 11%, finally peaking at nearly 50% in May 2021, as shown in **Fig. 2**.[3]

The bubble was not sustainable; by autumn of 2021, year-on-year revenue growth had dropped to less than 10%, and by the end of 2022 to a more realistic 5.2%, with most revenue growth coming from price increases rather than an increase in the number of visits.[4]

Three temporary or cyclical factors drove this increase in revenue.

Increased Disposable Income

Closed stores and product shortages offered fewer opportunities to buy, whereas government stimulus checks put extra money in peoples' wallets. At one point, the increase in per capita disposable income resulted in an average increase of more than 30% for the typical US household (**Fig. 3**).[5] Some used it to pay down debts or do home improvement projects. Others spent the extra money on their pets.

As the effects of these factors dissipate, the veterinary economy is returning to normal. The trend in disposable income has largely returned to what it was before COVID.[2]

Increased Time Spent at Home

Pet owners at home during lockdowns spent more time with their pets. Many noticed new pet needs, from fancier cat towers to additional veterinary care. In June 2020, fewer than half planned to cut back on pet supplies, despite the uncertainty.[6]

With owners beginning to return to the office, this driver of veterinary purchasing is also slowing.

Pent-Up Demand for Veterinary Care

At the peak of the pandemic, practices simply could not keep up with the increased demand for veterinary services. In 2020, changes to clinic procedures to reduce COVID exposure risks, public health measures, and staff illness meant that the practices saw fewer appointments per day than in previous years.[7]

This created a pent-up demand for veterinary care when the constraints eased. The year 2021 became a year of catching up, clearing the backlog of elective surgeries and overdue vaccinations. The average practice saw two to three more appointments per day in 2021, and on average, clients asked for more services at each visit.[7] This was a short-term surge, not a sustained or structural increase in demand.

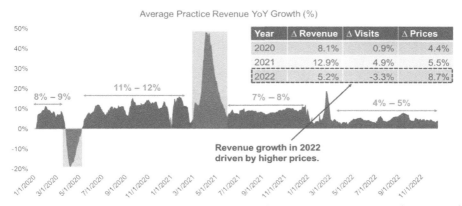

Fig. 2. Average practice revenue, year-on-year growth VetSource industry data. (*Courtesy of Sheri Gilmartin, VetSuccess, USA*).

A False Demand Narrative: The Adoption Boom

Throughout 2020 and 2021, we heard stories of a pet adoption boom: people spending time alone during lockdowns adopting pets for companionship, love, and laughter.[8]

Veterinarians braced themselves for waves of new puppy and kitten visits, parasites, and parvovirus cases. The tsunami did not last. What happened?

Now that the clouds of dog and cat hair have settled, we can look at longer trends. Shelters experienced a surge of dog and cat adoptions in 2019. In 2020, the shelter population dropped by 20,000 dogs and the number of fosters increased by 5000 dogs. But by September 2022, pet adoptions from shelters were lower than those in December 2019, before the pandemic hit.[9] There simply was no prolonged adoption boom.

With income, adoption, and time spent with pets returning to pre-COVID levels, and practices clearing their appointment backlogs, the trend in veterinary revenue growth seems likely to return to levels seen before the pandemic, in the range of 3% to 6% per year.

DEMAND FOR VETERINARY LABOR

The US labor market is on fire. Despite highly publicized (and significant) layoffs at tech companies such as Amazon, Google, and Twitter, job openings remain at an all-time high.[a][10] For the next 10 years, competition for labor will be one of the defining challenges across the US economy, as workers from the Boomer generation retire from the workforce.

Veterinary medicine is no exception. Veterinary job openings ballooned during the 18 months between May 2020 and November 2021 and began stabilizing again in 2022, with many more job openings in corporate practices than before the pandemic (**Fig. 4**).[11]

As competition for the best veterinarians increases, corporate practices in particular are offering signing bonuses, moving allowances, and whatever it takes to win the battle for veterinary talent.[4] Finding and keeping top-performing credentialed veterinary technicians and veterinary assistants is no less of a challenge.[4]

---

[a] Many of the highly publicized layoffs are happening in companies and industries that over-hired during 2021. Others are in industries dependent on venture funds. As inflation takes hold and interest rates rise, it becomes more expensive for them to borrow; cutbacks are inevitable.

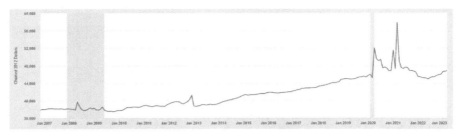

Fig. 3. Real disposable income per capita, January 2007 to March 2023. Blue line indicates real disposable personal income per capita. Shaded areas indicate US recessions. (*From* U.S. Bureau of Economic Analysis; fred.stlouisfed.org)

To react successfully, veterinary practice owners must understand the labor market.

Behind the Demand for Veterinary Labor

Three questions can shed light on the problem of demand for veterinarians.

- *Which practices are doing most of the recruiting?* Corporate practices and consolidators posted more than 2.5 times the number of jobs than did independent practices in mid-2022.[11] Did corporate hiring surge to meet their growth needs? Or have these practices hired too many people?
- *How much quitting happened during this time period?* The so-called Great Resignation affected veterinary medicine too. Pressures from the pandemic made it impossible to ignore the impact of burnout on departure rates in veterinary practice.
- *Are these new jobs or replacement hires?* This is the core question. New jobs indicate growth and expansion. Replacement hires are a signal that something is wrong; practice staff is changing but not growing.

A closer look reveals that much of the apparent demand is from replacement hires and inefficient practices.

VETERINARY PRACTICES ARE IN A RETENTION CRISIS

Even before COVID, veterinary medicine had a much higher rate of turnover than human medicine. The veterinarian turnover rate is twice that of physicians, and the rate of veterinary technician turnover is likewise higher than that of nurses and of veterinarians.[12–14]

TURNOVER

Turnover in a veterinary practice is like feline leukemia virus, weakening practice health year in and year out. If workers are always quitting, the practice is always hiring, retraining, and introducing someone new to the staff and the clients. That's costly, it is time-consuming, and it comes with an additional opportunity cost in the time existing staff could be generating income but are instead hiring and training new colleagues.

WHY ARE VETERINARIANS AND STAFF QUITTING?

In 2022, 40% of veterinarians surveyed told the American Veterinary Medical Association (AVMA) that they were thinking of leaving the profession.[15] The two most-cited reasons were about wellness: issues around mental health (32%) and number of hours required or work–life balance (29.4%).[15]

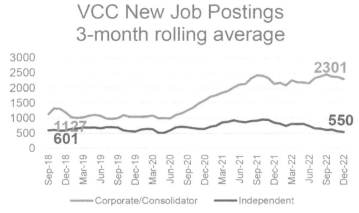

Fig. 4. AVMA veterinary career center new job postings, 3-month rolling average.

Veterinary medicine has a wellness problem, and it is driving employees away in droves!

STAFF BURNOUT IN VETERINARY MEDICINE

Veterinarian and veterinary technician burnout costs veterinary medicine nearly $2 billion annually in lost economic opportunity.[16] Burnt-out colleagues suffer from compassion fatigue, are at greater risk of illness, and are less productive in practice.[16]

As burnout and other mental health issues drive people out of the profession, turnover increases, bringing with it reduced clinic efficiency, staffing gaps, decreased ability to meet client needs, and further stress in the practice.

HIDDEN COSTS OF TURNOVER

Staff turnover drains more than money from a practice. In addition to seeing fewer appointments each day, practices pay hidden costs.

- Recruitment costs: From writing and posting the job advertisement to interviewing and negotiating contracts, recruitment takes time and money.
- Training costs: New staff members need training on processes and systems. Some may need training in particular skills.
- Learning curves: It can take a year for a new hire to fully integrate into a practice. During that time, everyone else has to support them, perhaps interfering with their own work. It is time well spent, but still has a cost.
- Loss of institutional memory: Every staff member who leaves takes with them the little facts that add continuity and improve workflows: from why the examination room is stocked a certain way to how to get the computer software to behave.
- Team culture: Every hire and every departure impact team morale and engagement. Positive and negative emotions are both contagious.
- Damage to the practice brand: The staff is part of every practice's brand. When a well-loved doctor or staff member leaves, clients wonder what is wrong in the practice. Reduced productivity from understaffing also affects a clinic's reputation.
- Loss of client relationships: Veterinary medicine is as much about people as it is about animals and medicine, with veterinarians and staff building close

relationships with clients. When a staff member leaves, the relationship is broken. A client may follow a favorite veterinarian or staff member to another practice.
- Productivity penalty: Understaffed practices are less productive. The practice does not run as efficiently. Everyone works harder, and clients notice a difference as appointments get backed up.
- Staff development disruption: In an understaffing situation, everyone has to pitch in to cover the basics. Agreements made with staff for additional training or development opportunities may have to go on hold, creating more dissatisfaction.
- Decreased satisfaction of remaining staff: Practices often ask remaining staff members to work extra hours when someone leaves. This disrupts lives, raises stress levels, and turns satisfied staff members into flight risks.

High turnover is more than a symptom of employee burnout: It hurts the practice culture, clients, and patients, and ultimately the bottom line.

PRODUCTIVITY

Increased demand for veterinary care will drive more business, and if not handled correctly, also creates more "busyness." That is why productivity is so important.

Productivity is doing more work in less time or taking less time to do the same level of work. Reduced productivity does the opposite.

Imagine training for a marathon by running on a treadmill. You can raise or lower the angle or change the belt speed, but you are still running on a flat surface with relatively little resistance. Now imagine moving that workout from the treadmill to the beach. Suddenly, instead of a flat belt you are running in sand: warm and beautiful, but deep and unstable. You work harder and take longer to run the same distance. The sand has reduced your running productivity.

Headlines about the reduced productivity of American workers are common. The US Bureau of Labor Statistics reported that nonfarm business sector labor productivity decreased 7.3% in the first quarter of 2022, the largest decline in quarterly worker productivity since the third quarter of 1947, when the measure decreased by 11.7%.[17] Even as overall hours worked increased 5.5%, output from the average American worker dropped 2.4%.[18]

At the same time, business unit labor costs—how much an average business pays its workers to produce one unit of output—increased 11.6%, the most since 1982, as hourly compensation increased 3.2%.[19]

Workers were paid more but produced less. Companies had to pay more for the same output. This is the impact of reduced productivity on a business.

When productivity declines in veterinary medicine, a practice cannot handle as many visits in a day as it used to. This was the situation in 2020, when veterinary practices saw nearly 25% fewer patients per hour per full-time equivalent (FTE) veterinarian (**Fig. 5**).[20]

The same principle applies to credentialed veterinary technicians and other staff members. Curb-side appointments require time to greet the client, explain the process, take the pet into the clinic, talk with the owner outside, and bring the pet back.

Compare that to the standard in-person appointment, when the veterinarian or technician can multitask, talking with the owner while conducting parts of the physical examination. Staff work harder to achieve the same outcome or run out of time in the day.

As noted above, turnover also reduces productivity. New team members are not as fast or efficient as those who have been with the practice for years, and burnout will slow anyone down.

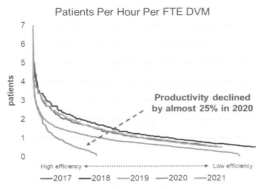

Source: AVMA Census of Veterinarians

Fig. 5. Patients per hour per Doctor of Veterinary Medicine (DVM) FTE. (With permission from the American Veterinary Medical Association (2023 AVMA Economic State of the Veterinary Profession).

Low Productivity Decreases Profitability

Inefficient practices experience a cascade of problems. As productivity spirals down, it brings team morale and engagement down with it. Employees have little interest in resolving problems. Disengaged employees look for new jobs.

Even the busiest employees are not productive if they are doing the wrong work. This is a common complaint of our credentialed veterinary technicians, although highly capable, many are limited to restraining pets, cleaning cages, and drawing up vaccines.

Poor productivity creates ripples of inefficiency, resulting in longer wait times for appointments and surgeries. Pandemic effects led to an extreme form of this backlog, but it will not go away if a practice is still inefficient.

Decreased practice productivity ultimately affects the quality of service a practice provides. Dissatisfied clients and patients vote with their feet, paws, claws, and wings.

Enhancing Practice Productivity

Attention to the productivity of the entire veterinary practice team can go a long way to take a practice from busy and struggling to busy and thriving.

Improving the performance of a nonproductive practice starts with understanding the problem: is there a genuine workforce shortage or a productivity hole? Successful treatment is impossible without the correct diagnosis.

The most efficient veterinary practices see up to 42% more patients per day per FTE veterinarian than their lower efficiency counterparts. This is the difference between a veterinarian seeing 21 patients vs. 12 patients in 1 day. At 5 working days per week that is over 2400 more patients per veterinarian per year.

According to an analysis by the AVMA, if 10,000 practices in the United States moved from low to high efficiency, the labor shortage would decrease by 3633 FTE veterinarians, 7838 FTE credentialed veterinary technicians and veterinary assistants, and 7133 FTE nonmedical staff (**Fig. 6**).[21]

Improving productivity is thus a large part of relieving veterinary medicine's perceived labor shortage.

To be clear, productivity is not about spending as little time as possible with each patient; this is not good veterinary care. Productivity is about making every moment spent with the patient count: leveraging each staff member's knowledge and skills,

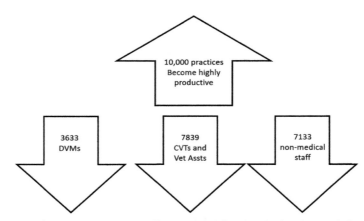

Fig. 6. Impact of improving practice efficiency on labor needs. (With permission from the American Veterinary Medical Association (2023 AVMA Economic State of the Veterinary Profession).)

so that each patient gets the care and attention they deserve while allowing the practice to meet its financial goals.

Moreover, improved productivity does not mean that business squeezes every ounce of output and effort from employees, leaving them exhausted. On the contrary, efforts to improve productivity should have the opposite effect, making it easier for employees to perform at their best and feel better about their work.

LABOR FORCE PARTICIPATION

Burnout, work–life balance, and other aspects of well-being are driving veterinarians away from practice. Although COVID might have accelerated the trend, more people have been leaving the US workforce than joining it for about 20 years.[22]

The Baby Boom generation began aging out of the workforce before the pandemic. Since they were born over a period of about 20 years, they were expected to leave work over a similar interval.

COVID generated an acute exit from the workforce by Baby Boomers and members of younger generations, too. Why?

Several factors contributed.

- Lack of affordable childcare, making it more expensive to work than to stay home and look after the children.
- The availability of stimulus payments and extended unemployment benefits during the pandemic, which provided a viable short-term option to working.
- Growing frustration that is leading workers to push back on employers and reject "the way it's always been" for the employed workforce.

New veterinarians have different career expectations. The old model of the individually owned practice is no longer every veterinarian's dream. New veterinarians value their lives outside of work and want time for their mental and physical health, families, and other interests. This does not make them any less dedicated as veterinarians, but it is changing the profession.

Regardless of the reason, the labor force participation rate is lower than before the pandemic; many workers who dropped out are not returning. The US economy needs about 2.5 million new workers just to get back to the pre-pandemic trend line.[23,24] Although we have enough people in our population, too few are either willing or able to enter the labor force. This has led to a record 12 million job openings across the economy.[10]

An Exodus of Veterinarians

Nearly 3000 veterinarians left veterinary medicine in 2021.[12] It is as if an entire national graduating class of veterinarians said "no thanks" to practice. After so much time, money, and energy spent on becoming qualified veterinarians, why are they opting out?

Overwork and burnout are major culprits. Veterinarians are working more each week. Between 2019 and 2022, the median number of veterinary work hours increased by 5 hours, to 45 per week.[15] Half of veterinarians work more than this, and it is not what they want.

In a 2022 survey, 24% of veterinarians indicated that they wanted to work fewer hours and would accept less compensation to do so.[15] These veterinarians are saying, in effect, "it's too much." The reality of veterinary practice does not match the expectations and wishes of members of the profession.

Bridging the Participation Gap: Myths and Opportunities

Practices need more people working more hours, but veterinarians want to work less. What is the solution?

Some segments of the veterinary world are calling for more veterinary schools and expanded class sizes, turning out more veterinarians.[25] This approach will add more veterinarians, but not for several years. Adding more veterinarians to inefficient practices will not solve the problem; it will, however, add to the single largest cost center for every veterinary practice: labor. This will have the unintended consequence of decreasing the affordability of veterinary care.

Other voices are calling for a mid-level practitioner, something equivalent to the nurse practitioner in human medicine.[26] Yet veterinary medicine already has support staff with an advanced skill set: credentialed veterinary technicians. Most of them are woefully underused. Adding another highly trained but underused staff member will not solve the problem.

What will work, and quickly, is improving the productivity of existing staff members, and welcoming back veterinarians who have recently left the profession, on terms that meet both their needs and those of the practice.

LOOKING TO THE FUTURE

Understanding underlying trends helps differentiate between normal business cycles of expansion and contraction and one-off factors, such as stimulus payments and lockdowns, and better prepare for the future.

Although the United States is emerging from the worst of the pandemic, systemic issues in the economy and the profession remain. Wise members of the veterinary profession will consider these when planning their futures.

Does the Recession Label Matter?

Economists, governments, and observers like to comment on whether or not a country's economy is in recession, defined as two consecutive quarters of shrinking gross domestic product (GDP) and a rise in the unemployment rate—or more practically, a time when the economy is not doing well, many people lose their jobs and businesses have trouble making money.

In many ways, whether or not a recession has been officially declared is immaterial. What matters at the level of veterinary practice is the decisions clients make about paying for veterinary care.

The strength of their bond with their pet, their relationship with their veterinarian, and the specific pet and condition in question matter. Most important may be how confident a client feels about their finances, at present and in the near future.

The Impact of Inflation

Inflation is more important for a practice's future financial health than pent-up demand. The Consumer Price Index is now as high as it has been since the 1980s.[27] Much of this is coming from increased prices for food and fuel, items for which it is difficult to economize. As prices rise but incomes do not, people are worse off in real terms.

Practices serving lower and middle-income communities may find themselves particularly affected by these larger economic forces, and by the level of confidence their clients have in the financial future. Even in middle-class households, as many as one in four or one in five dog owners say they cannot afford to take their dog to the veterinarians for care.[28]

In 2021 and 2022, the cost of veterinary care increased in line with overall consumer pricing, but the magnitude of that increase doubled. Between 2020 and early 2021, prices increased by 4.3%; from mid-2021 to 2022, prices increased by 8%. Wages are not keeping up, so households do not have as much money to spend.[27,29]

Your client's money simply does not go as far, and that is as true in the veterinary practice as it is in the supermarket. Pet owners must make difficult decisions about what they can afford to spend on their pets. They may delay some treatments or select less than the gold standard of care. One in five would purchase fewer pet medications if the economy worsens.[30]

The Demographic Drought Will Continue

New generations entering the workforce simply are not as big as the Baby Boom generation. As the Boomers retire, there will be fewer workers available.

The US veterinary labor market will remain tight for the foreseeable future. The demand for veterinarians and veterinary staff will remain, but training more veterinarians and creating another level of practitioner will not solve the problem. Adding people does not fix inefficiency, turnover, or a poor practice culture.

Productivity improvements are faster, easier, and more sustainable and provide a triple win. Improving pay, engagement, and the working environment increases staff retention. More efficient use of existing skilled workers can dramatically ease hiring pressure. Improving productivity also reduces the cost of care, improving affordability for pet owners.

WHAT CAN PRACTICES DO?

Although the macroeconomic trends are outside any practice's control, each practice's responses are not. Practices can take the following steps to improve their economic resilience.

Reduce and Eliminate Debt

In times of economic hardship or financial pressure, cash flow is king. Paying interest on loans adds no value to a practice. Money spent servicing debt is not available for anything else. Talk with your practice's financial advisor about reducing or eliminating any debt held within the practice.

Differentiate and Communicate

What is unique about your practice, and why does that matter to your clients? Find out exactly what brings clients to your practice, rather than the practice up the road. Differentiate your practice based on this unique value, and you will not have to compete on price; your clients will stick with you. Spread the word about what makes your practice special every time you communicate with clients or the community.

Innovate and Simplify

Change is challenging. It is not always easy to figure out a different way to do something you have always done, or to bring in a new technology or service. However, there is no better way to keep your practice relevant, healthy, and growing.

Ask staff members for input: How would they change your workflows or relieve bottlenecks and pain points? Use automations and electronic systems strategically to reduce administrative tasks. Leverage telemedicine within the evolving context of the Veterinarian-Client-Patient Relationship (VCPR). The right innovations can help yours become a high-performing practice.

Optimize Staff Responsibilities

Make the most of every team member's skill and interest. Put the right people in the right roles, with no one over- or under-skilled for their responsibilities. If one of your staff members has a particular interest in nutrition, let them develop and run a series of classes or provide nutrition consultations, reducing the load on a veterinarian and creating a new chargeable service. Staff optimization can increase staff engagement and reduce turnover.

If you're genuinely understaffed, consider different working arrangements to attract employees looking for a nontraditional schedule. Welcome options include split shifts, staggered working hours, part-time veterinarians, and more.

Build and Nurture Relationships

Veterinarians think first about building relationships with clients: they are the profession's reason for being. Clients who value your practice's specific qualities will bond and stay.

Pay equal attention to the culture and relationships within the practice. Your team spends all day together; make it a positive experience. Good relationships among staff create positive ripples, improving well-being, reducing turnover and burnout, and creating a more positive place for clients and patients.

Think about your relationships with your suppliers, with local businesses, and with service organizations like the police. Veterinarians have a long tradition of supporting Little League teams and providing care for K-9 officers. These weave your practice into the fabric of your community.

Build collegial relationships with other practices in your area. Leading and managing a veterinary practice can be lonely; it is good to know you can quickly get a second opinion or support if you need it. Never bad mouth the competition; it is unprofessional and does not reflect well on you.

Competing for Talent

Every practice will have to compete for talent in the tight veterinary labor market. Implementing these best practices will improve your chances of landing the best applicants.

- *Be transparent about the job and benefits:* From the job posting, to interviews, to onboarding, be clear and honest about your practice culture, your expectations, and the pay and benefits you offer. Transparency matters. Be as generous as you can, when hiring staff, you get what you pay for. Go for the best you can afford. The candidate who does not fit also deserves a quick and honest answer.
- *Embrace job freedom and flexibility:* Even in clinical practice, some work can be done from home or during nonstandard hours. Consider using split schedules, part time work, and relief veterinarians under long-term contracts. Encourage staff members and candidates who do not want a traditional schedule to suggest one. Be open to finding win–win solutions.
- *Recruit actively and creatively:* Every conversation is a recruitment opportunity. Always be ready to quickly describe your practice's differentiating factors, your culture, what you look for in a staff member and what you offer. Engage people where they are: Consider setting up a table at a community event or hosting a practice open house.

Easing the Pain from Inflation

Inflation is a major challenge to practice success, and one over which we have no control. Choose your responses to improve your practice's financial performance, no matter how big or small it is.

- *Understand how and when to change prices:* Pricing is both an art and a science. Blanket increases may cause more disruption and client complaints than increasing the cost of specific services. Make sure that your entire staff can discuss pricing honestly and sensitively.
- *Find other ways to reduce cost:* Review inventory turnover. Do you have the right mix of in-house versus prescribed products? Where do you source the products you sell or consume in the practice? Good supplier relationships can make the difference here. Always look for ways to improve practice efficiency, so that you can rely less on price increases to increase profits.
- *Use every opportunity to talk about the cost of care:* Clients understand that the cost of veterinary care is rising. They may not understand what drives those costs, and where the money goes. Although financial discussions can be uncomfortable, they build trust and help clients see the value in your services. Train every staff member to have these discussions; you never know when or where they will come up.
- *Welcome conversations about options along the spectrum of care:* The pet owner who never sees the veterinarian will never benefit from your care, no matter the price. Approximately 15% of pet owners do not visit the veterinarian because of high perceived cost or low perceived value.[28] Offering different levels of care, known as the spectrum of care, can give pets some much-needed medical care and add to practice revenues, but only if you and your staff are willing and able to talk about it.[31]

SUMMARY

The pandemic dramatically disrupted the world of veterinary medicine and indeed the entire world around us. One-time events, such stimulus payments and more shared time between owners and pets, exacerbated a series of cyclical factors like inflation that boosted the highs and depressed the lows.

Is there a labor shortage in veterinary medicine? Probably not, although it can feel that way, with more competition for a talent pool that wants to work less, and too many low-efficiency practices suffering from high staff turnover.

Fixing the productivity problem will make the biggest, most sustainable difference in the least time. Stop the hiring and training churn by making work more attractive, so staff do not burn out and quit. Prepare for systemic changes in the economy by watching trends and responding appropriately. Be flexible when something unexpected happens.

Despite these challenges, the future for the veterinary profession is encouraging. As in medicine, healing from an acute injury takes far longer than the injury itself.

After three strange years, expect the overall economic picture to continue normalizing to something closer to the world before COVID. The natural cycle of veterinary practice will reassert itself. The biggest question is around the impact of inflation, and whether your clients feel that they themselves are suffering from a recession, regardless of what any economist says.

ACKNOWLEDGMENTS

Marne Platt, VMD MBA, for support with writing and editing.

DISCLOSURE

M. Salois is the President of Veterinary Management Groups (VMG), a subsidiary of Covetrus. No other external funding was received in support of this manuscript.

REFERENCES

1. Surviving Recession. Veterinary Practice News Website. Published May 5, 2009. Available at: https://www.veterinarypracticenews.com/surviving-recession. Accessed April 5, 2023.
2. U.S. Bureau of Economic Analysis. Year on Year Percent Change in Personal Consumption Expenditures. Available at: https://fred.stlouisfed.org/series/DPCERO 1Q156NBEA. Accessed April 5, 2023.
3. VetSource. Veterinary Industry Tracker Website. Courtesy Sheri Gilmartin. Available at: https://vetsource.com/resources/veterinary-industry-tracker/.
4. Brakke Consulting. 2022 animal health Industry overview. Orlando, Florida: VMX; 2023.
5. U.S. Bureau of Economic Analysis. Real Disposable Personal Income Per Capita. Available at: https://fred.stlouisfed.org/series/A229RX0#. Accessed April 27, 2023.
6. American Pet Products Association. (2022) COVID-19 Pulse Study: Pet Ownership During the Pandemic. Volume 6, March 2022.
7. Salois, M. Presented at: American Veterinary Medical Association Veterinary Business and Economic Forum. October 14, 2021, online.
8. Erskine Chris. The latest shortage? Dogs and cats, as folks foster and adopt pets during quarantine. The Los Angeles Times; 2020. Available at: https://www.latimes.com/california/story/2020-04-02/requests-to-foster-and-adopt-pets-surge-as-coronavirus-keeps-us-at-home. Accessed April 5, 2023.
9. Petfoodindustry.com. Pandemic new pet boom myth busted; Adoptions lower 2021-22. Available at: https://www.petfoodindustry.com/articles/11748-pandemic-new-pet-boom-myth-busted-adoptions-lower-2021-22. Accessed April 5, 2023.

10. U.S. Bureau of Labor Statistics, Job Openings, Total Non-Farm, 12-01-2001 – 12-01-2022. Available at: https://fred.stlouisfed.org/series/JTSJOL. Accessed April 5, 2023.

11. American Veterinary Medical Association Veterinary Career Center, data courtesy of C. Hansen, personal communication.

12. Hansen, C. Presented at American Veterinary Medical Association Veterinary Business and Economic Forum. October 14, 2021, online.

13. Nursing Solutions Inc. (2022). 2022 NSI Nation Healthcare Retention & RN Staffing Report. March 2022. Available at: https://www.nsinursingsolutions.com/Documents/Library/NSI_National_Health_Care_Retention_Report.pdf. Accessed April 6, 2023.

14. Saley, C (2022). Survey: Nearly half of physicians changed jobs during the pandemic. June 27, 2022. Available at: https://chghealthcare.com/blog/physicians-changed-jobs-survey/. Accessed April 6, 2023.

15. Bain B, Hansen C, Oeddraogo F. (2023) AVMA report on the economic state of the veterinary profession. Schaumberg, IL: American Veterinary Medical Association Economics Decision; 2023.

16. Neill CL, Hansen CR, Salois M. The Economic Cost of Burnout in Veterinary Medicine. Front. Vet Sci. Veterinary Epidemiology and Economics 2022;9:81404. https://doi.org/10.3389/fvets.2022.814104.

17. U.S. Bureau of Labor Statistics. Nonfarm business labor productivity: Output per hour for all workers, January 2012 – October 2022. Available at: https://fred.stlouisfed.org/series/OPHNFB#. Accessed April 27, 2023.

18. U.S. Bureau of Labor Statistics, U.S. Department of Labor, The Economics Daily, Nonfarm business sector labor productivity decreased 7.3 percent in the first quarter of 2022 Published June 9, 2022. Available at: https://www.bls.gov/opub/ted/2022/nonfarm-business-sector-labor-productivity-decreased-7-3-percent-in-the-first-quarter-of-2022.htm. Accessed April 27, 2023.

19. U.S. Bureau of Labor Statistics, Press Release: Productivity and Costs: First quarter 2022, preliminary. Published May 5, 2022. Available at: https://www.bls.gov/news.release/archives/prod2_05052022.pdf. Accessed April 27, 2023.

20. Ouedraogo, F.B. The US Market for Veterinary Services. Presented at: American Veterinary Medical Association Veterinary Business and Economic Forum. October 14-16, 2021, online.

21. Ouedraogo, F.B. Improve Efficiency to Enhance Quality of Services, Increase Access to Animal Healthcare, and Build a Healthier and Stronger Workforce: Insights from 60 Independently Owned Companion-Animal Practices. Presented at: American Veterinary Medical Association Veterinary Business and Economic Forum. October 25, 2022, online.

22. U.S. Bureau of Labor Statistics, Labor Force Participation Rate, January 1, 1998 -February 1, 2023. Available at: https://fred.stlouisfed.org/series/CIVPART. Accessed April 6, 2023.

23. U.S. Bureau of Labor Statistics, Civilian Labor Force Level, January 1, 2011 - February 1, 2023. Available at: https://fred.stlouisfed.org/series/CLF16OV. Accessed April 6, 2023

24. Bain B, Hansen C, Oeddraogo F, et al. AVMA report on economic state of the veterinary profession. Schaumberg, IL: American Veterinary Medical Association; 2021.

25. Smither, S. Veterinaryteambrief.com website "Do we need more veterinary schools?" Published March 2015. Available at: https://files.brief.vet/migration/article/22261/tat_do-we-need-more-veterinary-schools-22261-article.pdf. Accessed April 7, 2023

26. Wugan, Lisa. "Is veterinary medicine ready for a mid-level practitioner?" VIN News Service. Published September 27, 2021. Available at: https://news.vin.com/default.aspx?pid=210&Id=10484775&f5=1. Accessed April 6, 2023
27. Stone K. VetSource Website. Finance. Do you know what your veterinary pricing practices are costing you?. Available at: https://vetsuccess.com/blog/do-you-know-what-your-veterinary-pricing-practices-are-costing-you/Accessed April 27, 2023
28. American Veterinary Medical Association (2022). 2022 AVMA Pet Ownership and Demographics Sourcebook. May 2022.
29. Federal Reserve Bank of Cleveland (2023). Median Consumer Price Index January 1, 1983 – February 1, 2023. Available at: https://fred.stlouisfed.org/series/MEDCPIM 158SFRBCLE. Accessed April 6, 2023
30. American Pet Products Association. (2022) COVID-19 Pulse Study. Pet Ownership During the Pandemic 2022;8.
31. Boatright, K. What is the spectrum of care? American Animal Hospital Association. Published October 28, 2022. Available at: www.aaha.org/publications/new stat/articles/2022-11/what-is-the-spectrum-of-care/. Accessed April 6, 2023

The Future of Small Animal Veterinary Practice

Lowell Ackerman, DVM, DACVD (Emeritus), MBA, MPA, CVA, MRCVS

KEYWORDS

- Pet-specific care • Genetic testing • Pet health insurance • Problem-free pets
- Consistency of care • Personalized medicine

KEY POINTS

- Pet-specific care (personalized medicine) will become more important as pet owners become more aware of its benefits and will expect veterinary practices to be able to provide such services.
- Pet owners will take a more active role in the care of their pets, with the goal of trying to raise problem-free pets, as much as possible.
- Access to care, and spectrum of care, will be important concepts for pet owners and veterinary teams.
- Consistency of care will become important to veterinary practices as they hope to be able to deliver an assured level of care to their clients.
- The veterinary workplace and its workforce will need to adapt to changing markets, and the veterinary pharmacy model will need to evolve to remain viable and profitable.

INTRODUCTION

Do we require a crystal ball to predict the future of small animal veterinary practice? Or do we need to use super-forecasting tools, time-series analysis, or econometric modeling? Perhaps, but projecting current trends into the future need not be so difficult if we realize that several factors are unlikely to change in the near to intermediate term (**Box 1**).

So, although it is difficult to be precise and there are always risks of unforeseen circumstances and economic shocks (such as the prospects of recession, war, climate change emergencies, or political crises), here are some reasonable predictions for the future of small animal veterinary practice.

EMBRACING PET-SPECIFIC CARE (PERSONALIZED MEDICINE)

In today's small animal veterinary practice, most protocols are species-based, designed in general to accommodate either dogs or cats (or any other species treated

Westborough, MA, USA
E-mail address: Lowell.Ackerman@gmail.com

Vet Clin Small Anim 54 (2024) 223–234
https://doi.org/10.1016/j.cvsm.2023.10.005
0195-5616/24/© 2023 Elsevier Inc. All rights reserved.

> **Box 1**
> **Factors likely to remain consistent in the years ahead**
>
> - Pet lovers will continue to want to bond with animals and share their lives with them.
> - Consumers in general will make spending decisions considering value, not just price.
> - Veterinary medicine, as a profession, will continue to draw those interested in a career working with animals.
> - Although the profession is not recession-proof, it is recession-resistant, and that is likely to continue in the future.
> - Pet owners will be most interested in actions to keep their pets healthy, even more than options for treating those pets when they are not well.

at the practice). However, in human medicine, contemporary models of care tend to focus on the individual based on specific risk factors. It is appreciated that some people come with specific genetic risk factors (eg, family history of heart disease), others might have tendencies based on their lifestyle choices (eg, smoking and alcohol consumption), and yet others may be predisposed to issues based on other preexisting situations (eg, risk of type 2 diabetes mellitus associated with obesity or the risk of certain adverse reactions for patients taking certain medications). This focus on the individual in human medicine is often referred to as personalized medicine, precision medicine, predictive medicine, or genomic medicine. In veterinary medicine, this approach is typically referred to as pet-specific care, lifelong care, or client-centric care.[1]

You might think that veterinary teams already practice pet-specific care with all support tending to be individualized for each patient, but most recommendations are relatively generic in nature, especially when it comes to prevention and early detection. Can all pets reasonably be considered "senior" at 7 years of age, or are there vast differences in anticipated lifespans between a Great Dane and a miniature poodle that should be reflected in such recommendations? Do we think there might be a difference in heart disease risk between a Cavalier King Charles Spaniel and a mixed-breed pet? Is the risk for cardiomyopathy, or polycystic kidney disease, equally distributed across all breeds of cats?

If we believe that pet owners are paying for value in the examination room, then we should probably also be prepared to accept that most owners expect that veterinary teams, as experts in the health care of animals, will counsel them appropriately as to the health care needs of their specific pet.[2] Is it reasonable for an owner to expect that when they pay for a professional evaluation that they are also paying for the team's expertise in apprising them of the specific care, risks, and assessments that would be appropriate for their particular pet, not just a physical examination and routine recommendations? For example, should the owner of an American cocker spaniel expect the veterinary team to be aware of glaucoma risk, and to recommend screening at the appropriate time? Should the owner of a Maine Coon Cat expect that the practice will consider cardiomyopathy risks and make appropriate recommendations? If we begrudgingly answer that clients are indeed entitled to this level of attention, then we need to do more to deliver better pet-specific care.[3]

Predicting that clients will want and expect such pet-specific care is not far-fetched, because many receive that level of care from their own physicians. Many have also experienced routine health risk assessments performed by health care professionals and have come to expect them as a part of personalized medicine. They are prepared to answer questions such as the amount of alcohol they consume, how much they smoke, whether they have a family history of heart disease or cancer, and other such questions that they realize are needed for them to receive personalized recommendations from the medical team. We can do the same for our patients, and at some point in the future, likely in the very near future, clients will come to demand it. If we were to ask many of them, they would likely indicate that they assume that this is happening already on a regular basis during their visits with veterinary teams.

It is not necessary to reinvent the wheel to provide pet-specific care for our patients.[4] Although it would be most convenient if such tools were incorporated into our practice management software, there are excellent resources already available to veterinary teams.[1] Health risk assessments have been created for both dogs and cats, examples are available online, or they can be developed easily with input from the hospital team.

In many cases, we do not have information on the family history of our patients, but breed predisposition can serve as a proxy for identifying individuals that warrant further screening.[5] Although glaucoma screening might have some utility in all pets, there are definitely certain pets at higher risk, in addition to those that demonstrate suggestive clinical signs.

One tool that also might be predicted to increase in utilization when it comes to pet-specific care is genetic testing. Unlike phenotypic testing (blood tests, imaging, and urinalysis, for example) that might reasonably be expected to contribute to a diagnosis, genetic disease testing is meant to help determine risk. So, a pet may have a genetic mutation or marker that indicates it has a heightened risk for developing a condition (eg, cardiomyopathy, glaucoma, and polycystic kidney disease), but it is not a foregone conclusion that the pet will actually experience debilitating aspects of the condition. This is not because the genetic tests are error-prone (far from it), but that it takes more than just a genetic mutation or marker to cause disease; there are often many redundant systems that can keep the potential problem subclinical, some markers may be linked to disease risk but are not causative, and there may be environmental factors that are important in disease expression.[6] There is a colorful phrase sometimes used to illustrate this point, which is "genetics loads the gun, but environment pulls the trigger." The reason why we are eventually likely to perform more genetic testing is that it can help identify risks in pets as early as 1 day of age, results do not vary with age, it can be done in pets that are entirely asymptomatic, and it helps us identify those pets that might be more carefully assessed with more specific tests going forward. For example, a young pet with a genetic marker indicating increased risk for cardiomyopathy will not necessarily develop clinical cardiomyopathy with certainty, but it can definitely be flagged as a potential candidate for more in-depth cardiac screening at the appropriate time. For those not familiar with such laboratory analysis, genetic testing is readily available and quite affordable; a panel of hundreds of genetic tests can be run on a single sample (blood or saliva), typically for about the cost of a set of radiographs.

The nice thing about pet-specific care is that it is valued by clients as being the most appropriate care for their pets. It is also a great conversation starter, and facilitates discussions of prevention, early detection, and management that might otherwise not happen until the pet may already be experiencing problems. It can also be very profitable for practices, and very fulfilling for staff, to focus on keeping pets well rather than waiting for pets to have problems before intervention occurs.[7]

Emphasis on Ways that Pet Owners Can Help Keep Their Pets Problem Free

Although veterinary teams have primarily focused their attention on the diagnosis and treatment of diseases in pets, pet owners instead have focused on the notion of wanting to keep their pets as healthy and happy companions—so-called problem-free or almost perfect pets.[8,9] They adopted their pet as a loving family member with whom to share their lives and not as a work project that demands inconvenience and investment.

The concept of "problem-free" pets is really the flip side of the coin regarding the pet-specific care model, applicable to pet owners. However, for veterinary teams to win over the hearts and minds of tomorrow's pet owners, they will need to acknowledge its importance.

The situation is not unlike any consumer purchase. Whether you buy a car, a computer, or a television, you expect that it will perform as expected for its anticipated lifespan, with minimal inconvenience and few crises. For a car, you expect that you will need to do regular maintenance, oil changes, and other interventions according to a predefined schedule, but if confronted with unexpected issues, at some point the perceived value of that vehicle is diminished. Similarly, you expect your computer to just work as anticipated. You are likely prepared to install security software and back up your files regularly (hopefully on an automated schedule), but unforeseen crashes and glitches can seriously affect your satisfaction with the device. Perhaps not surprisingly, there can be a similar frustration when unsuspecting pet owners need to deal with problems with their pets that nobody told them might reasonably be anticipated. They would benefit from having a "Maintenance Schedule" for their pets and that comes with pet-specific care and promoting the concept of problem-free pets. For an example of a maintenance schedule, please see pet-specific care for the veterinary team.[1]

You might wonder what this has to do with predicting the future, but helping pet owners maintain problem-free pets has not been a priority for the profession but will likely be in the future if veterinary teams hope to play a vital role in this lucrative marketplace. Problem-free pets may be a bit of a misnomer because we can never completely eliminate issues with pets, but it is a worthwhile aspiration for veterinary teams to conceptionally consider what they can do professionally to help pet owners get the most enjoyment possible from their pets, with minimal adverse consequences.

Interestingly, trying to keep pets' problem-free is not only great for pet owners but also fulfilling for veterinary teams and profitable for veterinary hospitals, so it is worth consideration. If the veterinary profession does NOT embrace this concept, then *non-veterinary alternatives* surely will, because consumer spending on this approach is likely to dwarf that spent on disease treatment.

When one considers the recommendations that could be done to keep pets problem-free, it becomes clear that some of those are not necessarily given due diligence by veterinary teams today.[10] They include prepurchase counseling, behavioral counseling and training, appropriate nutrition and weight management counseling, and implementing home dental care programs. If just a few of these programs are implemented, they could make a big difference to pet owners and pets alike and put the veterinary team front and center in discussions of wellness care.

For example, although our large animal counterparts have long played an important role in prepurchase examinations, this has not really been the case for small animal teams, and we typically enter the picture after a pet has already been acquired. This puts the veterinary team at a distinct disadvantage and may change the perception of our advice from advocacy to antagonism. Nobody wants to learn that they may have made a bad purchase, especially for a living creature that will likely be part of their lives for well over a decade. Just imagine the difference if veterinary teams had been part of the process, helping prospective pet owners select an appropriate pet (breed, age, and sex), purchase it from a reliable source, and request appropriate information about the health status of that pet and other members of its family. Pet owners would not only be willing to pay for this valuable veterinary service, but they would also likely pay a premium to purchase something more likely to grow up to be a problem-free pet.

The same could be said for preemptive behavioral counseling. There is no need to wait for pet owners to report incidents of destructive behavior, house-soiling, or even fear, anxiety, and stress (FAS) when visiting the veterinary hospital. These can all be better dealt with proactively with the advice of the veterinary team.[11] Because pets are often abandoned or rehomed when they display problem behaviors, this is extremely important to maintaining the human–animal bond, and also keeping these clients as loyal customers of veterinary practices.[12] Helping establish suitable training regimens from the start, and guiding pet owners through the process of quickly identifying and correcting problems (appropriately) could be more lifesaving than cancer treatment later in the pet's life.

Dealing with FAS in pets presenting to veterinary practices is extremely important, because it affects client, patient, and staff satisfaction with those interactions and can affect client willingness to seek veterinary services, as well as what care they might be prepared to provide at home. Initiatives such as Fear Free (fearfreepets.com) provide excellent training and resources for veterinary teams and have clearly demonstrated the value of such approaches. When pets are not stressed when visiting the veterinary hospital, pet owners are more at ease in bringing their pets in, and veterinary teams have a much easier time dealing with those pets in a variety of situations. A by-product of this approach is that the same principles can be used by pet owners at home to overcome resistance to such routine tasks as bathing, cleaning ears, brushing teeth, administering medication, or trimming claws. When pets willingly accept our interventions, they are much more likely to be considered problem-free pets.[8] This makes them better companions for their caregivers and much better patients for veterinary practices.

SETTING PET OWNERS UP FOR SUCCESS FROM THE START

The veterinary profession has extraordinary capabilities and yet is often constrained by pet owner limitations, and veterinary practices that deal with this effectively will have a noticeable advantage in the future. Practices that fail to address this will continue to be constrained and may even suffer setbacks in being able to deliver needed care.

It is unfortunate that many pet owners do not have realistic expectations about the care and costs associated with pet ownership. It is also unfortunate that most veterinary teams do not actively participate in better informing clients of those needs. The result is often frustration on the part of veterinary hospitals and pet owners, and pets not always receiving the care that they need.

The problem begins with the fact that not all pet owners regularly use veterinary services and expands from there. The "medicalization rate" refers to the percentage of dog and cat owners that regularly seek veterinary services, and it can vary widely between species, and with a number of factors, including geography, socioeconomic status, and individual circumstances and preconceptions. It can also vary significantly as a function of the human–animal bond.[12] There are still a considerable number of pet owners who do not seek regular veterinary care. This not only reflects a significant business opportunity for the profession, but improvements can often be achieved with existing technology and personnel.

Because there are many potential limiting factors in the ability of pet owners to use veterinary services, there has been renewed interest in so-called access to care and spectrum of care. Access to care can be difficult to assess and correct, but such barriers can be economic, geographic, cultural, or informational. Some pet owners might have financial limitations, others might experience language barriers, some may work shifts that do not allow them to be available to bring pets in during regularly scheduled business hours, others might have to rely on public transit which limits being able to transport pets, some just might not realize that their pets require regular veterinary team attention, and some just do not know the breadth of services that veterinary medicine can provide (I did not know they had dermatologists for pets!).

For those clients who do have access, some will want or need options that can fit their financial situations.[13] Although most veterinary teams tend to gravitate toward the most comprehensive care as a "gold standard," it is appreciated that quality care can be delivered across a spectrum of costs and still attain acceptable outcomes, as is often necessary in human medicine.[14] Similarly, if someone needs a watch (or a vehicle, or a hotel room, or clothing), they can select options that fit their budgets. When it comes to timepieces, they could spend a few dollars, or thousands, or they could just use their mobile device to tell time. Although each option has its advantages and disadvantages, it would be difficult to argue that there is only one option for getting the job done. The goal of the spectrum of care is to offer pet parents the appropriate level of care depending on their pet's condition and owner preferences and to ensure that owners have access to the right resources to make informed decisions about their pet's health. The practices of the future that at least partially solve these aspects of access to care and spectrum of care will no doubt reap the benefits of their actions.

One of the main advantages of considering spectrum of care in veterinary medicine is that it allows for a tailored approach to treatment (pet-specific care, as described above). Another benefit of the spectrum of care approach is that it allows for cost-effective yet still acceptable options. This can help reduce the overall cost of care while still providing an appropriate level of care for the animal's condition, which ideally will improve service utilization rates. With appropriate counseling and informed consent, clients can understand the tradeoffs inherent when making choices and may be better at accepting risks and less than optimal outcomes.[15] Providing a spectrum of care does not require veterinary teams to provide services below their standards of care, only to considering alternatives to a binary, all-or-nothing approach to medicine.

Setting appropriate expectations should happen during puppy and kitten visits or preferably even before (prepurchase counseling). When clients understand the likely future health care costs and recommendations for their pets, they can use appropriate "risk management strategies" to plan accordingly. Veterinary teams can greatly assist by discussing typical costs of lifelong care for pets (often significantly higher than most pet owners realize), as well as the specific costs anticipated for a pet based on its particular circumstances and risk factors (eg, hip dysplasia assessment and glaucoma screening). It can also be helpful to describe potential unforeseen elements that cannot necessarily be planned, such as a trip to an emergency clinic, perhaps the need for referral to a specialist at some point in the future, and costs associated with long-term management of things like periodontal disease, allergies, arthritis and a variety of other things that are not uncommonly encountered in pet care.

The consideration of risk management strategies, including pet health insurance, is extremely important in helping pet owners plan for unforeseen situations. When fully implemented, strategies to promote pet health insurance make it much more likely that pet owners can follow recommendations for care, without being limited by financial constraints. For pet health insurance to be a useful solution for pet owners, veterinary teams need to counsel them on the types of features to look for in a policy (such as chronic care provisions and coverage of inherited conditions), recommend examples of policies that would meet such criteria, advise that policies should be initiated early so that nothing is considered preexisting and exempt, and correctly positioning insurance not as a method of saving money, but of providing peace of mind in being able to deal with unexpected circumstances.[16] We do not insure our cars or homes with the idea that it will save us money, and the same is true for pet health insurance. Pet health insurance continues to grow at a fast pace, year-over-year, but in some countries, it is starting at such a low base that such rapid growth may not always be discernible.

Although pet health insurance is designed to deal with unanticipated expenses, many pet owners are also eager to manage their anticipated expenses. Many already use "subscription services" for a variety of amenities, including entertainment streaming, meal kit delivery, memberships, and software licenses; there are even subscription services for pet products and experiences. Many consumers, especially younger consumers, find it easier to budget anticipated monthly expenses rather than pay larger amounts on a periodic basis. Retailers find that customer satisfaction is higher with such services, as are renewal rates. Veterinary practices also use such subscription services, which they sometimes refer to as "wellness plans," but any type of service that has predictable costs can be paid for with such payment plans. Subscription plans help consumers pay for anticipated services, but it is extremely important that veterinary practices clearly explain the basket of goods and services that are covered by such plans and that everything else not specified in the plan is excluded and must be paid for separately. Pet owners must realize the difference between insurance and subscription plans, and blurring those lines is not advised.

CONSISTENCY OF CARE

Veterinary medicine is one of those last bastions of "rugged individuality" in which clinicians value their ability to practice how they want without being told what they should do for case management. In fact, there may be some rebelling against working for corporate practices that require adherence to certain protocols. Such freedoms may seem liberating, but they come at a cost. It is impossible to promise clients that the hospital is providing an exceptional level of care, when that level of care is inconsistent between the different clinicians providing services! The lack of consistency not only confuses clients, when they experience different staff members at the same hospital giving different recommendations, but it is also confusing for the paraprofessional and front office staff who must keep track of what each clinician is likely to have recommended to a client.

For now, most hospitals tolerate this freedom, sometimes referred to as a "cowboy mentality," and even many corporate consolidators may promise that when they take over a practice that nothing will be changed. However, in the future, it is very likely that more consistency of care will be required, even if doctors are still afforded considerable leeway in their approaches.

In some cases, it may be litigation, the threat of litigation, or mandates from governing bodies that will promote the use of standards of care. In other cases, hospital teams themselves may want to embrace standards of care that help memorialize best practices. This not only ensures the level of care for clients and pets but also facilitates training for staff members so they better understand their roles and can also play a more active part in discussing cases with clients or communicating between clinicians.

Having standards of care in place is not only helpful in defining the level of care practiced at the hospital, but there are very real business advantages as well. When clinicians can reach a consensus on specific standards of care, they can also hopefully reach a consensus on which first-line products would be needed in inventory to fulfill those standards. For example, there might be a standard of care for integrated parasite control in dogs, and hospital teams can decide which should be the preferred products to use with that standard. These products would be in the hospital formulary and stocked as inventory. Clinicians would still have the freedom to select other products that meet the same standard but are not first-line choices and could order these for the client for home delivery from pharmacy partners or write a prescription. This lowers inventory costs and helps keep the pharmacy profitable.

It is important for hospital teams to appreciate that having standards of care, and providing consistency of care, are not meant to impede anyone's freedom; they are meant to assure clients and staff of the level of care they can expect at the hospital. This is something that our human physician counterparts do with regularity. Although they provide care personalized to the individual, they rarely deviate from recognized standards of care, or they would need to be prepared to accept responsibility and accountability if they strayed from such norms.

Standards of care are important in medicine and are not meant to constrain freedom, but to recognize generalized evidence-based realities. Clinicians can still offer clients personalized solutions based on their individual circumstances, but it is a worthwhile level-setting endeavor to start from a standard of care and have a conversation with clients or veterinary team members about why a particular situation might benefit from some deviation from such a standard. Standards of care also do not mean a cookie-cutter approach to medicine. They are just a reflection of guidelines that exist based on what is known about a specific condition or circumstance. Most guidelines are created by veterinary organizations or specialty boards/colleges, are typically free for members of the profession to access, and represent an evidence-based consensus of what is known about a topic.[1] Successful practices in the future are likely to embrace such standards, as is the case in human medicine.

REIMAGINING THE VETERINARY PHARMACY

For many veterinary practices worldwide, dispensing represents a significant portion of hospital revenue, and this is both a good thing and a bad thing. What seems clear, however, is that the future promises more, not less, competition, and veterinary pricing models will need to evolve accordingly.[17] In many countries, veterinarians have a relative monopoly over the sale of pharmaceuticals, but there are consumer and legislative pressures to make such products available more widely from other providers. Eventually, market forces are bound to win out, so it is important to be proactive in positioning dispensing appropriately.

Veterinary medicine is not the only profession to have to deal with this loss of exclusivity. Long ago our physician counterparts relinquished most dispensing to pharmacists, and more recently eye care professionals have had to contend with more retailers selling glasses and contact lenses on a prescription basis. Consumers have appreciated the convenience of being able to "comparison shop," and competition has driven down prices, even as regulatory agencies have endeavored to ensure and maintain quality in the marketplace.

Because dispensing represents such a large share of revenue in small animal practice, it can be terrifying to contemplate such a loss of income, but this need not be the case. The pharmacy can still be very profitable for practices if they make some needed changes to their processes.

The first step is to limit the pharmacy to those products that are absolutely needed to meet the hospital's standards of care. Most veterinary hospitals have a relatively small retail footprint, so will never be able to compete with large retailers in terms of their ability to buy in bulk and sell in high volumes. Accordingly, veterinary hospitals need to be very selective in what they stock to those products that make sense and for which they have a competitive advantage (eg, injectables), where convenience for clients allows those products to be sold for a premium, or those that are needed to provide required services (eg, emergency drugs).

Many veterinary pharmacies are bloated with too many products and although this surplus may generate a lot of revenue for the hospital, it does not necessarily mean that this service is profitable. When hospitals are squeezed by outside competition, they need to practice smarter, not harder, and this often means limiting rather than expanding inventory. Hospital pharmacies will be most profitable when they limit inventory to that which can be justified based on standards of care, competitive advantage, value pricing, and taking steps to improve compliance[17] (**Box 2**).

In some cases, when a recommendation for medication is made but a client expresses interest in getting the prescription filled elsewhere, this is sometimes regarded by hospital teams as disloyalty. However, this is not really the case if we consider things logically. After all, the client paid for the evaluation, and once a medication recommendation was made, it is completely reasonable for them to consider their options for where they can get the most value for that purchase. This is no different from visiting an eye care professional, being told that you need glasses or contact lenses, and then taking a prescription and shopping it around until you get the best deal

---

Box 2
Ways to increase the profitability of the veterinary pharmacy

- Create a formulary that prioritizes dispensing to those products recommended in hospital standards of care.

- Embrace consistency of care standards to avoid product class duplication, increase familiarity with specific products by hospital teams, and such selectivity may allow more favorable purchase terms from manufacturers and distributors.

- Partner with an online pharmacy to provide products that are not in the formulary, are not profitable for the hospital to dispense, or cannot be competitively priced. It is often possible to receive an incentive payment in such partnerships, which provides income but requires no ordering and carrying costs for those items.

- Use injectables when medically prudent to do so, which provides convenience to clients, and for which compliance can be guaranteed.

- Emergency drugs are not "shopped" and can be sold at a premium. There is no need to price them using the same methods used for products that have rapid turnover.

- Prioritize products that are licensed for the species being treated, for the purpose intended, and avoid stocking products that would promote extra-label drug use (eg, human-labeled drugs, generics, and biosimilars). Prioritize drugs labeled for use in the species being treated and according to label recommendations.

- Price products sensibly so prices reflect value delivered. This is rarely accomplished with markups.

- Counsel clients about the medications being dispensed, why they were chosen, potential side effects, monitoring required, and whether the medication is intended to cure or control the problem being addressed. If clients do not see the value in your recommendations, they may very well seek out the cheapest option available elsewhere.

possible. In the future, our clients are likely going to have more choices, not less, so it is important that we are not offended when clients want to explore their options. Our goal should be value delivery along with cost-competitiveness, so pricing is less of a determining factor. We can still win in this space, but not by simply marking up the cost of medications to unjustified levels. Hospitals should stock products that fit within their standards of care, are profitable to dispense, or for which there is some other competitive advantage. For everything else, it is worth working with a partner pharmacy that will provide a commission to the hospital for the sale and arrange home delivery for the pet owner.

CHANGING MODELS OF VETERINARY PRACTICE

For decades, veterinary practices were relatively small endeavors, with such types of businesses sometimes referred to colloquially as "mom & pop" operations. This is still true in many parts of the world, but particularly in North America and Europe, corporate-owned practices are increasingly more common.[18] The pace of consolidation continues to grow, along with the number of players in the veterinary space.

There is no reason to suspect that consolidation efforts will slow down in the future, and even more consolidation is likely given the cannibalism of smaller corporate groups by larger ones and that is likely to continue.

Theoretically, corporate practices should be more profitable because of economies of scale and scope, but such efficiencies are not always evident. Similarly, one might surmise that they could succeed by branding practices that the public might associate with good experiences, such as is done with most franchise businesses, but this is also not a foregone conclusion.

In the future, some corporate-owned practices are most likely to succeed because they can provide a consistent experience for pet owners and veterinary team members. Most practices purchased by consolidators tend to be larger with three or more veterinarians, have a certain amount of up-to-date equipment, decent employee benefits, and the ability to provide mentorship (which is valued by inexperienced staff), and they have the financial wherewithal to establish compensation and benefit packages that will attract professional and paraprofessional talent. In the future, this may be a deciding factor in their ability to endure and continue to grow.

In the future, it is also likely that successful veterinary practices will need to better cater to the needs of the pet-owning public, especially representatives of millennials and Generation Z. To accomplish this, business models will need to flex to other services that may not always require bringing pets into the clinic for every encounter.[19] It is likely that virtual care options and remote interventions will be needed, along with different tiers of service representing a spectrum of care and professional versus paraprofessional service alternatives.[20]

CHANGES TO THE WORKFORCE

One of the easiest things to predict in veterinary practices is that change is inevitable, yet many practices are not necessarily prepared for such realities. We can reasonably expect that such changes will be magnified when it comes to the workforce. There is now an acute awareness of "burnout" in the profession, and the very real risk of mental health disorders and even suicide.[21] We are seeing evidence of "quiet quitting," staff being overwhelmed during and after the pandemic, and no real evidence that things are going to go back to the way they were before.

It can reasonably be inferred that successful practices of the future will need to have developed mechanisms to deal with this reality.[22] Expect that wages, schedules, and benefits will need to reflect that staff should be able to have a reasonable work–life balance and fair compensation for the value they provide.[23] Harassment should not be tolerated in practices, and there will need to be ways to reasonably resolve conflicts in the workplace.

For the profession to thrive in the future, it will be important to recognize the contributions of paraprofessionals and provide career ladders for them to advance and use their skills.[24] It will also be critical to recognize different tiers of accomplishment not only between credentialed versus noncredentialed technicians/nurses but also a hierarchy of veterinary assistants, technicians/nurses with 2-year versus 4-year degrees, those with master's degrees, and those that have attained veterinary technician specialties status. These different tiers of accomplishment should be accurately reflected in differentiated wage strata, as an incentive for these critically important staff members to be appropriately vested in the profession.

No prediction of the future is complete without alluding to advancements in technology. It is likely that there will be more interest in artificial intelligence (AI), as well as opportunities for remote monitoring (eg, collars capable of transmitting real-time data, and glucose-monitoring devices). The most likely change anticipated is for practices to embrace more telehealth opportunities where it becomes seamlessly interwoven into the practice workstream.[25] We should also expect that tomorrow's clinicians will embrace better clinical reasoning than just following routine approaches, whether assisted by AI, telehealth, or appropriate training and mentorship.[26] Perhaps there is not so much a shortage of veterinary professionals and paraprofessionals worldwide, but rather an imperfect utilization of the talent that already exists. Accessing that capacity through technology would be a worthwhile goal, as would providing reciprocity of licensure across jurisdictions to reflect comparable professional credentials.

SUMMARY

Although the future of veterinary practice is bright, there are some challenges that seem unavoidable. Many can be dealt with effectively, but some practices will have a harder time adapting than others.

DISCLOSURE

No apparent conflicts of interest.

REFERENCES

1. Ackerman L. Pet-specific care for the veterinary team. Hoboken, NJ: Wiley-Blackwell; 2021.
2. Donnelly AL. Meeting the Needs of Pet Parents. [book ed. In: Ackerman L, editor. Pet-specific Care for the veterinary team. Hoboken, NJ: Wiley-Blackwell; 2021. p. 311–4.
3. Weinstein P. Creating a pet-specific user's manual. [book ed. In: Ackerman L, editor. Pet-specific Care for the veterinary team. Hoboken, NJ: Wiley-Blackwell; 2021. p. 391–8.
4. Nicholas JC. Strategies for Success with Pet-Specific Care. [book ed.]. In: Ackerman L, editor. Pet-specific Care for the veterinary team. Hoboken, NJ: Wiley-Blackwell; 2021. p. 775–8.
5. Boss N. Breed Predisposition. In: Ackerman L, editor. Pet-specific Care for the veterinary team. Hoboken, NJ: Wiley-Blackwell; 2021. p. 193–8.
6. Ackerman L. The Genetics of Disease. Pet-specific care for the veterinary team. Hoboken, NJ: Wiley-Blackwell; 2021. p. 141–6.

7. Dicks MR. Financial Benefits of Pet-Specific Care. [book auth.]. In: Ackerman L, editor. Pet-specific Care for the veterinary team. Hoboken, NJ: Wiley-Blackwell; 2021. p. 819–24.

8. Ackerman L, Ackerman R. Problem Free Pets. The ultimate guide to pet parenting. Dermvet Publishing; 2020.

9. Ackerman L, Ackerman R. Almost Perfect Pets. A proactive guide to selection, health care and pet parenting. McFarland & Company Publishers; 2022.

10. Ackerman L. Proactive Pet Parenting. Anticipating pet health problems before they happen. Problem Free Publishing; 2020.

11. Landsberg G, Radosta L, Ackerman L, editors. Behavior Problems of the Dog and Cat-E-Book. Elsevier Health Sciences; 2023.

12. Lue TW, Pantenburg DP, Crawford PM. Impact of the owner-pet and client-veterinarian bond on the care that pets receive. J Am Vet Med Assoc 2008; 232:531–40.

13. Khuly P. Affordability of Veterinary Services. [book ed.]. In: Ackerman L, editor. Pet-specific Care for the veterinary team. Hoboken, NJ: Wiley-Blackwell; 2021. p. 83–6.

14. Haworth D. Opportunities and challenges of providing services for low-income clients. [book ed. In: Ackerman L, editor. Pet-specific Care for the veterinary team. Hoboken, NJ: Wiley-Blackwell; 2021. p. 399–402.

15. Block G. Providing Cost-Effective Care for Those in Need. [book ed. In: Ackerman L, editor. Pet-specific Care for the veterinary team. Hoboken, NJ: Wiley-Blackwell; 2021. p. 835–8.

16. Ackerman L. Pet Health Insurance. In: Ackerman L, editor. Pet-specific care for the veterinary team. Hoboken, NJ: Wiley-Blackwell; 2021. p. 843–8.

17. Ackerman L, editor. Blackwell's five-minute veterinary practice management consult. Third Edition. Hoboken, NJ: Wiley-Blackwell; 2020.

18. Mamalis LA. Corporate Veterinary Practices. In: Ackerman L, editor. Blackwell's Five-minute veterinary practice management consult. book ed. Hoboken, NJ: Wiley-Blackwell; 2020. p. 62–3.

19. Weinstein P. Challenges to the Profession. [book ed. In: Ackerman L, editor. Blackwell's Five-minute veterinary practice management consult. Third Edition. Hoboken, NJ: Wiley-Blackwell; 2020. p. 6–9.

20. DeWilde C. Improving Client Engagement Through Technology. In: Ackerman L, editor. Pet-specific Care for the veterinary team. Wiley-Blackwell; 2021. p. 347–52.

21. Ackerman L. Feel Something, Say Something, Recognizing stress within the veterinary profession. AAHA Trends 2022;38(11):50–4.

22. Prendergast H. Leveraging Staff. [book ed.]. In: Ackerman L, editor. Blackwell's Five-minute veterinary practice management consult. Third Edition. Hoboken, NJ: Wiley-Blackwell; 2020. p. 200–1.

23. Brogdon R. Engaging Staff. [book ed. In: Ackerman L, editor. Blackwell's Five-minute veterinary practice management consult. Hoboken, NJ: Wiley-Blackwell; 2020. p. 204–5.

24. Felsted K. Employee-Related Costs. [book ed. In: Ackerman L, editor. Blackwell's Five-minute veterinary practice management consult. Third Edition. Hoboken, NJ: Wiley-Blackwell; 2020. p. 178–9.

25. Ackerman L. Virtual Care (Telehealth). In: Ackerman L, editor. Pet-specific care for the veterinary team. Hoboken, NJ: Wiley-Blackwell; 2021. p. 59–64.

26. Englar RE, Dial SM. Low-cost veterinary clinical diagnostics. Hoboken, NJ: Wiley-Blackwell; 2023. p. 354pp.

Cost of Care, Access to Care, and Payment Options in Veterinary Practice

Jules Benson, BVSc, MRCVS[a,b,*], Emily M. Tincher, DVM[a,b]

KEYWORDS

- Spectrum of care • Access to care • Inflation • Innovation • Stratification
- Diversification • DEI • Cost of care

KEY POINTS

- 25% to 50% of US cats and dogs do not receive any veterinary care on an annual basis
- The role of the human–animal bond in human health makes access to veterinary care a One Health issue
- The cost of care continues to increase above the level of inflation and is the primary barrier to accessing veterinary services
- A spectrum of care approach aims to provide a continuum of acceptable care while remaining responsive to client expectations and financial limitations
- The diversification of care models available to pet owners (ie, stratification) could provide a systemic way to provide more care to more pets
- Current financial solutions increase access to care but greater innovation is necessary to provide access to a more diverse audience

INTRODUCTION

Most veterinarians (95%) think that all pets deserve access to veterinary care[1] but 25% to 50% of pets do not receive regular veterinary care.[1] Amid increasing pet ownership and increasing costs of veterinary care, a combination of potential solutions might be found through the greater adoption of a spectrum of care approach,[2] by introducing new models of veterinary care, and through the evolution of payment solutions.

ACCESS TO CARE
Barriers to Accessing Veterinary Care

At least 25% to 50% of more than 150 million pet cats and dogs do not receive any veterinary care on an annual basis in the United States,[1] with cats disproportionately

[a] Nationwide® Mutual Insurance Company; [b] Nationwide Insurance (Pet) PO Box 182965, Columbus, OH 43218, USA
* Corresponding author. Nationwide Insurance (Pet) PO Box 182965, Columbus, OH 43218.
E-mail address: j.benson@nationwide.com

Vet Clin Small Anim 54 (2024) 235–250
https://doi.org/10.1016/j.cvsm.2023.10.007
0195-5616/24/© 2023 Elsevier Inc. All rights reserved.

vetsmall.theclinics.com

affected. These estimates vary, and reaching a population of pet families who do not access veterinary care is challenging. Coronavirus disease 2019 (COVID-19) irregularities notwithstanding, multiple data sources from 2020 through 2023 suggest that although year-over-year revenue is increasing across veterinary practices, visits are decreasing, with an increasing proportion of pet parents presenting their pets for urgent care because the proportion of pets receiving regular care is decreasing.[3,4]

When a demographically representative sample of US pet owners was surveyed, more than 1 in 4 pet owners (28%) experienced a barrier to accessing veterinary care. The top barrier, finances, will be discussed in "The Cost of Care" section. Additional resource constraints include time, language barriers, cultural differences, transportation, and availability of veterinary services. Veterinary service deserts continue to expand across the United States, driven partially by a workforce crisis affecting all areas of the profession, especially veterinarians and credentialed technicians. Both geographic locations and hours of service availability have been affected.

Is Owning a Pet a Privilege?

In a 2018 survey of 771 veterinarians, only 27% agreed with the statement, "Everyone, regardless of circumstances, should be able to own a pet."[1] These results may suggest that pet ownership is viewed as a privilege by many veterinary health-care teams, who may think that only those who can afford certain levels of veterinary care should be able to own pets. However, the positive benefits of the human–animal bond should be acknowledged for all pet owners, including families with limited financial (or other) resources. Pet owners will continue adding pets to their families whether the veterinary profession approves or not, and alienation or judgment felt by the pet owner presents another barrier to obtaining veterinary care. The combination of the documented value of the human–animal bond and zoonotic diseases (eg, intestinal parasites and rabies) make increasing access to care a One Health concern. Methods to meet pet families where they are while acknowledging that pet ownership is a responsibility will be discussed in the "Spectrum of care" section.

The Human-animal Bond

Research from organizations such as the Human Animal Bond Research Institute (habri.org) highlights the benefits pets and families bring to each other. These evidence-based benefits include the development of positive social behaviors in children, improved wellness for people with dementia, reduced loneliness, and decreases in blood pressure.[5]

The Role of Diversity, Equity, Inclusion, and Belonging

Although the benefits of being around animals are well documented, often those who benefit most from having a pet face the most barriers when it comes to accessing the veterinary care they want for their pets.[1]

COST OF CARE
Introduction

The cost of veterinary care has long been a primary source of tension between pet families and veterinary health-care teams and is a major barrier to accessing veterinary care. This section aims to explore costs as a barrier to care, the drivers behind cost increases, and how these drivers are experienced by pet families.

The Cost of Care as a Barrier to Veterinary Care

Of the more than 1 in 4 Americans who have faced a barrier to veterinary care, 80% of them identify cost as a cause.[1] Specifically, the 2021 Economic Well-Being of U.S

(United States) Households (SHED) study identified that only 32% of adults surveyed would be able to cover a US$400 emergency expense by using cash or its equivalent.[6] It is likely that increases in the cost of care will continue to challenge pet families across the economic spectrum, with an increasing number of pet families exploring alternatives to regular care as a result (eg, moving to sporadic care and using tele-health services).

Drivers of the Increasing Cost of Care

Increasing cost of care is driven by interrelated factors including increased prices of specific goods and services, the ever-increasing availability of new diagnostics and treatment, and increased access to more facilities with advanced levels of care.

Cost inflation: the increasing costs of goods and services

Cost inflation measures the change in cost for specific goods and services. For example, if a practice increases the cost of a routine examination from US$60 to US$66, the cost has inflated by 10%. In calculating the consumer price index (CPI), the Bureau of Labor Statistics measures the cost of more than 80,000 items across more than 200 categories every month.[7] One of these categories is "Veterinarian Services." The sum of items across all 200 categories are grouped together as "All Goods."

Fig. 1 shows the annual CPI for veterinarian services plotted against the CPI for All Goods. During the past 20 years, Veterinarian Services inflation has outpaced All Goods inflation significantly almost every year.

Although each year in the chart above may not reflect an enormous difference, over time, this has contributed to a dramatic difference in how far a dollar goes. **Fig. 2** shows how purchasing power from January 2002 to April 2023 has changed in terms of what US$100 could buy. Specific to Veterinarian Services, the same items that could be bought for US$100 in 2002 would require US$276 in 2023, a 61% increase compared to All Goods at US$171.

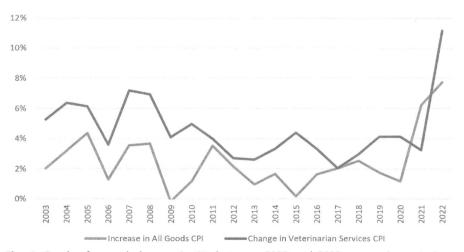

Fig. 1. Graph of annual changes in CPI between 2003 and 2022, comparing veterinary services CPI to all goods CPI. (*Source*: Consumer Price Index. U.S. Bureau of Labor Statistics. Updated January 18, 2023. Accessed May 21, 2023. https://www.bls.gov/cpi/questions-and-answers.htm.)

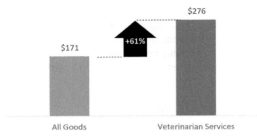

Fig. 2. Graph showing the change in relative cost of goods between 2002 and 2023, comparing veterinary services CPI to all goods CPI. (*Source*: Consumer Price Index. U.S. Bureau of Labor Statistics. Updated January 18, 2023. Accessed May 21, 2023. https://www.bls.gov/cpi/questions-and-answers.htm.)

The drivers for the increasing cost of veterinary goods and services fall into the following categories.

- *Staffing costs*: The competitive nature of the veterinary labor market has been well documented[8–11] in the years preceding this publication. American Veterinary Medical Association data show that compensation for new graduates increased by almost US$20,000 from 2021 to 2022,[12] and hefty signing and retention bonuses have become more common.[13,14] Nonveterinarian staff members have also taken the opportunity to negotiate for more favorable terms.[15]
- *Adapting to changing practice economics*: With a pervasive loss of pharmacy revenue and increasing staffing costs, many practices are taking the opportunity to rightsize the prices of services such as examination fees, surgery time, and even telemedicine.
- *Increased cost of consumables and drugs to veterinary providers*: A combination of COVID-19 supply-chain hangover, baseline inflation, and dramatic increases in key items lead to pass-through costs for consumers.

New diagnostics and treatments
Even if veterinary practices were to freeze prices of current goods and services, the cost of care for pet families in most practices would still increase because of advances in diagnostics, treatments, and preventatives. Two case examples in **Figs. 3** and **4** demonstrate how changes in clinical protocols result in significant increases in the cost of care. Although both cases draw from historical examples, recent analyses continue to support this trend—Vetsource (vetsource.com) highlights that one of the drivers of higher cost of care is more items per invoice than in previous years.[16]

Increased access/referral to advanced care facilities
Increased demand for specialty veterinarians during the past several decades[17] has led to the expansion of emergency and referral facilities. In the 1980s, most boarded specialists were employed by veterinary teaching hospitals but the growth of referral practice means that the majority are now employed in private practice. Although it has long been possible to find emergency and referral practices in the urban and suburban areas of large United States, it is now increasingly difficult to locate small-to-medium-sized cities without at least one referral center, something that was not true 30, or even 15, years ago.

This explosion of specialized care has resulted in increased access to advanced level care. Although this improves a form of "access to care," it also introduces some challenges.

Case 1

Signalment: 3-year-old male neutered Labrador Retriever, 12-hour history of vomiting every couple of hours, eating and drinking, BAR

Invoice in 2006		Invoice in 2008	
Exam	$50	Exam	$50
Radiographs	$150	Radiographs	$150
Metoclopramide inj.	$28	Cerenia inj.	$75
SQ fluids	$23	cPL snap test	$65
5lb bag of GI diet	$15	SQ fluids	$23
		5lb bag of GI diet	$15
	$266		**$378**

Change in cost to consumer		+ $112	+ 42%

The cost of care for a vomiting dog increased by 42% because of the availability of new diagnostics and treatments.

Fig. 3. Case study showing the inflation of veterinary care costs between 2006 and 2008 in a vomiting dog.

Case 2

Signalment: 4-year-old female spayed Pit Bull presenting for annual examination

Invoice in 2012		Invoice in 2014	
Exam	$60	Exam	$60
Rabies vaccine	$35	Rabies vaccine	$35
DHPPL vaccine	$30	DHPPL vaccine	$30
4Dx SNAP test	$65	4Dx SNAP test	$65
HeartGard x 6 months	$60	HeartGard x 6 months	$60
Frontline x 6 months	$90	NexGard x 6 months	$150
	$340		**$400**

Change in cost to consumer		+ $60	+ 18%

The cost of annual prevention increased by 18% because of the availability of new preventives.

Footnotes: NexGard (afoxolaner) is an oral isoxazoline flea and tick medication released by Merial in 2013. It was the first of the new class of isoxazoline drugs; highly efficacious and offering greater convenience than prior topical treatments like Frontline (from the same manufacturer).

Fig. 4. Case study showing the inflation of veterinary care costs between 2012 and 2014 for canine wellness.

- *Increased cost of care*: With more advanced levels of care comes higher costs. Bigger facilities, more specialized staff, advanced equipment, and new therapies all carry a bigger price tag for goods and services.
- *Decrease in the availability of intermediate care options*: Referrals from primary care are driven by a combination of (1) referral care being more accessible, (2) industry-wide education and marketing that prioritizes advanced-level care, and (3) the fear of liability around providing a "standard of care." An effect of this is that fewer primary care veterinarians are offering treatments or procedures that fall into what could be described as intermediate-level care. Examples might include perineal urethrostomy, gastric dilatation and volvulus surgery, or cruciate ligament lateral suture stabilization. Some specialists report that common, more complex medical cases such as maintenance of epilepsy[18] are being referred to them. This can place pet families in the position of choosing between a high-cost referral or basic/no care, with limited intermediate options.

Summary

For all of the reasons detailed above, costs will continue to be the primary barrier for pet families wishing to access veterinary care. Veterinary medicine is often referred to as a "recession-resistant" industry,[19–21] and, coming out of COVID-19, it is still experiencing a supply–demand curve that tilts in its favor.[22] However, without finding solutions to address care costs that leave an increasing number of pet families behind, we cannot hope to (1) fulfill our mission of providing some care for more pets and (2) reap the economic benefits of a diverse population who are looking for cost-effective pet health-care solutions.

SPECTRUM OF CARE
Introduction

One way to increase access to care is for veterinary health-care teams to embrace a spectrum of care approach to clinical practice.[2] As defined in the Journal of the American Veterinary Medical Association, a spectrum of care approach "aims to [provide] a continuum of acceptable care while remaining responsive to client expectations and financial limitations (**Fig. 5**)."[23] It combines evidence-based medicine with a pet family's emotional, physical, and financial resources, then communicates a range of care options from basic to advanced to them without judgment (**Fig. 6**).

A Spectrum of Care in Clinical Practice

Pet family goals, values, and resources
Pet families are diverse in their needs for veterinary care, in their experience of a human–animal bond, and in the resources they have available for pet care. Identifying their needs can prove challenging, especially when faced with pressures for efficiency in the examination room. Teams that heavily lean on a one-size-fits-all approach to pet health-care recommendations, often with a bias toward advanced-level care, can find themselves struggling with efficiency, contentious client relations, staff-wide moral distress, and decreased compliance or loyalty. Pet-centric, family-centric, and external factors contribute to the known, unknown, and voiced and unvoiced needs of each pet evaluated for care.[24]

In response to this challenge, Nationwide (https://www.petinsurance.com/veterinarians/spectrum-of-care/) partnered with Rehavior (https://rehavior.com/) to identify subconscious drivers of motivation through empirical evidence.[25] Three primary viewpoints emerged, with nearly equal distribution of demographics within

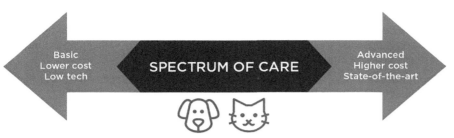

Fig. 5. Diagram showing how basic and advanced care options across a spectrum of care. (*Adapted from* Fingland RB, Stone LR, Read EK, & Moore RM (2021). Preparing veterinary students for excellence in general practice: building confidence and competence by focusing on spectrum of care, Journal of the American Veterinary Medical Association, 259(5), 463 to 470. Retrieved Jul 1, 2023, from https://doi.org/10.2460/javma.259.5.463.)

each viewpoint (eg, race, ethnicity, household income, marital status, and gender identity).

- *Convenience*: This group prefers the easiest option, perhaps opting for a single treatment over repeated visits to avoid stressing their anxious pet or juggling a busy family life, even if it is more expensive.
- *Choice*: This group wants to hear all the available options, and they do not want the most expensive listed first. Families that identify with this viewpoint often choose advanced or intermediate levels of care and lean heavily on evidence-based medicine for their decision but trust is built and maintained by their veterinary team providing them with a full range of options.

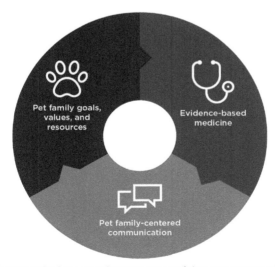

Fig. 6. Diagram showing the key considerations in applying a spectrum of care in veterinary practice. (*Adapted from* Stull, Jason W et al. "Barriers and next steps to providing a spectrum of effective health care to companion animals." Journal of the American Veterinary Medical Association vol. 253,11 (2018): 1386 to 1389. https://doi.org/10.2460/javma.253.11.1386.)

- *Cost*: Financial constraints are most pressing for this group. They often select more basic or intermediate levels of care, and they are the most concerned about being judged by the veterinary health-care team, highly valuing when they are shown clinical empathy.

Regardless of group, all pet families highly prioritized their pets' health, and deeply disliked being presented the most expensive option first.

Evidence-based medicine

A spectrum of care approach begins with an assessment of the evidence-based medicine applicable to the pet presented for care. This is accomplished by combining the available scientific evidence with the clinical expertise of the veterinary team to identify a range of diagnostic and treatment options, from basic to advanced, as is demonstrated in **Fig. 7**.[26] The range of options available from a particular veterinary health-care team is influenced by veterinarian factors (eg, technical skill and expertise) and practice factors (eg, equipment and working hours). Additional options along a spectrum of care are often available at other locations, discussed more in "Stratification of Care" section. More outcomes-based research to better quantify the chances of success and potential drawbacks, especially for basic and intermediate care options, is needed in veterinary medicine.

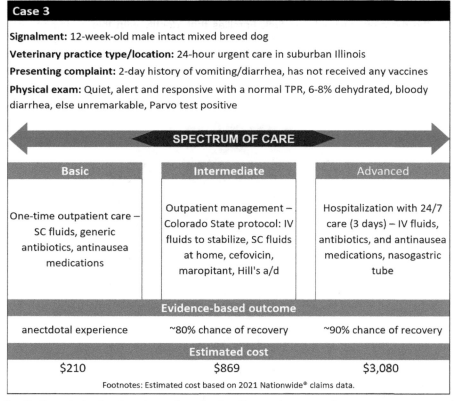

Case 3

Signalment: 12-week-old male intact mixed breed dog

Veterinary practice type/location: 24-hour urgent care in suburban Illinois

Presenting complaint: 2-day history of vomiting/diarrhea, has not received any vaccines

Physical exam: Quiet, alert and responsive with a normal TPR, 6-8% dehydrated, bloody diarrhea, else unremarkable, Parvo test positive

SPECTRUM OF CARE

Basic	Intermediate	Advanced
One-time outpatient care – SC fluids, generic antibiotics, antinausea medications	Outpatient management – Colorado State protocol: IV fluids to stabilize, SC fluids at home, cefovicin, maropitant, Hill's a/d	Hospitalization with 24/7 care (3 days) – IV fluids, antibiotics, and antinausea medications, nasogastric tube
Evidence-based outcome		
anectdotal experience	~80% chance of recovery	~90% chance of recovery
Estimated cost		
$210	$869	$3,080
Footnotes: Estimated cost based on 2021 Nationwide® claims data.		

Fig. 7. Case study showing the options for treating canine parvovirus across a spectrum of care. (*Data source from* 2021 Nationwideclaims data.)

Pet-family centered communication

Although there are often a range of treatment and diagnostic options offered in veterinary practices, the most advanced option is often still preferentially recommended, sometimes resulting in pet families feeling shamed or judged if they did not choose this option. By seeking first to understand with communication techniques such as open-ended questions and reflective listening, combining the evidence-based options with pet family goals and resources, a spectrum of care approach involves communicating options in a nonjudgmental way, using the skill of clinical empathy.

Strong evidence from human medicine suggests that clinical empathy is associated with improved patient satisfaction, increased adherence to treatment, and fewer malpractice complaints, as well as increased physician health, well-being, and professional satisfaction.[27]

"Standard of Care" Versus "Gold Standard Care"

In the United States, most state practice acts require that veterinarians practice in compliance with a standard of care, a legal term defined as, "care required of and practiced by the average reasonably prudent, competent veterinarian in the community."[28] Regulations do *not* require that all veterinarians recommend the most advanced or intensive care, often described as "gold standard care."

It is recommended to avoid using these 2 terms interchangeably because this can reinforce the idea that the most advanced care is always the best care.

Spectrum of Care and Practice Productivity

From a productivity and profitability standpoint, it may seem counterintuitive for practices to adopt a spectrum of care approach where basic and intermediate levels of care may be recommended instead of advanced care. However, intermediate care options can increase production in a general practice setting. There is some evidence that general practices are considering ways to increase management of high-production medical cases and procedures (eg, orthopedic procedures such as cranial cruciate ligament or fracture repair) without referral while maintaining strong clinical outcomes.[29] Additional research is needed to quantify the long-term impact of meeting pet families where they are across a spectrum of care in cases that decrease average client transaction (ACT) by evaluating other practice metrics (eg, increased frequency of visits and retention year-over-year).

STRATIFICATION OF CARE
Introduction

Stratification in companion animal veterinary medicine describes the diversification of care models available to pet owners. With an estimated 25% to 50% of pets currently not receiving veterinary care on an annual basis[1] (and an unknown number receiving sporadic care), stratification is one of the systemic ways to provide more care to more pets.

What Problems can Stratification Address?

The process of stratification across an industry can be viewed as honing in on increasingly specific solutions that address the various market needs. In veterinary medicine, this means care models that take advantage of one or more of the following.

- *Increasing accessibility*
  - *Lowering or subsidizing cost*: many accessible care models rely on some measure of being attractive through increased affordability (often in addition to

convenience and/or consumer experience). Most models that deliver lowered costs to consumers achieve this through increased efficiencies, economies of scale, reduction in the range of services offered (with resulting decreased overhead), or through subsidization.

(Studies support that subsidized care models can increase access to care without affecting the business of for-profit care models.)[30]

- o *Increasing physical accessibility*: decreasing physical barriers to care addresses a primary problem identified by pet families. This can be achieved by colocating with another business (eg, big box stores), creating locations in areas that are currently care deserts, or assisting with or eliminating the need for transportation of pets.
- o *Increasing remote accessibility*: modalities like tele-triage, telemedicine, and teleconsulting are still in their relative infancy but are increasing rapidly. Despite what could be interpreted as a conservative approach by organized veterinary medicine[31] and a constantly shifting regulatory environment around the veterinary–client–patient relationship, the traits of digital-enablement, availability, convenience, and cost-effectiveness are attractive to large portions of the pet owning population.[32,33] (Note: at-home testing is an area of remote care that is nascent at the time of writing.)
- *Providing a narrow range of common or desired services*
  - o *Preventative only*: the most common example is vaccine clinics. Whether these take place in the parking lot of a pet store or are run by a local private practice, they address one of the pain points that many pet families feel: being able to provide the most basic level of preventative care without incurring the cost of a full-service veterinary visit.
  - o *Incremental care*: by limiting the range of goods and services available (eg, limited in-house diagnostics, no in-house pharmacy, and no capability for surgery), incremental care facilities can provide the majority of care for the most common conditions without the overhead that can drives up costs. Current incremental care models are often housed in large retail locations (eg, big box stores).[34]
  - o *Dedicated urgent care*: for cases that cannot wait for an appointment with their general practice but are not sick enough to require a 24/7 emergency service or hospitalization (eg, ear infections, vomiting, diarrhea, and lameness). Urgent care models often have limited hours and can be associated with general or emergency practices or be entirely separate.
  - o *Other niche areas of practice*: dedicated businesses that focus on specific areas of high or increasing demand in general practice are already becoming a reality. End-of-life care has seen sustained growth,[35] and general practice (ie, nonspecialty) dentistry and surgery are already available in some markets.[36]

    Note: specialty practices that use boarded professionals were not included in this list—this is a relatively mature area of stratification that continues to grow.

Barriers to Stratification

It is worth noting that there are still considerable barriers to widespread stratification. In the authors' opinions, the greatest hurdles will be as follows:

- *Creating sustainable models*: creating new models that are profitable will take investment and patience.

- *If you build it, will they come?*: building a model with the needs of the customer in mind is essential but the process of identifying how to move customer behavior to new models can be a challenge. For example, survey results might show that shoppers at a grocery retail location would find it convenient if veterinary services were available there. However, the practicalities of bringing their pets there may bring challenges that were not addressed in the survey: for example, are pets allowed in the grocery portion of the store so that they can easily combine veterinary appointments with everyday shopping?
- *Staffing*: staffing any veterinary facility with veterinarians, technicians, and support staff has been incredibly challenging for the past few years and shows little sign of relenting. With increases in compensation across much of the industry, this adds to the already-considerable obstacle to creating profitable alternative care models.

It may be that it will take a combination of patient investors (or corporate money), a change in the behavior of pet families, and the maturation of the past few years' veterinary staffing initiatives (eg, new veterinary and technician schools and expanding class sizes) to accelerate the expansion of stratification.

Summary

Increasing long-term access to care requires growing profitable businesses. Pet ownership and veterinary services have reached a critical mass such that stratification—taking advantage of efficiencies of scale and evolving our care models—is the logical next step in meeting the needs of pet families.

FINANCIAL OPTIONS FOR PET FAMILIES
Introduction

The earlier sections detail some of the systemic changes that could help make veterinary care more accessible and more affordable for pet families. Whatever changes occur, budgeting for care or paying for unexpected care will continue to be a challenge for pet families and veterinary health-care teams to navigate together.

Financial Options for Pet Families Planning Ahead

There are several financial solutions for pet families who wish to increase their ability to budget for planned and/or unexpected veterinary expenses.

Pet insurance
Pet insurance is a highly regulated financial industry that primarily provides coverage for pet health expenses. Around 3% of pets in the United States are estimated to be covered by a pet health insurance plan at the time of writing.[37] Although this may be significantly lower than the proportion of insured pets in other countries such as the United Kingdom (~25%)[38] or Sweden (~80% of dogs),[39] data from the North American Pet Health Insurance Association (https://naphia.org/) show that the US market has seen consistent growth (>20% year over year).[40] Published data show that US clients with insured pets visit more often, spend more, and are more likely to be retained year over year.

In order to significantly increase access to care, pet insurance models will need to evolve, offering products that offer the following:

- A range of price points, coverages, and reimbursement options
- Transparency and ease-of-use
- The ability to meet families where they are through a diversity of entry-points

Wellness plans

Wellness plans create a contract between a pet parent and either a single veterinary provider, a commonly owned group of providers, or a network of providers. Well-run wellness plan programs have demonstrated the ability to provide better care for pets, produce more practice revenue, and improve client satisfaction.[41] These plans offer predictable payment terms for defined goods or services during the course of a year that may include the following:

- Examinations: many plans offer either uncapped or a set number of examinations for wellness ± illness visits throughout the year.
- Wellness care: services included span from only providing core vaccines to a full range of wellness care
- Discounts and loyalty programs: some wellness plans will provide discounts on care not covered under the plan (eg, accident or illness care), discounts on goods or services with partner companies, or pet wellness incentive programs.

Although wellness plans have been most common (and successful) in large hospital groups (eg, Banfield Pet Hospital) who are able to scale the administration, technology implementation, financing and purchasing, there are an increasing number of solutions that lower the barriers to administration and implementation for smaller groups or for independent practices.

Personal savings

A "pet savings account," which keeps the pet family in control of balances and disbursement, is a popular concept with an unknown level of utilization. The pros and cons of a pet savings account are relatively simple: pro—it keeps the pet family in control of their money and has no fees or administration; pro—if the money is not used, it stays with the pet family; con—it takes time to save, and veterinary costs can be large and/or unexpected; and con—requires a level of fiscal discipline.

Financial Options for Pet Families Facing Unplanned Veterinary Costs

For many of the reasons cited in the earlier sections, pet families facing unexpected and unplanned-for veterinary expenses continues to be a challenge faced by families and practices every day. The most common payment solutions are summarized as follows:

Personal savings, credit card, friends, and family

Pet families with sufficient savings, credit, or flexible friends and family may choose to manage costs this way, although many still use the options mentioned in the following sections. Regarding friends and family, crowdfunding has increased in popularity but presents obvious problems in collecting money for urgent procedures.

In-practice credit solutions

Credit solutions that can offer fast approval, low (or no) interest, and minimal administration have been popular in medical offices for decades, for good reason. There are 2 popular forms of veterinary financing available in the United States:

- Line of credit (eg, CareCredit): a credit card with interest rate and repayment options that vary with the applicant's credit score, the credit limit requested, and repayment options. The line of credit can be used for eligible fees or services at other locations (eg, pharmacies and other vet offices).
- Short-term loan (eg, Scratchpay): applicants apply for a loan when a veterinary expense is incurred. Multiple loans can be applied for if additional financing is needed.

Both solutions have some commonalities:

- Applicant screening: both credit solutions use an applicant's credit rating to assess terms and repayment options available (although credit rating may not be the only factor). In both cases, notification of approval status usually occurs quickly.
- Processing fees paid by the practice: Scratchpay cite a flat 5% processing fee for veterinary providers on their website[42]; CareCredit fees are not published but base rates are reported to be comparable to Scratchpay with longer repayment plans or lower interest rates resulting in higher processing fees.[43]

Although the area of financial services is notoriously difficult to break into, there continues to be scope to disrupt this space.

Practice payment plans

Accepting deferred payment feels like a heart-warming, community-oriented way to do business but most practices no longer offer this option due to poor experiences with nonpayment. For practices looking to balance any potential lost payments against the certainty of incurring credit processing fees, there are solutions that seek to decrease the administrative and technology burden of implementing in-practice payment solutions.

Charitable solutions/financial aid

For pet families experiencing financial hardship, there are numerous charitable organizations that accept grant applications. REACH Animal Care Program through the American Veterinary Medical Foundation[44] (https://vcare.avmf.org/) accepts applications from veterinarians on behalf of clients experiencing financial hardship.

Summary

To substantially increase access to care, innovation within and outside of the financial solutions currently available will be required. With finances being such a key part of the pet family experience, a working knowledge of the available tools is essential for veterinary health-care teams, as will be an understanding of the evolution of these solutions.

CLINICS CARE POINTS

- Have a staff meeting to discuss values around the responsibilities of pet ownership. If some on the team think owning pets should only be accessible by some, what is the minimum baseline? Are examination room communications in line with practice values?
- Identify the community-specific and practice-specific factors stopping your practice from being more accessible—better understanding access to care can be as simple as working out what is getting in the way of seeing more pets (or more of the right pets) in a day.
- Consider how general practices can improve access to intermediate-level care. Managing more complex medical and surgical cases at the primary care level may improve access to care and fit general practice business models of profitability.
- Create opportunities to better understand the expectations of pet families regarding veterinary care. Understand that "gold standard" recommendations often clash with these expectations.
- For existing clinics, clearly differentiate yourself from other businesses by creating a compelling, mission-driven value proposition for pet families. This might include

identifying and developing niches that work for you and your team, aligning with your mission, creating opportunities for efficiency, and increasing access to care.

- "Investigate for yourself" is not the advice that pet families are looking for from veterinary health-care teams when it comes to financial solutions. Despite the advent of Google and large language models such as ChatGPT, the veterinary practice remains (by far) the most trusted source for pet advice.

DISCLOSURE

Both authors are employed by Nationwide Mutual Insurance Company.

REFERENCES

1. Access to veterinary care coalition, *Access to veterinary care: barriers, current practices, and public Policy.* Faculty Publications and Other Works – Small Animal Clinical Sciences; 2018.
2. Stull Jason W, Shelby JA, Bonnett BN, et al. Barriers and next steps to providing a spectrum of effective health care to companion animals. J Am Vet Med Assoc 2018;253:1386–9. https://doi.org/10.2460/javma.253.11.1386, 11.
3. Veterinary Industry Tracker. Vetsource. Updated March 24. 2013. Accessed June 19, 2023. Available at: https://veterinaryanalytics.com/veterinary-industry-tracker/.
4. Veterinary Trend Watch. VetWatch. Accessed June 19, 2023. Available at: https://www.vetwatch.com/.
5. Research: Understanding the human-animal bond. Human Animal Bond Research Institute. Updated August 18, 2018. Accessed July 1, 2023. https://habri.org/research/.
6. Economic Well-Being of U.S. Households (SHED). Board of Governors of the Federal Reserve System. Updated August 22, 2022. Accessed May 21, 2023. Available at: https://www.federalreserve.gov/publications/2022-economic-well-being-of-us-households-in-2021-dealing-with-unexpected-expenses.htm.
7. Consumer Price Index. U.S. Bureau of Labor Statistics. Updated January 18, 2023. Accessed May 21, 2023. Available at: https://www.bls.gov/cpi/questions-and-answers.htm.
8. Fierce competition over veterinary labor. American Veterinary Medical Association (AVMA). December 01, 2021. Accessed May 21, 2023. https://www.avma.org/javma-news/2021-12-01/fierce-competition-over-veterinary-labor.
9. Veterinary labor demand remains strong during COVID. American Veterinary Medical Association (AVMA). December 03, 2020. Accessed May 21, 2023. https://www.avma.org/javma-news/2020-12-15/veterinary-labor-demand-remains-strong-during-covid.
10. Veterinarian employers require innovative solutions to attract, retain staff members. American Veterinary Medical Association (AVMA). October 25, 2022. Accessed May 21, 2023. https://www.avma.org/news/veterinarian-employers-require-innovative-solutions-attract-retain-staff-members.
11. Thin workforce, burnout lead to curtailed veterinary services. VIN News Service. December 7, 2022. Accessed May 21, 2023. https://news.vin.com/default.aspx?pid=210&catId=3115&id=11269744.
12. AVMA report on the economic state of the veterinary profession, 2023, Veterinary Economics Division, 2023. Available at: https://ebusiness.avma.org/ProductCatalog/product.aspx?ID=2094.

13. What is happening with bonuses in veterinary practice? VIN News Service. April 27, 2022. Accessed May 21, 2023. Available at: https://news.vin.com/default. aspx?pid=210&catId=14426&id=10912435.
14. 2023 Vet med hiring and retention trends. American Animal Hospital Association. December 18, 2022. Accessed May 21, 2023. Available at: https://www.aaha.org/ publications/newstat/articles/2022-12/2023-vet-med-hiring-and-retention-trends/.
15. Veterinary technicians being paid more but still face concerns about wages, burnout, debt. American Veterinary Medical Association. Updated February 14, 2023. Accessed July 1, 2023. Available at: https://www.avma.org/news/veterinary-technicians-being-paid-more-still-face-concerns-about-wages-burnout-debt.
16. Let's separate facts from feelings: The data behind emerging veterinary trends. Vetsource. Updated November 15, 2022. Accessed May 21, 2023. Available at: https://veterinaryanalytics.com/blog/lets-separate-facts-from-feelings-the-data-behind-emerging-veterinary-trends/.
17. Specialists in short supply. American Veterinary Medical Association. September 26, 2018. Accessed May 22, 2023. Available at: https://www.avma.org/javma-news/2018-10-15/specialists-short-supply.
18. Time for GPs to Take Back Skills They Gave Away to Specialists? Dr. Andy Roark. May 23, 2023. Accessed Jun 1, 2023. Available at: https://drandyroark.com/take-back-skills/.
19. Surviving Recession. Veterinary practice news. May 5, 2009. Accessed Jun 3, 2023. Available at: https://www.veterinarypracticenews.com/surviving-recession/.
20. Pet health 'has proven to be recession resistant': Zoetis CFO. Yahoo! Money. Aug 10, 2022. Accessed Jun 3, 2023. Available at: https://money.yahoo.com/pet-health-recession-resistant-zoetis-cfo-164147497.html.
21. Why The Pet Industry Is Recession-Proof. The Motley Fool. November 11, 2021. Accessed Jun 3, 2023. Available at: https://www.fool.com/investing/2021/11/02/ why-the-pet-industry-is-recession-proof/.
22. Are we in a veterinary workforce crisis? American Veterinary Medical Association. August 25, 2021. Accessed June 3, 2023. Available at: https://www.avma.org/ javma-news/2021-09-15/are-we-veterinary-workforce-crisis.
23. Fingland RB, Stone LR, Read EK, et al. Preparing veterinary students for excellence in general practice: building confidence and competence by focusing on spectrum of care. Journal of the American Veterinary Medical Association 2021;259(5):463–70. Retrieved Jul 1, 2023.
24. Brown CR, Edwards S, Kenney E, et al. Family Quality of Life: pet owners and veterinarians working together to reach the best outcomes. Journal of the American Veterinary Medical Association 2023. https://doi.org/10.2460/javma.23.01.0016.
25. Nationwide Mutual Insurance Company. Internal research. December 2023. Data on file.
26. Venn Emilee, Preisner Karolina, Boscan Pedro, et al. Evaluation of an outpatient protocol in the treatment of canine parvoviral enteritis: Outpatient treatment protocol in parvoviral enteritis. J Vet Emerg Crit Care 2016;27. https://doi.org/10. 1111/vec.12561.
27. Derksen F, Bensing J, Lagro-Janssen A. Effectiveness of empathy in general practice: a systematic review. Br J Gen Pract 2013;63(606):e76–84.
28. Dyess v. Caraway. 190 So.2d 666. 1966.
29. Cruciate ligament surgery in general practice. Covetrus. March 23, 2018. Accessed July 1, 2023. Available at: https://northamerica.covetrus.com/resource-center/ blogs/orthopedics/orthopedics/2018/03/23/cruciate-ligament-surgery-in-general-practice.

30. Haston RB, Pailler S. Simulation of the effect of low-cost companion animal clinics on the market for veterinary services. American Journal of Veterinary Research 2021;82(12):996–1002. Retrieved Jun 3, 2023, from.
31. Veterinary groups launch new coalition to advance telehealth for patient care. American Veterinary Medical Association. 2022. Accessed June 3, 2023. Available at: https://www.avma.org/news/press-releases/veterinary-groups-launch-new-coalition-advance-telehealth-patient-care.
32. The Virtual Vet Will See You Meow. The New York Times. April 7, 2023. Accessed Jun 3, 2023. Available at: https://www.nytimes.com/2023/04/07/health/vet-pet-health-telemedicine.html.
33. Smith SM, George Z, Duncan CG, et al. Opportunities for expanding access to veterinary care: lessons from COVID-19. Front Vet Sci 2022;9:804794. https://doi.org/10.3389/fvets.2022.804794.
34. Veterinary care for all. American Veterinary Medical Association. August 14, 2019. Accessed July 1, 2023. Available athttps://www.avma.org/javma-news/2019-09-01/veterinary-care-all.
35. Lap of Love: End-of-Life Pet Care. Veterinary Advantage. July 10, 2022. Accessed June 4, 2023. Available at: https://vet-advantage.com/vet_advantage/lap-of-love-end-of-life-pet-care/.
36. Pet Talk: Vancouver veterinarian opens new clinic offering affordable dental care. Available at: Oregonian. July 26, 2013. Accessed June 4, 2023. Available at: https://www.oregonlive.com/pets/2013/07/pet_talk_vancouver_veterinaria.html.
37. Section #2: Total pets insured. North American Pet Health Insurance Association. Updated May 3, 2023. Accessed June 23, 2023. Available at: https://naphia.org/industry-data/section-2-total-pets-insured/.
38. Pet insurance: Learning from the UK. Veterinary Practice News. February 13, 2020. Accessed June 23, 2023. Available at: https://www.veterinarypracticenews.com/pet-insurance-learning-from-the-u-k/.
39. Pet insurance for all: Sweden's experience. VIN News Service. October 2, 2019. Accessed July 1, 2023. Available at: https://news.vin.com/default.aspx?pid=210&Id=9305364&f5=1.
40. Section #1: Gross Written Premium. North American Pet Health Insurance Association. Updated May 3, 2023. Accessed July1, 2023. Available at: https://naphia.org/industry-data/section-1-gross-written-premium/.
41. Volk JO, Hartmann G. How wellness plans grow veterinary practice. J Am Vet Med Assoc 2015;247(1):40–1. https://doi.org/10.2460/javma.247.1.40.
42. What does it cost to offer Scratch Pay? Scratch. December 11, 2020. Accessed July1, 2023. Available at: get.scratchpay.com/faqs/offer-scratchpay-cost-fees.
43. Dedicated support you can rely on for your business. CareCredit. December 1, 2021. Accessed July 1, 2023. Available at: www.carecredit.com/providers/faq/.
44. REACH™ animal care program. American Veterinary Medical Foundation. Updated May 17, 2023. Accessed July1, 2023. Available at: https://www.avmf.org/grants-and-scholarships/reach-animal-care-program/.

The True Benefits of Veterinary Practice Ownership

Check for updates

Dan Markwalder, DVM*

KEYWORDS

- Acquisition • Business acumen • De novo • Veterinary practice ownership

KEY POINTS

- Now is a great time to be a practice owner.
- Owning your own practice has many benefits.
- Business acumen is critical to own a successful veterinary practice.
- Mentorship is one of the most important aspects of practice ownership.

INTRODUCTION

Is the era of independent practice ownership over? As I talk with many new graduates, the belief that they can own a veterinary practice seems to be behind us. Although veterinary medicine has a strong history of independent ownership, the trend of ownership favors corporate entities, from private equity to independent wealthy families. Many think this is the future of veterinary medicine. Yet, I have traveled to the majority of US veterinary schools, and I always finish my student presentation with this question: "Who would like to own and operate a veterinary hospital 1 day?" The vast majority of students raise their hands. I have been a veterinarian for 32 years. I have been an owner and partner in more than 20 veterinary hospitals during the last 3 decades, most recently selling my interest to join a national veterinary company, aiming to bring new veterinarians into practice ownership. Since becoming a veterinarian in 1991, I believe now is the best time to consider practice ownership.

THE REASON FOR MY OPTIMISM

Reasons behind this optimism include the following:

- As of 2023, the United States is home to 32,000 veterinary practices,[1] and the vast majority is independently owned.

Mission Veterinary Partners
* Corresponding author. 20450 Civic Center Drive, Southfield, MI 48076.
E-mail address: Dan.Markwalder@mvetpartners.com

Vet Clin Small Anim 54 (2024) 251–263
https://doi.org/10.1016/j.cvsm.2023.10.008
0195-5616/24/© 2023 Elsevier Inc. All rights reserved.

- The average veterinary practice uses 2.4 full-time equivalent veterinarians and has an annual revenue of less than US$1.2 million dollars and a profit margin that is unappealing to nonindependent buyers.
- A large number of boomer veterinarians are retiring, accelerated by coronavirus disease 2019 (COVID-19)—leaving a large number of practices available for purchase. How will the demand for pet care be met by the next generation of veterinarians? Studies show that millennial pet parents will be as good as, if not better than, the boomer pet owners who propelled the appeal of veterinary medicine in the corporate acquisition model. Moreover, millennial pet partners want the same level of health care for their pets as they receive from their personal health-care providers.

I believe that corporate consolidators have been not only beneficial but also essential to independent ownership as we look to the future of practice ownership.

A TALE OF 2 VETERINARIANS

Fasten your seatbelts—we will discuss the why, what, and how of practice ownership. However, first, I will share the tales of 2 veterinary practice owners—one an older practitioner and one a young practitioner—from different times.

Dr Dan Markwalder:

Dr Dan (Purdue, 1991), as he is referred to by most of his clients, wanted to be a veterinarian from the age of 6, and at age 15, he worked at his first veterinary hospital. Dr Dan was unsuccessful in his first veterinary school application attempt but he managed to prevail the second time around. During veterinary school, Dan had one goal—to eventually start and own a practice. Upon graduation, he spent 1 year in a 3-veterinarian practice, learning all about general small animal practice. In 1992, newly married, he moved his family to northwest Illinois to spend 8 months as a relief emergency veterinarian and full-time small animal practitioner. The major reason: no lender was willing to loan him enough money to begin a practice.

In March 1993, Dan opened his first de novo practice in the far suburbs of Chicago, Illinois. The 1200-square-foot facility had only 2 examination rooms, and the surgical suite doubled as the radiology room. The entire buildout cost about US$40,000. His first-year revenue was US$1million—with Dan working 75 hours a week with a beeper attached to his hip.

During the next 10 years, Dan eventually moved to a newly built, 4500-square-foot facility and started a second practice after his first kennel attendant graduated from veterinary school. Unlike his first practice, Dan's second practice was not financially successful. Dan realized that the issue was not the location, lack of marketing (which was nonexistent), or quality of medicine. The issue was Dan, who was not the type of leader the practice and teams needed. Fortunately, he found 2 mentors who helped him develop the leadership and business skills to be a successful practice owner. Dan fell in love with building and acquiring hospitals and developing a mentoring program that brings veterinarians into practice ownership. At the age of 55 years, Dan sold his practices to a corporate entity. As we approach more than 25 years of corporate ownership, Dan believes the time is right to combine a new generation of independent owners with the corporate advantages of scale to compete in the war on talent, innovation, and progressive medicine.

Dr Cody Creelman:

Dr Cody Creelman grew up on a beef cattle ranch in Northern Alberta, Canada. When he was 16 years old, a classmate suggested he sign up for a high school work experience program at the local veterinary clinic. From the moment he walked in, Dr Creelman was immediately hooked on the profession.

Pursuing his dream, Dr Creelman attended the University of Alberta, applying to veterinary school 4 times before being accepted. After graduating, Dr Creelman took a position at a beef cattle practice. Two years after taking the job, Dr Creelman was offered a partnership in the practice, and discovered a new aspect of the profession he loved—business management. Although the learning curve was steep, Dr Creelman helped grow the practice and dreamed of further expansion and diversification.

In 2014, he founded a mixed animal practice group and acquired 5 clinics across Alberta and Saskatchewan. In 2019, partnership issues led Dr Creelman to leave his 8 practices, and although he felt lost and uncertain about his future, his passion for veterinary medicine continued to burn bright. Optimistic about the future, Dr Creelman established a new type of practice that was built on innovation, customer experience, and an exceptional practice culture. Fen Vet was born.

Dr Creelman knew he could not acquire an existing practice that perfectly aligned with his mission and core values, so he opted to start a de novo practice. Fen Vet in Airdrie, Alberta opened in 2021 with 1 veterinarian, 2 veterinary technicians, a client care coordinator, and Dr Creelman. In the first year, the practice grossed US$1.7 million, and plans started for another Fen Vet location in downtown Calgary.

Dr Creelman's vision is to continue investing in Fen Vet's growth for as long as possible, and dreams that Fen Vet will evolve into an employee stock ownership plan. Fen Vet provides a completely different experience for pet owners and veterinary professionals. Fen Vet currently uses 34 team members, including 10 veterinarians, and in April 2023, 17 local veterinarians were on a waiting list, eager to work at the practice. In May 2023, Fen Vet launched a second location. The 4100-square-foot clinic has 7 examination rooms and a full medical team. Dr Creelman views operating the Fen Vet brand as his career's final chapter and hopes to expand the brand organically during the next 30 years.

NOW IS A GREAT TIME TO BE A PRACTICE OWNER

According to the American Veterinary Medical Association (AVMA), 40% of independent veterinary practices will be looking to sell in the next 5 years.[2] A vast majority of these hospitals will not be acquired by one of the national companies. I refer to these types of practices as "fixer-uppers"—they may be in a desirable geographic area but they have not always received the enhancements necessary to run and operate a practice for the future, such as capital expenditures for ultrasonography, laser, dental radiography, and electronic medical records. In many cases, they have little to no marketing plans and have inefficient operation models. As a result, the profitability is low. These practices have revenues of less than US$1 million with little to no updates in equipment during the last 10 to 20 years. They have less than 1200 active clients, and a low average client transaction. Laboratory revenues may be less than those of a well-managed practice.[3] Real estate may be in a desirable location but the building may need to be remodeled. So, why should you consider this type of practice? Simply put, the ability to secure capital to make the necessary changes such as new equipment, remodeling, and an electronic medical record system. The potential for these locations is remarkable if you provide a well-thought-out marketing plan to generate new clients, practice high-quality medicine, increase wellness testing compliance, increase dental procedures, and offer additional veterinary services. I personally partnered in 8 similar acquisitions during the middle to late 2000s. The practices had an average gross revenue of US$750,000, less than 10% profitability. After purchase, we were able to grow year-over-year revenue by an average of 32% with an average profitability of 22%. The average cost of acquisition for the goodwill (ie, client base) was US$500,000. This means I was able to acquire the practice goodwill for US$500,000 with a profitability of US$50,000 to US$60,000 and turn each into a US$2.8 to US$3.0 million dollar practice with an average profit of US$625,000 within 5 years. Moreover, it is not uncommon to receive 100% financing for goodwill from many lending institutions.

MENTAL WELL-BEING

Lack of mental well-being is a concern among veterinary clinicians and paraprofessional team members. Merck and others have documented higher levels of stress, burnout, and depression within the profession.[4] A study conducted among veterinarians in the Netherlands demonstrated that "the mean percentage of respondents from graduation years 2009 to 2014 who left practice within 5 years of graduation was 16.8%,"[5] with lack of adequate compensation one of the top reasons. An AVMA study (**Fig. 1**) that included 1217 practice owners and 1414 associate veterinarians showed that practice owners have higher compassion scores and lower burnout scores compared with associates.[6] However, practice owners and associates had high secondary traumatic stress. The COVID-19 pandemic may have contributed to this increase. The conclusion of the study seems to support the notion that practice ownership is beneficial to a veterinarian's quality of life. Higher compensation, more oversight over work schedule, and a better work environment may contribute to an improved overall mental well-being.

FINANCIAL WELL-BEING

The financial benefits of practice ownership are well documented. Practice owners are compensated about 2 to 3 times more than associate veterinarians. A practice owner should be compensated for their veterinary production, management fees, the distribution of profits generated by the practice, and fair market rent for the lease of the building or space the practice occupies. For example, let's assume that a veterinarian owns 100% of a practice that generates US$1.5 million in a given year, and they produced US$750,000. At a production rate of 20%, the owner receives compensation of US$150,000. Moreover, the owner works 5 hours per week in management-related duties, receiving an additional US$15,000. The profitability of the practice is around 15% of US$1.5 million, earning the owner another US$225,000. Finally, the practice owner owns the real estate and receives another US$90,000 per year in fair market rent for the building. The veterinary owner receives a total compensation of US$480,000. An associate would need to produce US$2.4 million for a similar salary!

Ownership is also a great way to quickly eliminate educational debt. For example, if you secure a US$1 million loan at a 6% fixed interest rate with a 20-year term to purchase a veterinary practice and real estate, your monthly payment would be approximately US$7300. Let us say you generate US$1 million in revenue for the practice and produce US$850,000 in production. After expenses and loan payments, your profit is US$150,000 (15%). You also make US$850,000 × 20%, or US$170,000, in production, US$15,000 for management fees, and US$150,000 in profit, for a total compensation of US$335,000. If you have a US$400,000 educational loan and pay US$100,000 per year, you can repay this loan in less than 5 years!

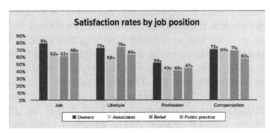

Fig. 1. Satisfaction rates by job position. With permission from the American Veterinary Medical Association (2023 AVMA Economic State of the Veterinary Profession).

Practice ownership gives you a marketable asset for the future. Similar to owning a home or a stock, you should gain a significant return on your investment when you eventually sell the practice. Veterinary medicine has one of the highest returns on investment for all health-care fields. For example, let us say you own a practice that grosses US$3.5 million dollars in revenue per year and US$600,000 in earnings before interest, taxes, depreciation, and amortization (EBITDA). Historically, practices were valued at a multiple, usually 4 to 6, or cap rate of the EBITDA. However, it is not uncommon to see higher multiples in competitive markets. If a multiple of 10 is applied to this example, the practice could sell for US$6 million. Even before the recent increase, a low multiple (US$600,000 × 4) would result in a value of US$2.4 million dollars. If you also own the real estate, you can either sell it to the buyer or a third-party real estate company or continue as a property owner and receive monthly rent payments. In contrast, a practice with US$3.4 million in annual revenue but only US$350,000 in EBITDA at a multiple of 4 is now valued at US$1.4 million. Protecting your practice's profitability is important for a future return on your investment.

TAX BENEFITS

Practice ownership also provides tax benefits. As a business owner, you purchase equipment to help produce income for your practice. The Internal Revenue Service allows you to write off some or potentially all of the equipment cost[7] by a depreciation method, and then deduct a portion of the amount from your hospital earnings, thereby reducing your tax burden.

Although you may have a 5-year loan on the equipment, you may be able to receive a tax deduction of 100% of the equipment cost in the first year, helping you to free up cash. For example, let us say you spend US$100,000 on equipment, and you will repay the 5-year loan at US$25,000 per year, including principal and interest. In the first year, you can deduct the full value of the equipment (US$100,000) from your earnings subject to taxes. Although you paid only $25,000 on the loan, you reduced your total profit subject to taxes by US$100,000. You can also deduct other expenses, such as continuing education, computer equipment, licensure, and other business-related expenses. In addition, you can employ a family member, and deduct their wages. Incorporated practices may also receive some tax benefits at the state level. Finally, as a practice owner, you can establish a retirement plan, which can be a great long-term benefit for you and your employees. Tax credits may be available if you open a new plan. Please consult an accountant or attorney to ensure you understand how to best afford your practice and yourself of these tax benefits.

LEADERSHIP AND CULTURE

Unfortunately, many veterinarians are detracted from ownership because the position requires leadership and business skills. Although many veterinarians may claim that ownership management duties led them to sell,[8] there are countless examples of founders who did not have formal leadership education but went on to lead successful companies. Formal training in leadership and business is not required for you to own a veterinary practice but much like being a veterinarian, a desire to be a great leader and an ability to learn and grow are essential. Questions to ask yourself if you want to develop the necessary leadership skills as a future practice owner include the following:

1. Do I want to create a vision and core values in an organization?
2. Do I want to be a person of influence?

3. Do I want to motivate and lead a group of individuals toward a common goal?
4. Do I have the appetite to learn and grow?
5. Do I love people and want them to grow and develop?

If you answered yes to these questions, you could and should lead a practice. Motivation is the key, and skills can be learned. To be an effective leader, you must be willing to have an insatiable appetite to grow, learn, and empower others toward a common vision. My own leadership path involved asking others to help and mentor me from a business and leadership front. Many resources are available today that allow an aspiring practice owner to develop leadership and business skills needed to succeed (see Resources list).

Additionally, nothing is more satisfying than creating a thriving culture among individuals in a practice. Culture is the shared behaviors and values that drive your work as an organization or hospital, making you different from the rest. Culture gives you a competitive advantage for operational performance as measured by team member retention through empowerment, engagement, and development. This reinforces your brand and gives you the ability to recruit and attract the best talent.

STANDARDS OF CARE

Consider a scenario where you can practice the level of care and medicine that is consistent with your beliefs and standards. As a practice owner, you have this freedom. You can choose which heartworm preventives to offer, decide that every surgery patient will receive an IV catheter and the latest pain management protocol, and that your practice will offer telemedicine. You are in the driver's seat.

You can also decide what practice type you want to own. Does urgent care or emergency medicine interest you, or do you prefer preventive and wellness care? Your personal preferences will help you decide which type of practice you should consider as a practice owner. You might prefer a practice that offers instant access to advanced diagnostics, from ultrasonography to computed tomography, or you might prefer preventive care, and wish to refer complicated medical and surgical cases. It is also important to establish standards of care to attract veterinarians best suited for your practice and ensure consistency of care for the patients and clients you serve.

MENTORSHIP

As a practice owner and leader, your number *one* job is not to provide the organization's vision, mission, and core values, or to create systems and processes. Although these factors are essential for the practice's success, your *most* important job is to recruit and retain the best talent. In other words, a practice owner must be a talent magnet. Most practices are currently in a talent war, making recruiting exceptional veterinarians difficult. However, the key to successful practice ownership is to grow by growing others. In her monumental book, *Multipliers*, author Liz Wiseman describes what a leader (ie, practice owner) must do to have a successful and productive team, be a genius maker, and be a multiplier as opposed to a diminisher (**Fig. 2**).

Many hospitals win the talent war by having a strong commitment to mentorship and team development, helping to attract and retain the best talent. We know that new graduates are willing to forgo the large signing bonuses if their employer has a strong commitment to mentorship. In addition, many high school graduates who have decided not to go to college are willing to take a veterinary assistant position if the employer will help them develop the necessary skills to become a credentialed technician.

THE FIVE DISCIPLINES OF THE MULTIPLIER

	DIMINISHERS	MULTIPLIERS
SEE	**THE ASSUMPTION** "People won't figure it out without me"	**THE ASSUMPTION** "People are smart and will figure it out"
DO	**THE DISCIPLINES** **1. The Empire Builder** Hoards resources and underutilizes talent **2. The Tyrant** Creates a tense environment that suppresses people's thinking and capability **3. The Know-It-All** Gives directives that showcase how much they know **4. The Decision Maker** Makes centralized, abrupt decisions that confuse the organization **5. The Micromanager** Drives results through their personal involvement	**THE DISCIPLINES** **1. The Talent Magnet** Attracts talented people and uses them at their highest point of contribution **2. The Liberator** Creates an intense enviornment that requires people's best thinking and work **3. The Challenger** Defines an opportunity that causes people to stretch **4. The Debate Maker** Drives sound decisions through rigorous debate **5. The Investor** Gives other people ownership for results and invests in their success
GET	**THE RESULT** $<50\%$	**THE RESULT** $2\times$

Fig. 2. The 5 disciplines of the multiplier.

PURPOSE AND DIRECTION

Author and speaker Simon Sinek became a phenomenon in the leadership culture when he published his first book, *Start With Why*. In a 2009 Ted talk, that had more than 60 million views, Sinek describes his Golden Circle. In the center is the why, next is the how, and finally, the what. Sinek goes on to explain that most companies know what they do and how they do it but few know why they are doing it. This purpose or passion is the driving force for the most successful businesses. So, start with your why. Why do you want to be a practice owner? Understand that no one buys into an idea or project until they know why it exists. Your why will give you fulfillment in all the activities associated with ownership and allow others, including clients and team members, to be inspired to join your efforts. This foundation is essential to inspire client loyalty in a competitive marketplace.

BUSINESS ACUMEN

A little-known secret is that you must be well versed in business acumen to be a successful practice owner. Although helpful, you do not need years of experience or a degree in business to be successful in practice ownership. A veterinary professional must be willing to learn and surround themselves with people who have demonstrated past success in the business realm. You must ask yourself if you are willing to develop the skills necessary to be a successful practice owner. This requires time and a willingness to learn.

Other questions to consider include the following:

- Are you passionate about finance, ready to dive into profit and loss statements and other financial metrics?
- Are you interested in developing systems and processes for your team?

- Are you passionate about marketing?
- Are you interested in technology and communication?
- Are you passionate about human resources, compensation, and benefits?
- Are you interested in inventory management and facility maintenance?

This may seem overwhelming but these are key aspects of practice ownership. However, you do not have to be passionate about all these areas. You can seek out people who are gifted in these areas and provide the necessary oversight. The best practice owners are leaders who understand their strengths and are willing to backfill with individuals who counterbalance where they may not be gifted or do not want to progress. Developing business acumen is essential for your success as a practice owner, and you must know who to hire when needed and how to make the right decisions to take your practice to the next level.

FULFILLMENT AND SATISFACTION

Practice ownership has additional benefits. You can take time away from the practice while still receiving income associated with being an owner (ie, a nonproducing member of the practice). Done correctly, practice ownership can afford you a healthy work–life balance. For some, practice ownership creates a legacy that lives well beyond their time as a practice owner. Others are more interested in practicing medicine at a level that gives them pride, and some want to tap into the passion of entrepreneurship and create something unique, such as a brand that fills a need in the marketplace.

RETIREMENT

You will eventually retire from veterinary medicine. If you are a practice owner, you will hopefully receive some return on the asset you created. Your practice will have economic value that typically includes the goodwill, inventory, and equipment. Someone (ie, the buyer) will put a value on these assets. Most people's retirement assets lie in their home and retirement fund, whereas a large portion of a practice owner's wealth comes from selling their practice. Furthermore, if you own the practice's real estate, you can generate ongoing income through rent.

THE FUTURE

Veterinary medicine's future looks bright. The compounded annual growth rate is expected to be more than 5% for the next few years and to continue at 3% to 5% thereafter.[9] Millennial and Gen Z pet acquisitions will continue to drive demand for veterinary services. In addition, younger generations who choose to have pets will increase demand for veterinary care. A 2021 survey conducted by Idexx Laboratories found that from a sample of 2000 American pet-owning adults.

- Eighty-eight percent said that their pet's health is as important to them as taking care of their own health.
- Eighty-six percent agreed that taking good care of their pet means they have regular visits with a veterinarian.
- Eighty-one percent would adjust their personal budget to pay for care their veterinarian recommended if they did not have the money to cover it.[9]

Innovation is a friend to veterinary medicine. Advancements such as pharmaceuticals, early diagnostic testing, and cancer screening help increase the level of care desired by pet parents. In addition, according to the US State of Pet Health report, dogs are now living an average of 11.8 years, which is up from 11 years in 2013, and 10.5 years in 2002.[10]

WHAT DOES PRACTICE OWNERSHIP LOOK LIKE TODAY?

There are similarities and vast differences between practice ownership in the past and ownership today. Twenty-five years ago, most practice owners sold to 1 or 2 of their associate veterinarians. Today, national companies are willing to buy at a much higher rate, and practice owners more commonly sell to corporations. If you desire to be a sole practice owner, I think purchasing a single practice with an annual gross revenue less than US$1 million dollars is the most economically viable option as you are not competing with corporate groups that have inflated the fair market value of larger practices. This also creates an opportunity to grow the practice into a business that is desirable by corporate groups, which will materially change the valuation dynamics, creating significant equity upside on top of the annual profits you generate. Depending on your long-term ownership plans, and if you wish to sell at some point in the future, that may or may not be important to you but regardless of your plans, it is an important variable that you should understand.

Being a sole owner allows you a great deal of independence. You are in charge. However, you will also have all of the responsibility. You make the decisions, you secure the funding, and you oversee all vital roles.

Partnerships today can take many different forms. They can involve one or more veterinarians or nonveterinarians. Partnerships between veterinarians who have different strengths in the veterinary field can be advantageous. Partnerships can also be beneficial when one veterinarian is interested in leadership and management and the other is more passionate about medicine. Increasingly, I have witnessed veterinarians partnering with nonveterinarians, such as veterinary technicians and practice managers, to open or acquire a practice. With all partnerships, crucial decisions must be considered, such as the following:

- What percentage of ownership will each partner have?
- What roles will each partner have within the practice?
- How will important decisions be made?
- What will your hiring and firing practices entail?
- What level of medicine will you practice?
- How will you determine what capital equipment purchases are needed?
- How will you handle and compensate your team members?
- What are your practice's core values?
- How will you reconcile disagreements?

Increasingly, partnerships are made between veterinarians and national companies (ie, joint ventures). This allows the owner to tap into the larger company's resources, such as better drug and supply costs, and established marketing and human resource departments. They have experience in building and construction management and can likely secure capital equipment at a lower cost than an average single veterinarian or independent practice owner. The disadvantage is that a national company may not be willing to purchase a practice in your geographic region. A private equity-backed company may want to sell to another company in a short period, which may allow you a greater upside in a shorter period. However, you may not want to hold onto your shares in the hospital for as long as your partner desires. These issues must be reconciled during the early stages of partnership.

Things to consider before becoming a practice owner include (**Table 1**) the following:

1. Do I want a partner? If so, why? What will this person bring to this partnership?
2. Do I want to be a solo owner? If so, what areas of ownership will I need to backfill?

Table 1
Considerations for prospective practice owners

Solo Owner	Partnership with 2 or More Veterinarians	Partnership with a Nonveterinarian	Partnership with a National Company
Do I want to be a leader or find a leader for my practice?	Will one of us be the primary leader of the practice?	Who will be the primary leader of the practice?	What does the partnership look like?
What are my areas of strength and weakness as a leader/owner?	What are each of our strengths and weaknesses on a medical front?	How will we divide nonmedical tasks of the practice?	What autonomy will you have within your practice?
How much time will I be able to devote to the nonmedical tasks of the practice?	Percentage of ownership for each	Percentage of ownership for each	When are we looking to sell and how does this affect my equity?

3. How long do I want to be an owner or partner?
4. What does the ideal partner for me look like?

HOW TO BE A PRACTICE OWNER TODAY

Once you have decided to become a practice owner, you will need to decide whether you want a de novo practice or an acquisition. A de novo is a new start-up hospital, whereas an acquisition is the purchase of an existing hospital in your desired geographic market. So, you must decide: Do I acquire an existing hospital or start from scratch?

See **Tables 2** and **3** for the pros and cons associated with de novo and acquisition models.

Once you have decided to either purchase or start a practice, I recommend developing a Business Plan, which is a step-by-step written document that will serve as a road map for your plans to own and operate a successful veterinary practice (see Resources list). This is essential to secure funding from a lender. If you do not know how to get started, artificial intelligence and ChatGPT can help you create business and marketing plans.

The next step is securing funding. In the case of an acquisition, a valuation should be performed on the practice. A valuation is usually performed by a third party to determine the value of the practice's goodwill, inventory, and equipment. The real estate is generally handled as a separate transaction. You should meet with a commercial lender to determine the best route of financing for your needs. Options include a standard commercial or a small business loan. Most commercial loans have 10 to 15-year

Table 2
Pros and cons of practice acquisition

Pros	Cons
• You acquire the goodwill (ie, client base)	• You acquire the practice's reputation
• Existing team	• You acquire the team
• Real estate, equipment, and inventory	• Outdated facilities/equipment
• Turn-key	• Old lease
• Quicker return on investment	• Quality of medicine and culture
• Positive cash flow	• Change management

Table 3	
Pros and cons of opening a de novo practice	
Pros	Cons
• You can choose where you go	• No client base
• Not paying a high multiple	• Negative cash flow
• Create/design your own practice	• Longer development time
• Fill a void in an underrepresented area	• Budget is essential
• Higher upside return on investment	• Unknown events can cause slower ramp up
• Your team, your standards, and your vision	

repayment terms, which you must consider as you calculate the practice's profitability projections.

MEETING WITH AN ATTORNEY FOR INCORPORATION

Please do not skip this part in your practice ownership journey. An attorney is essential for several aspects of ownership, such as drawing up partnership operating agreements, and reviewing leasehold agreements and other real estate considerations. Finally, an attorney will counsel you on how to incorporate your practice and help you determine whether to form a limited liability corporation, a C-corporation, or an S-corporation. They will help you draft the bylaws and articles of incorporation for your veterinary practice. You should hire an attorney early in the process and consider them an essential member of your team.

FINDING AN ACCOUNTANT

Financial health is an essential part of veterinary practice ownership. An accountant can assist you with payroll and generate important financial documents such as balance sheets and profit and loss statements. I recommend you set up your general ledger with the American Animal Hospital Association (AAHA) chart of accounts, which is standard in the veterinary industry and will help you assess the different revenue buckets and expense items as you look at your profit and loss statement to assess your practice's financial well-being. Your accountant can generate reports, such as payroll deductions, taxes, and reporting needed by your lender, and help you with tax matters. An accountant should be a close advisor who not only generates necessary reports but also meets with you periodically to review the reports.

CONSTRUCTION MANAGEMENT

Either early on, in the case of a startup, or potentially during the life of your practice ownership, you may engage in new construction to remodel or expand. You will need to become familiar with veterinary construction from a buyer/planner standpoint. I would encourage you to seek out continuing education on veterinary construction management—not only from a client perspective but also considering the practice's efficiency, flow, and operations. You must become familiar with the materials currently used in veterinary construction and consider details such as how to reduce noise and odor in a veterinary facility. I recommend using architects and general contractors who have experience in veterinary construction.

SUMMARY

If you dream about owning your own veterinary practice, now is a good time to take steps to make that goal a reality. Find a mentor to act as a guide and be willing to develop business and leadership skills to navigate the process. Practice ownership has numerous benefits if you are willing to put forth the effort and make the investment, and many routes are available to help you realize your dream.

CLINICS CARE POINTS

- Owning your own practice has many financial and well-being benefits.
- Although you do not need a business degree to open a practice, you do need to be well versed in business acumen to have a successful veterinary practice.
- To own a practice, you must make decisions such as if you want a de novo practice or an acquisition, if you want a partner, and what type of partnership you want.
- Mentorship is vitally important to attract and retain top talent.
- Corporate consolidation in veterinary medicine provides opportunities for independent owners.

DISCLOSURE

None.

REFERENCES

1. AVMA Economic and Business Committee, 2023.
2. 2021 AVMA Census of Veterinarians.
3. Brakke Consulting, John Volk, telephone call from author.
4. Merck Animal Health Veterinary Well Being Study 2020.
5. Sonneveld D, Goverts Y, Dujin C, et al. Dutch veterinary graduates leaving practice: A mixed-method analysis frequency and underlying reasons. Vet Rec 2022; 192(2):e2178.
6. Ouedraogo F, Lefebvre S. Benefits of practice ownership among US private practice veterinarians extend to professional quality of life. JAVMA 2022;260(15): 1971–8.
7. Internal Revenue Service Publication 946 (2022), How to Depreciate Property. Section 179.
8. Packaged facts, 2022.
9. IDEXX. Perspective on companion animal industry trends. 2022.
10. Global Animal Health Association. Global State of Pet Care: Stats, Facts and Trends. 2022. Available at: https://www.qrillpet.com/blog-and-news/pet-health-trends-pets-are-living-longer-than-ever. Accessed June 8, 2023.

FURTHER READINGS

Bennetts L. The Feminine mistake: are we giving up too much? 2008.
Cantanzaro TE. Building the successful veterinary practice, vol. 1, 1997.
Covey SR. The 7 habits of highly effective people, 30th anniversary edition 2016.
Financial and productivity pulsepoints. ed. 10. AAHA Press; 2019.
Frankel L. Nice girls don't get a corner office 2004.

Gerber ME, Weinstein P. The E-Myth veterinarian 2015.

Gladwell M. Blink: the power of thinking without thinking 2007.

Goleman D. Emotional intelligence: why it can matter more than IQ. 10th anniversary edition 2005.

Goleman D. Working with emotional intelligence 2000.

Johnson S. Who moved my cheese? An amazing way to deal with change in your work and in your life 2006.

List LM. Buying a veterinary practice. AAHA Press; 2006.

List LM. Starting a veterinary practice. AAHA Press; 2006.

Lundin SC, Paul H, Christensen J. Fish! A proven way to improve morale and improve results 2020.

Opperman M. The art of veterinary practice management 2014.

Prentiss C. Zen and the art of happiness 2006.

Rath T, Clifton D. How full is your bucket? Expanded anniversary edition 2004.

Ruiz DM. The four agreements: a practical guide to personal freedom 1997.

Stein SJ, Book HE. The EQ Edge: emotional intelligence and your success 2011.

U.S. Small Business Administration. Write your business plan. 2023. Available at: https://www.sba.gov/business-guide/plan-your-business/write-your-business-plan–helpful resource to help write your business plan. Accessed June 13, 2023.

The Progressive Veterinary Practice

Natalie Marks, DVM, CVJ

KEYWORDS

- Artificial intelligence • Digital marketing • Feline medicine • Low stress
- Progressive practice • Shared decision making • Spectrum of care

KEY POINTS

- Veterinary practices must continually evolve to meet the needs of the ever-changing pet owner demographic.
- Veterinary practices have evolved to include various practice types and a spectrum of appointment types to provide more accessible and comprehensive care for patients.
- Modern marketing and communication methods are essential to appeal to today's veterinary clients.
- Pet owners should be educated about their pet's anticipated cost of care and different available payment options.
- Practices should strive to improve care offered to cats and help cat caregivers understand the importance of feline health care.

INTRODUCTION

The practice of veterinary medicine dates back to 9000 BC, when sheepherders used basic medical skills to treat their flocks. Thousands of years later, the first brick and mortar veterinary practices were established, with companion animals eventually receiving medical care equal to, or better than, that of farm animals.

Veterinary medicine has changed significantly over the past decades. Only 50 years ago, a typical veterinary practice was made up of a single veterinarian who owned a small building along with a microscope, an X-ray machine, and basic surgical tools. They likely had a small staff who were trained on the job. Veterinarians of this era treated everything that came through the door, from new puppies to emergencies. However, veterinary medicine mainly focused on dogs, with the occasional feline patient considered an afterthought. These practices were created (from layout, to medicine, to tools, to communication) for dogs only, which explains why practices have struggled to engage cat caregivers for so long.

MarksDVMConsulting, 3830 North Bell Avenue, Chicago, IL 60618, USA
E-mail address: drnataliemarks@gmail.com

Vet Clin Small Anim 54 (2024) 265–276
https://doi.org/10.1016/j.cvsm.2023.10.011
0195-5616/24/© 2023 Elsevier Inc. All rights reserved.

vetsmall.theclinics.com

In contrast, today's typical small animal veterinary practice includes at least two veterinarians, two credentialed veterinary technicians, and several additional support staff,[1] and a suite of modern diagnostic equipment. In addition to general practices, many communities have emergency and specialty practices, with veterinary specialists who can provide diagnostics and treatments rivaling that of human medical care.

In general practice, the pendulum has swung back toward veterinary medicine's origination: preventive care. In particular, veterinarians are helping cat caregivers understand that veterinary care, and especially preventive care, is essential for their feline family members. Unfortunately, many cat caregivers have misunderstandings about feline pets (eg, cats are easy pets, cats do not need veterinary care because they live indoors, cats do not visibly show pain, cats are independent and do not need care). Progress has been made, but less than two out of five cats in the United States currently receive routine veterinary care,[2] which means there is still a long way to go.

Veterinary practices have realized the importance of their patients' emotional health and reducing fear, anxiety, and stress to make veterinary visits more pleasant, and consider their patients' needs when planning for facility layout and design. The importance of caring for each pet's complete health status is now understood.

Today's pet owner has different expectations than those of even 10 years ago. Of the 86.9 million pet owners in the United States, 16% are Gen Z and 33% are Millennials[3] who expect more personalized care for their companions and want to have an experiential journey at their veterinary practice. Most of today's pet owners (85% of dog owners and 76% of cat owners) consider their pets to be family members,[4] and many are willing to provide comforts, such as fresh or home-cooked pet food, pet insurance, and specialty medical care to ensure their pet lives a long, healthy life. They want to have a relationship with their pet's veterinary care team and expect to communicate regularly with them through multiple channels.

Veterinary practices must continually evolve to meet the needs of the ever-changing pet owner demographic. They must be forward-thinking and innovative to create ways to build client relationships and improve the care provided.

Of equal importance, practices must strive to meet the emotional and physical needs of their team members and should prioritize team well-being. Practices should intentionally foster a welcoming and inclusive environment for all clients and team members. Although well-being initiatives are partially driven by the current challenges within the veterinary industry, such as staffing shortages, the costs associated with staff retention, and the enormous time and financial investment of training new team members, they are long overdue.

With so much change behind us, it is obvious that the future of veterinary medicine is ever evolving. Successful practice management requires constant understanding of dynamic industry trends, and continuous consideration of the needs of the current and future generation of pet owners.

VETERINARY PRACTICE TYPES

Whereas the traditional veterinary practice was a one-stop model, with the veterinarian seeing all types of appointments, from wellness visits to sick pets, to emergencies, and from dogs and cats to birds and rats, modern veterinary practices are often more specialized. As veterinary medicine has advanced, some veterinarians have decided that they can practice better medicine by offering fewer services to fewer patients. Some practices become certified in certain areas of interest, such as Cat Friendly Hospital or Fear Free Certification.

In addition, the dynamic nature of veterinary medicine makes it difficult for a veterinarian to keep up with all of the available diagnostic and treatment options. New developments, such as monoclonal antibody therapy, and gene therapy for cancer treatment, are beneficial to pets, but may not be adopted by general practice veterinarians for a variety of reasons. Practices may lack adequate time to research new technology, train their teams, and implement new workflows. They may also lack understanding about how to make the technology profitable for their practice or may be hesitant to adopt technology that is not yet widely accepted. However, these advancements are hugely beneficial to pets, and specialty-type practices can allow pets access to the full range of available care.

Species-Specific Veterinary Practices

Although most veterinary practices still care for multiple species, some practices focus on cats or exotic pets. This allows the veterinary team to hone the handling skills needed to provide low-stress care for a particular species. Cats-only hospitals, for example, reduce the anxiety associated with encountering, or maybe just smelling, dogs in the facility, which helps cats to relax. The veterinary team can focus on developing the skills needed to handle cats in ways that avoid unnecessary stress. Other ways these practices cater to cats include.

- Having no lobby, to avoid cats having to acclimate to several spaces.
- Using pheromones to promote relaxation.
- Using examination rooms for multiple purposes (eg, diagnostic rooms) to avoid transferring patients to other areas.
- Removing smells and sounds that are noxious to cats.
- Including enrichment items, such as cat trees, shelving, toys, and high-value treats.
- Using towels as restraint aids.

Some practices that see multiple species designate separate canine and feline waiting areas and examination rooms, which can also help reduce stress and anxiety.

Low-Stress Veterinary Practices

It is no secret that veterinary visits can cause pet's significant stress. One study showed that dogs demonstrated a 16% increase in mean blood pressure and an 11% increase in pulse rate, and a higher number of dogs panted, during veterinary visits compared with at home.[5] Progressive practices should make additional efforts to reduce visit-related stress for pets and clients. From practice design to handling techniques, every aspect of a patient's journey should be considered to make the experience more pleasant. In addition to species-specific areas, low-stress practices often design their waiting areas and examination rooms to appeal to cats and dogs. Including items that a pet associates with past positive experiences can help put them at ease and reduce anxiety. For example, a feline examination room may be designed as an indoor "catio," with elevated perches, pheromone diffusers, and enticing cat toys. A canine examination room may be designed as a dog park, complete with benches and a fire hydrant. Lobby-less practices will be a trend of the future, where concierge-style treatment will include ushering clients from their vehicle directly into an examination room. Other design elements that can contribute to a positive visit include

- Playing classical music for dogs, and classical or reggae music for cats.
- Using soft pastel colors on the walls, floors, and furniture.

- Avoiding fluorescent lighting, which can cause a noxious, low-grade hum that animals can hear.
- Providing traction (eg, rugs, floor runners) on hard floors, to prevent slipping.
- Adding elevated surfaces for cat carriers, because cats are most comfortable on vertical surfaces.

Many practices who wish to incorporate low-stress methods complete Fear Free training courses to earn Fear Free Certification. Certification is available for individual team members and practices through https://fearfreepets.com.

Service-Specific Veterinary Practices

Instead of every practice providing full-service veterinary care, many practices now provide specialty or niche care. Emergency practices are often open 24/7, which removes the need for general practices to fit in emergencies between regular appointments. Additionally, emergency veterinarians are specially trained, and can often provide higher-level care. Many urgent care practices have opened to fill the gap between day practices and after-hours emergency and specialty hospitals.

Specialty practices employ board-certified veterinary specialists who can handle more difficult cases, which allows general practice veterinarians to focus on wellness care and minor illnesses. Other niche practices, such as dentistry or behavior practices, offer specific care. These types of practices typically do not offer wellness care. This is beneficial for many reasons; it preserves the referral partner relationship and allows board-certified veterinarians to focus on their area of specialty.

On the other hand, wellness care practices focus on routine wellness and preventive care, such as routine examinations, preventive diagnostics and screening, vaccines, and parasite prevention. These practices cover a pet's routine wellness care, but do not offer illness care, and typically refer sick pets to another local practice.

Open-Concept Veterinary Practices

This emerging trend in veterinary practice design allows pet owners to accompany their pets throughout the appointment journey. Open-concept practices feature a large, open examination and treatment area instead of typical examination rooms and a restricted treatment area. Pet owners stay with their pet throughout the visit and are encouraged to spend time with their hospitalized pets. This model can foster stronger veterinary-client relationships because it allows the pet owner to observe every aspect of their pet's care and understand the associated value.

How Advanced Technology Benefits Progressive Veterinary Practices

Regardless of practice type, technological advancements can improve efficiency and reduce veterinary team burden. Most practices use practice management software, but few take full advantage of the many time-saving tools, such as digital forms, SOAP templates, inventory management, or key performance indicator tracking. Full use of practice software allows practices to become virtually paperless, which improves efficiency and reduces waste. Integrations between veterinary software and reference laboratory studies, veterinary distributors, and other industry partners can also save veterinary team members valuable time, and automations provided with diagnostic equipment can improve efficiency. Although these tools often require an initial time investment, truly progressive practices understand the long-term value and embrace efficiencies provided by technology. The time savings reduces veterinary team stress and allows veterinary teams to be more productive.

VETERINARY PRACTICE MARKETING AND COMMUNICATIONS

A client's and patient's journey begins long before they enter a practice. Instead of loyally visiting the town veterinarian, today's veterinary client considers many factors before carefully selecting a veterinary practice that fits their needs. To remain relevant and competitive, progressive practices must appeal to clients through a variety of digital channels.

Marketing

Digital marketing has become increasingly important and will continue to play a large role in communicating with existing and potential clients. More than 75% of consumers search for a company's Web site before visiting their physical location (https://visualobjects.com/digital-marketing/blog/benefits-of-local-seo).   Likewise, pet owners looking for a veterinarian typically perform an online search and review the top search results. Therefore, a practice's Web site should be visually appealing, well-organized, and user-friendly, or the potential client may quickly move to another site.

Today's veterinary client wants to build a relationship with their veterinary health care team. So, a practice's Web site should highlight their services and values to attract the type of clients they wish to serve. For example, a low-cost clinic typically serves a different clientele than a specialty hospital, and their Web site should clearly reflect their mission. Practices that are Cat Friendly Certified or Fear Free Certified should highlight such certifications on their Web site to advertise their niche expertise to potential clients. Web sites that feature personal images instead of stock photographs, and that highlight the practice's team members and their values help potential clients get to know the practice, and help the practice begin to connect with the client. Practices should carefully select photographs, ensuring to include all species they care for, and especially cats, to reinforce that all pets need regular veterinary care. Photographs should showcase the patient journey, highlighting such things as physical examinations, the treatment area, and the kennel area, and should include any specific strategies that set the practice apart from others.

To appear in a searcher's results, a veterinary practice must have a Web site with good search engine optimization (SEO). Many factors affect SEO and Web site performance, and progressive practices often consult an SEO expert or veterinary marketing agency to help them develop a successful SEO strategy.

General SEO strategy involves including keywords on the Web site that pet owners are likely to search for, and regularly posting unique content. Many practices regularly publish blogs as a way to increase SEO, establish a digital content library, and educate pet owners. Blogs also allow practices to highlight cat care, and topics should equally address canine and feline health issues.

Social media provides another way for practices to present their personality and brand to potential clients, and contemporary veterinary marketing includes posting to social media platforms, such as Facebook, Instagram, and TikTok. A good social media strategy typically includes a combination of educational posts, photographs, and videos to help pet owners get to know a practice. Thoughtfully planning a content calendar, instead of randomly posting when the opportunity arises, helps ensure practices post regular, valuable content that appeals to pet owners. Practices can also align with organizations, such as the American Veterinary Medical Association, American Association of Feline Practitioners, and American Animal Hospital Association, to provide relevant educational resources directly on their Web site.

Some practices hire a veterinary marketing company, whereas others hire or appoint a marketing manager. This team member is responsible for coordinating Web site updates, blog writing and posting, and social media content management. Elevating a team member to a marketing manager position is a wonderful way to empower veterinary professionals who are more creative in this area than in traditional management. Veterinary marketing managers can work remotely or hold a hybrid position, which allows for greater flexibility and job satisfaction.

Client Communication

Today's client wants to be able to communicate quickly and efficiently with their veterinary team. Thus, client communication has evolved from telephone-based conversations to a multitude of digital options. A variety of communication platforms are available, and some practice management software includes email and texting capabilities. Because 99% of texts are opened (95% within 3 minutes of being sent[6]) texting, in particular, can allow for efficient two-way communication when decisions must be made quickly, such as with hospitalized patients, or during surgery, and is much better than playing telephone tag.

Instead of calling a practice to ask a question or schedule an appointment, clients can now text the practice or schedule online, which is more efficient for clients and veterinary team members. Digital communication also allows clients to quickly request prescription refills at any time.

App-based client communication platforms allow practices to share a branded app with their clients. Most client-veterinary communications can occur within the app, including

- Texting
- Video chatting
- Tele-triage
- Telemedicine appointments
- Sending push notifications
- Scheduling appointments
- Requesting prescription refills

Although clients want to be able to access their veterinary team at all hours, work-life balance is critical to maintain veterinary team member well-being. Progressive practices often partner with a veterinary telehealth company to provide after-hours advice and guidance to clients needing immediate help. Efficient practices also effectively use tele-triage services during lunch breaks, staff meetings, or on days they are short-staffed, to increase productivity.

CONTEMPORARY APPOINTMENT OPTIONS

A traditional veterinary appointment involved a pet owner calling and making an appointment, bringing their pet to a brick-and-mortar facility, and then staying throughout the appointment. Options for contemporary veterinary appointments range from fully in-person visits to virtual care.

Tele-Triage

Tele-triage provides a way for veterinary team members to advise pet owners about whether their pet requires a veterinary appointment, and whether an in-person or virtual appointment is appropriate. Pet owners call, text, or video chat with a designated team member who provides guidance. Many digital platforms provide the capability for clients to send photographs and synchronous or asynchronous video, which can allow a team member to help them make decisions regarding their pet's care. However, this is still a fluid topic in veterinary medicine with the ever-changing landscape of tele-health, the Veterinary-Client-Patient-Relationship (VCPR), and each state's version of the practice act. In my opinion, priority should be taken to solve the ongoing issues around legality and delivery of tele-health services; it is a critical piece surrounding access to care.

Virtual Appointments

Virtual appointments became a necessity during the pandemic, and progressive practices continue to offer them because of the convenience they provide clients and veterinary teams. Virtual appointments are helpful for clients who have transportation issues or who cannot physically bring their pet in. They are also valuable for pets who experience significant anxiety or who become aggressive during veterinary visits. Virtual visits allow veterinarians to see more patients and provide care for pets who may not otherwise visit a veterinarian. Rechecks can be performed more efficiently in many cases, and some situations, such as dermatology issues and inappropriate urination in cats, lend themselves to this format. Virtual appointments are appropriate in many other situations, such as

- Behavioral consultations
- Minor medical issues
- Skin conditions
- Nutritional consultations

Virtual visits also provide work-from-home opportunities for veterinary team members.

Virtual visits are especially helpful for cats who become stressed during veterinary visits, or whose owners are hesitant to take them out of their normal environment. Although in-person visits are necessary to maintain a veterinary-client-patient relationship and provide hands-on care, issues that arise between these visits can often be addressed during a virtual appointment. The Veterinary Virtual Care Association provides model telemedicine regulations, including guidelines for establishing a veterinary-client-patient relationship.[7]

Hybrid Appointments

Drop-off appointments, curbside care, and other options provide a spectrum of opportunities for practices to meet pet owners' needs. Veterinary practices can provide video feed of the pet's examination so the pet owner can be involved, and the veterinarian can help them understand what is needed for the pet's care. These alternatives particularly appeal to Millennial and Gen Z pet owners, who are three times more likely to value telemedicine and curbside care.[4]

Low-Stress Appointments

Veterinary practices have made significant progress toward making veterinary visits less stressful for pets, and particularly cats. Low-stress handling techniques, clinic design, and environmental considerations now allow veterinarians to provide care for previously reactive animals. Many cat caregivers skip veterinary visits because they are concerned about the stress the appointment will cause their cat, and addressing this issue is another step in the right direction to ensure cats receive regular veterinary care.

Carrier training is a critical component of low-stress client education, because carrier-related stress (particularly for the cat caregiver) is a primary reason cat caregivers do not seek veterinary care.[8] Practices should help clients understand how to desensitize cats to their carrier by leaving the carrier out and encouraging interaction with the carrier. Carrier training has important implications beyond veterinary visits, such as preventing escape through an open door and when people visit, and during emergencies.

Concierge Appointments

Some progressive practices are moving toward a concierge-style experience for pet owners. Instead of the client interacting with a client service representative (CSR) and multiple other support staff, a designated team member, who is often referred to as a veterinary health coach, guides the client through each part of the visit, from check-in to payment. This style of service helps bond the client to that team member and helps them feel valued by the practice.

Tele-Consulting

Modern technology allows general veterinary practitioners the ability to consult with veterinary specialists about difficult cases. Fewer veterinarians are going into specialty roles, and many areas do not have easy, logistical access to specialty care, which limits clients' access to advanced diagnostics and care. Under the guidance of a specialist, a general practice veterinarian can perform the necessary diagnostics to reach an accurate diagnosis and initiate treatment. When a patient does require referral, the work-up that has been done can save time for the specialist and the client. Veterinary specialists are available for consultation via several different platforms and through many reference laboratories.

How Contemporary Appointment Options Benefit Veterinary Teams

Tele-triage, virtual visits, and other telehealth options provide additional opportunities for veterinary team members to work remotely. Whereas traditional appointments require CSRs to sit behind a desk, more progressive options allow for fewer in-person CSRs. Remote CSRs can facilitate tele-triage conversations, answer text messages and emails, and return telephone calls.

Some practices use virtual CSRs, with the client talking to a remote team member through a screen in the lobby instead of an in-person CSR. The remote CSR can check in the pet, converse with the owner, and alert the owner when they can move to the examination room.

ALTERNATIVE VETERINARY APPOINTMENTS

In addition to the appointment types a practice offers, veterinary team roles and patient care are also shifting to increase efficiency and offer a better experience for pet owners.

Physical Examination

Progressive practices strive to use veterinary team members to their full potential while maximizing efficiency. Whereas the veterinarian once performed the entire patient examination, veterinary technicians now often perform a preliminary physical examination and convey the results to the veterinarian. The veterinarian can then approve diagnostics, which the technician will perform, allowing the veterinarian to review the results before they see the patient.

Elevating veterinary technicians to a higher role in the practice by allowing them more responsibility has multiple benefits. Technicians are more invested in the practice and enjoy greater job satisfaction when they are used to their full potential. Additionally, reducing the veterinarian's time in the examination room allows them to run several rooms at once and focus on more complex duties, such as analyzing diagnostic testing results and formulating treatment plans.

Wellness Care

Over the last several decades, veterinary medicine has shifted from treating sick pets to preventing diseases from developing. Wellness care has become increasingly important as veterinary practices help pet owners understand the value of preventive medicine. Vaccines have long been the mainstay of wellness care; however, vaccine protocols are now customized according to a pet's lifestyle and risk factors. American Animal Hospital Association canine vaccination guidelines[9] and American Animal Hospital Association/American Association of Feline Practitioners feline vaccination guidelines[10] advise that many core vaccines should be given every 3 years instead of annually. Instead of vaccinating on a given schedule, some practices offer titer testing to minimize the number of vaccines administered over a pet's lifetime.

Many people travel with their pets, whether to warmer states for the winter or internationally for business. Different locations present different infectious disease threats and may warrant different vaccination protocols. Additionally, travel, vector migration, and cross-country rescue and adoption has made many "regional" diseases more widespread, and asking open-ended history questions about an animal's lifestyle is more important than ever.

Parasite prevention is an important component of wellness care. Dogs and cats should receive year-round heartworm, flea, and tick prevention. Pet owners often understand the value of parasite prevention for dogs who go outside, but may fail to understand why cats, and particularly indoor-only cats, also need parasite prevention. The fact that a significant number of heartworm-positive cats live indoors, and that mosquitoes can easily gain access to clients' homes, show that cats also need year-round protection. Additionally, few cats are truly indoor-only, because exposure to pathogens can easily occur via windowsills, housemates, clothing and shoes, and vectors.

Ticks transmit several infectious diseases, many of which are zoonotic. Migration of new tick species and emerging vector-borne diseases make tick prevention critical for all pets, including indoor cats.

Wellness Diagnostics

Whereas blood work was once performed only on sick pets to reach a diagnosis, it is now recommended for all pets to establish baseline values, detect trends, and diagnose subclinical disease. A complete blood count, chemistry including symmetric dimethylarginine, and urinalysis should be performed annually for adult pets, whereas more extensive testing is often recommended for senior pets.

With recent advancements in DNA testing, there are now several companies that analyze a dog's or cat's genetic profile. Knowing which breeds contribute to a pet's genetic makeup can help veterinarians better understand which diseases a pet may be at risk for, so they can tailor screening tests throughout the pet's life. Additionally, some DNA companies screen for genetic health conditions, letting pet owners and veterinarians know whether a pet has a genetic predisposition for specific diseases.

Sick Pet Diagnostics

Historically, veterinary diagnostics were limited to the tests that could be performed in the practice. Today, through veterinary reference laboratories, veterinarians have access to hundreds of tests that can provide further information about a pet's health status. As an added convenience, some reference laboratories provide integrations with practice management software, so results are automatically uploaded into the correct patient's medical record. Although some diagnostics, such as radiographs or exploratory surgery, obviously must be performed in-house, many tests, such as fecal analysis and basic blood work, can be sent out to save veterinary practices time and money. Some reference laboratories also provide pathologists and specialists who veterinarians can consult for guidance on complicated cases. Veterinarians can also consult various specialists, from radiologists to surgeons, to help them provide more comprehensive care for their patients.

Digital and artificial intelligence–driven advancements have revolutionized veterinary diagnostics. For example, digital radiography has replaced film-based techniques, and endoscopy allows for minimally invasive imaging. Most current laboratory analyzers rely on artificial intelligence to evaluate samples, from urine to blood. Additionally, some laboratories offer digital cytology services, where slide images are digitally submitted, evaluated by a clinical pathologist, similar to having a virtual clinical pathologist, and results sent to the practice.

Shared Decision Making

The idea of a veterinarian presenting gold standard diagnostic and treatment options in a one-direction delivery method, and the client accepting the plan without question is an outdated view. Today's clients want to understand all the options available to their pet, referred to as spectrum of care, so they can make the decision that best fits their needs, beliefs, and budget. Seasoned veterinarians may initially struggle with this concept, because we were taught to deliver gold standard recommendations and wait, versus having a collaborative care discussion. Shared decision making is a collaborative approach that involves the client in all decisions regarding a pet's health care. It depends on mutual respect and communication and requires the veterinary team to accept the client's decisions without judgment.

PAYMENT OPTIONS

Today's clients want to know what costs will be associated with their pet's care, and do not want to be surprised by an expensive invoice. They also want convenient payment options that help them afford their pet's care.

Cost-of-Care Conversations

Cost-of-care conversations should ideally start before or at the latest during the first puppy or kitten visit. At that point, veterinary practices should prepare the new pet owner for costs associated with care during the first year, and beyond. It is helpful to provide clients a handout or resource that outlines routine wellness care, including spay or neuter surgery, and the associated costs. Cost-of-care conversations should continue throughout the pet's life, so the owner knows what to expect.

These conversations should also include information about different financial resources clients can use to help them pay for their pet's care, such as a pet savings account, pet health insurance, or a health care credit card.

Pet Health Insurance

Many pet health insurance companies offer plans to help pet owners cover the cost of care. Most companies offer accident and illness plans, and many offer riders that cover wellness care. An insurance plan allows pet owners to approve emergency or illness care without having to consider their budget, which ensures pets receive the care they need. Insurance allows veterinarians to provide higher-level care and reduces stressful situations, such as clients being unable to afford care and economic euthanasia.

Progressive practices understand the benefits of pet health insurance and have intentional conversations with their clients about insurance. One study revealed that younger pet owners (ie, owners between 18 and 34) were more than twice as likely to purchase a pet insurance policy,[11] which may indicate that pet insurance will continue to become more commonplace.

Third-Party Payment Options

A 2022 Synchrony Lifetime of Care study found that nearly half of pet owners underestimate the cost of pet care, and an unexpected bill of $250 causes significant stress for one out of four pet owners.[12] Several third-party payment options provide a means for clients to provide essential care without paying the full amount upfront. A health care credit card, such as CareCredit, allows clients to cover their pet's veterinary bill, and then pay the credit card company directly over time. Other companies, such as Scratchpay, approve pet owners for short-term loans, with the lender paying the veterinary practice directly and then collecting payment from the client over several months or years.

Digital Payment Options

Today's clients expect secure, convenient payment options that are more efficient than standing in line to pay a receptionist. In fact, Millennial and Gen Z clients are 2.5 times more likely to value online billing.[4] Digital payment options save time for clients and veterinary team members and decrease waiting room congestion. Mobile payment options allow clients to pay in the examination room, in their car, or from home. Cashless options, such as contactless payment systems and mobile wallets, also allow for faster transaction processing. Processing fees for these services sometimes preclude their use by veterinary practices, but companies that allow practices to apply the fee to the client's invoice may make these options more reasonable.

SUMMARY

Veterinary medicine is an ever-evolving field, which gives practices endless opportunities to learn, grow, and improve. Practices that embrace change and constantly raise their standards of care can build lifelong client and pet relationships and improve their teams' fulfillment and well-being. Looking forward to the future allows practices to anticipate new trends and welcome progress.

CLINICS CARE POINTS

- Progressive practices constantly evolve to appeal to today's pet owner, and pet owners of the future.
- Digital marketing is essential to reach and build relationships with pet owners.
- Practices should take advantage of digital tools and artificial intelligence–powered advancements to increase efficiency and provide the best care possible.
- Practices benefit from offering a variety of contemporary appointment options to meet the needs of every pet owner.

- Practices should emphasize wellness care, including customized vaccine protocols, year-round parasite prevention, and wellness diagnostics.
- Practices should continuously discuss cost of care and payment options with clients to ensure pets receive the care they need.

DISCLOSURE

I have nothing to disclose.

REFERENCES

1. AVMA. 2018 AVMA Report on The Market for Veterinary Services. 2018.
2. Bir C, Ortez M, Widmar N, et al. Familiarity and use of veterinary services by US resident dog and cat owners. Animals 2020;10(3):483. Available at: https://www.ncbi.nlm.nih.gov/pmc/articles/PMC7143178/#B1-animals-10-00483. Accessed May 10, 2023.
3. Pet Industry Market Size, Trends & Ownership Statistics. American Pet Products Association. 2023. Available at: https://www.americanpetproducts.org/press_IndustryTrends.asp. Accessed May 10, 2023.
4. AVMA. 2022 AVMA Pet Ownership and Demographics Sourcebook. 2022.
5. Bragg R, Bennett JS, Cummings A, et al. Evaluation of the effects of hospital visit stress on psychological variables in dogs. JAVMA 2015;246:2. Available at: https://avmajournals.avma.org/view/journals/javma/246/2/javma.246.2.212.xml. Accessed May 10, 2023.
6. Text Request. 2023 State of Business Texting Report. Available at: www.textrequest.com/blog/texting-statistics-answer-questions/. Accessed May 10, 2023.
7. Veterinary Virtual Care Association. VVCA Model Telemedicine Regulations. Available at: https://vvca.org/. Accessed May 10, 2023.
8. Fear Free. Study shows cat carrier training reduces stress. 2023. Available at: fearfreepets.com/study-shows-cat-carrier-training-reduces-stress. Accessed May 10, 2023.
9. AAHA. 2022 AAHA Canine Vaccination Guidelines. 2022. Available at: https://www.aaha.org/aaha-guidelines/2022-aaha-canine-vaccination-guidelines/home/. Accessed May 12, 2023.
10. AAFP. 2020 AAHA/AAFP Feline Vaccination Guidelines. 2020. Available at: https://catvets.com/guidelines/practice-guidelines/aafp-aaha-feline-vaccination. Accessed May 12, 2023.
11. Access to Veterinary Care Coalition. Access to Veterinary Care: Barriers, Current Practices, and Public Policy. 2018.
12. Synchrony. Lifetime of Care Study. 2022. Available at: http://petlifetimeofcare.com/. Accessed May 10, 2023.

Leadership in Veterinary Practice

Dave Nicol, BVMS, Cert Mgmt, MRCVS

KEYWORDS

- Leadership • Vision • Culture • Performance management

KEY POINTS

- A clear working definition of leadership is essential as a starting point for growing leadership competency effectively. Further, there are four areas all leaders should focus their attention on: vision crafting, building the team, culture farming, and performance management.
- For senior leaders, articulating a clear practice vision (vision crafting) is crucial. Many veterinary practices lack a well-communicated vision, affecting commitment. Successful vision crafting involves creating authentic Purpose, Mission, and Values statements and guiding team alignment. Providing the basis for organizational performance.
- Performance management focuses on continuous performance improvement through clear goal setting followed up with three essential meetings: annual planning, quarterly progress reviews, and weekly "BAAM" sessions for accountability. Effective leadership also values real-time feedback, emphasizing positive reinforcement over criticism.

INTRODUCTION AND BACKGROUND

I have always been fascinated by people and relationships, possibly even more so than the ubiquitous desire for every vet to explore the animal kingdom.

From my earliest days as a bright-eyed schoolboy/wannabe vet, hanging on every word the vet uttered, or as a shelve stacker in the local supermarket, it was obvious that the quality of the work was greatly impacted by the happiness and harmony of the people tasked with doing the work.

I recall vividly the impact it had when a much-loved senior manager in the supermarket I worked left and was replaced by his deputy, who was more of a bully than a manager. This aggressive style manager utterly changed the "vibe," as I would have called it then, resulting in many errors as fearful school children tried to avoid his wrath. It was not long until most of us found other places to earn our pocket money! And so the pattern continued as I entered the veterinary realm; each practice I visited as a student had a different "feel." Some were happy places where people seemed

VetX International, Ridgeland House, 165 Dyke Road, Brighton, BN3 1TL, England, United Kingdom
E-mail address: drdavenicol@gmail.com

Vet Clin Small Anim 54 (2024) 277–291
https://doi.org/10.1016/j.cvsm.2023.10.002
0195-5616/24/Crown Copyright © 2023 Published by Elsevier Inc. All rights reserved.
vetsmall.theclinics.com

to like each other, and the day went smoothly. Others were chaotic and messy. People would literally and figuratively get in each other's way. The former clinic was a place you would be happy to return to. In the latter, you could not wait to get back to university.

As a graduate veterinarian entering the workforce, it was again apparent that the actions of leaders could lift individuals and teams or knock them down. Several times I witnessed both things occurring.

As I progressed in my career, I hoped to learn from each of these experiences and in many ways, a desire to build on the work of others drives me forward. Since those informal days of curiously studying the human side of veterinary practice, I have managed or owned several veterinary practices. I have experienced success and frequent failure in many attempts at business. Taken hours of formal and informal education in business and leadership and currently own two practices, one a traditional brick-and-mortar clinic in London. The other is a mobile hospice practice serving locations across the United Kingdom.

I have met with, interviewed, or consulted with hundreds of practice owners and published research on veterinary leadership. I have been a terrific leader for some and an appalling leader for others. As time has gone on, I hope that there are fewer of the second category!

Each day of trying to be the best leader I can, I learn more about the subtle art of being the type of leader veterinary teams need. You may notice that I used relatively soft words when describing how my workplace experience felt. I was, of course, alluding to culture, and it is no accident that such fluffy words appeared. Instead, it demonstrates a central truth about leadership. We all know it matters, but we have very little idea of what it means. Such is the nature of leadership, as many describe it.

But unless we let go of this notion, we will continue making appreciative noises yet not taking the concrete actions required to be effective leaders.

Let us start by being clear that this is a subject of the utmost importance. Poor leadership is extremely bad for your practice. There is absolutely no shortage of evidence to support this fact.

In 2007, for example, Skogstad and colleagues published a paper entitled *The Destructiveness of Laissez-faire Leadership Behavior* in which the concept that the oft-quoted "Laissez-faire" style of leadership (previously purported to be a totem of high trust) was, in most cases, simply an abdication of any leadership responsibility.[1] Such a dereliction of duty resulted in hugely damaging effects on performance and team well-being.

In another meta-analysis, researchers found a strong correlation between destructive leadership behaviors and a host of negative outcomes, including lower job satisfaction, decreased job performance, higher turnover, and increased workplace bullying and conflict.[2]

These and countless more studies consistently demonstrate the considerable negative impacts poor leadership can have on both employee well-being and overall organizational performance. This might lead you to also conclude that leading effectively would be a top priority for any practice owner. Yet in the course of my research, I have been able to demonstrate that almost three-quarters of those responsible for managing the veterinary practices in which they work reported that they struggled to find time for leadership priorities.[3]

What follows in this article is my attempt to bring some pragmatic clarity to your understanding of what leadership is and is not. What tools are available to you, the leader and how you might effectively use these tools to improve both your employee experience and practice performance?

As you read, you will note that I use various words to describe the business entity. Sometimes, I call it a practice, and other times an organization. This is because veterinary medicine has changed so dramatically in the last decade that readers will come from various practice backgrounds working in different sectors and refer to things slightly differently. Therefore, the most frequent word I use to describe the business entity is an "organization" because regardless of size, age, sector or ownership structure, this word fits well. You can mentally insert whatever word fits your reality best, be it practice, clinic, corporation, shelter, or nonprofit.

I also mention some businesses and individuals by name. These are all people I know well and have either business or personal relationships with. I say this for full transparency. Although each has permitted me to use their names and organizations as examples, there were no inducements, financial, or otherwise, to do so. They were selected simply on relevance to the discussion, excellence in their fields, and because I can confidently say they are what they appear to be.

WHAT IS LEADERSHIP?

Run a search on Google, and you will find a plethora of articles and resources, which use broad and lofty-sounding descriptions of leadership. Such articles will be read similarly to what follows.

Leadership is a crucial factor that drives the performance, growth, and success of an organization. It involves the ability to inspire, influence, and guide individuals toward achieving common goals.[4] Leadership sets the direction and tone of an organization and can affect everything from employee morale and productivity to customer satisfaction and overall business outcomes.

Research shows a significant correlation between leadership and organizational performance. For instance, a meta-analysis conducted by Judge and Piccolo[5] found that transformational leadership—characterized by inspiring, intellectually stimulating, and considering employees as individuals—was strongly associated with positive organizational outcomes, including increased employee job satisfaction and performance.

Moreover, leadership is integral to fostering an innovative and adaptive organizational culture. A study by McKinsey[6] found that 86% of executives identified leadership as a critical determinant of organizational innovation.

In the context of change management, effective leadership plays a pivotal role in steering the organization through uncertain and complex business environments. In a survey by the Project Management Institute,[7] 84% of project managers agreed that leadership competence is critical for successfully driving strategic initiatives.

In conclusion, leadership matters in delivering successful organizational outcomes as it influences employee performance, innovation, and the ability to navigate change effectively. The right leadership can turn an ordinary organization into an extraordinary one, underpinning its long-term success and sustainability.

All of which may well be true, but does not it all seem rather theoretic, dry, and lacking in specificity? It is as if it was written for the benefit of a pompous CEO presiding over a Global Fortune 500 Company. You can virtually see them casually leafing through the pages of Harvard Business Review!

But what does this have to do with the running of a veterinary practice? I personally think such texts do more harm to leadership by putting people off than inviting them in to learn more.

The truth is that leadership does matter. In fact, I believe a lack of leadership skills is the single greatest problem at the heart of the epidemic of burnout we face in veterinary medicine today.

Low-skill leaders myopically focused on either clinical outcomes or financial outcomes have dropped the ball when it comes to the number one job of every leader—"people care."

The result? Too many professionals are working in practices where they fail to thrive and consequently burn out too fast and are often lost to the profession for good.[8] What is required is more a set of tools and less an ethereal definition of leadership. Because everyone in a leadership role can learn how to wield the tools required to lead brilliantly. And when they do, they will contribute to the creation of stable, sustainable, and attractive places to work.

So here is my working definition of leadership:

Leadership is the process by which a group of people are brought together and work to accomplish a meaningful, shared objective sustainably.

There is a lot to unpack in that sentence, and doing so will reveal more about the specific responsibilities of leaders. But before we do, a word on one of the greatest impediments to good leadership; a blight I call Hamster Wheel Syndrome.

Hamster Wheel Syndrome

You may note in my opening words a reluctance to reference a sole person, a commander-in-chief, as the leader. Although I fully acknowledge that such a role is incredibly important, beyond the smaller start-up practice with three to four people working in close harmony, there is no reality that a practice can operate effectively with one person shouldering all of the responsibilities of leadership and clinical practice. If we were to take a moment to list out the various jobs this would entail, it might read as follows:

Vision crafting—the process of articulating your reason for existence!

Culture farming—the intentional actions required to curate a healthy culture

Hiring—the process of talent acquisition

Performance management—the process of talent management

Standards of care—defining how we do the clinical work

Financial management—making sure the organization does not run out of cash.

Clinical caseload—the day-to-day work that pays the bills

Personal development—doing the work of one's own professional skill development

And these are just a few of the things you have to accomplish; furthermore, there is no mention of commitments outside of work, such as family, friends, and hobbies.

To attempt to bear such a weight inevitably results in poor performance in almost all areas. The exception is clinical work, which tends to dominate, but almost always to the detriment or abandonment of all others. This is the state into which almost all clinical leaders fall, and I refer to it as getting stuck on the Hamster Wheel.

"Hamster Wheel leaders" struggle under two flawed concepts

1. "For others to follow me, they must respect me, and the best way to accomplish that is to be the best at everything. This is especially true of my clinical work." Naturally, it follows that others will ask such a totem for help when they get stuck. And here comes the problem, rather than help them, the leader in question does the work for the individual because "It'll just be faster and better if I do it myself." Et voila! The trap is sprung, and now the hapless leader falls into a pattern of taking ownership of everything. Not only does this kill any hope of ever making time for leadership activities but also prevents the growth in others needed to allow for effective delegation.

2. This clinical work is the most important work that anyone can do. It is easy to see why leaders make this error. Clinical work brings immediate reward in the form of revenue and the "good feels" that come with clinical progress. Everything happens quickly, and it feels like you are doing important work. All of this would be true were it not for the fact that your job title also includes leader, not just clinician. Leadership work, and I am talking about the big picture stuff we will talk about shortly, is a far more valuable activity than clinical work because it is leveraged, that is, the energy you put in becomes amplified several times over as other people improve (skills and efficiency) due to your effort.

These two schools of thought are very hard to overcome, so ingrained into the veterinary psyche they have become. A helpful thought to recall if you suffer from this condition is as follows.

When you became a vet, you took a Hippocratic Oath that went along the lines of "It shall be my constant endeavor to ensure the health and welfare of animals committed to my care."

Perhaps, as you take up the mantle of becoming a leader, you might be well advised to take another oath as follows, "It shall be my constant endeavor to ensure the health and welfare of the PEOPLE committed to my care." It is not only good for your people, as they will have more space to grow as you make space for others to become excellent. It is also good for you as the weight on your shoulders, in time, decreases as the skills in others increase.

A classic win–win, but it does take a leap of faith, a large dollop of patience, and the right people on your team.

Nonnegotiable Leadership Actions

There are in fact, far too many things to cover in one short article to fully capture the multifaceted nature of leadership. And one could tackle the issue from many angles.

For example, is leadership about how we do our work, or is it about the nature of the work itself? In truth, it is both. The leader of any organization has a job description in common with every other role. But given the senior nature of the role, how the leader chooses to conduct themselves will inevitably set the tone for how the entire organization behaves.

To that extent, we can broadly classify leadership work into two categories: activities (deciding what we are all going to do) and behaviors (deciding how we will all behave as we complete the activities).

The beautiful thing about leadership is that the most important activities you are responsible for result in the quality of the activities everyone else focuses on and the development of the broader behaviors displayed by the team. For the remainder of this article, we refer back to our list of activities required of the leader. Specifically, vision crafting, culture farming, building the team, and performance management.

Two of these subjects are covered in other chapters of this edition Veterinary Practice Profitability-You Have to Measure It to Manage It: Building A Veterinary Practice Team and Chapter 16: Workplace Culture. As such, we will address the remaining two critical leadership action areas, which are vision crafting and performance management.

VISION CRAFTING

Top of every senior leader's list must be the creation and articulation of the practice vision. This is what I consider a strategic (or big picture) leadership activity.

In my 2021 report, *Leadership Actions & Their Effect on Veterinary Practice Culture*, we learned that little more than half of all veterinary practices have a recognized vision. The data also revealed a difference in perception between practice owners, of whom more than 60% claimed to have a vision in place, whereas only 38% of practice managers believed this to be the case. I have no reason to believe one group is lying. Instead, the likely reason for the discrepancy is simply a failure of the practice owner to effectively share and articulate what the vision is. In short, even in the clinics that took the time to create a vision, the level of commitment to that vision is low. How can someone be committed to something when they do not know it exists? This is a huge mistake; a clinic lacking a clear vision has no means to stand out or compete in the battle for human attention (from potential employees and potential customers). Such clinics are doomed to be average at best, competing on tangible properties like location, facilities, and salary offers. Although each of these things matters when it comes to talent, sadly, none ranks highest on the scale of things that matter most to employees.

In today's employer market, individuals want to work in places where they feel appreciated; they can do work with purpose and work in teams where values are shared. Such things are derived only from a well-crafted vision.

Crafting Your Vision Statement

Many people promote the "Vision, Mission & Values" approach to vision crafting, but this seems problematic for the following reasons. Such statements inevitably seem to lack substance. The vision is often lofty and vague. The mission feels more like a rewording of the vague vision, leaving us none-the-wiser what the actual organization objective is. Finally, the values are frequently what I would kindly describe as aspirational. That is to say, they bear no resemblance to the real values the workforce displays each day.

In short, this is an entirely fictitious document. One that no one buys into and is therefore quickly consigned to the "box ticked" bottom of the leader's desk drawer.

Jim Collins, in his book Beyond Entrepreneurship: Turning Your Business Into An Enduring Great Company,[9] provides a vastly improved way of creating an organizational vision. A good vision, he states, is formed by having a purpose statement (that clearly defines why you exist), a mission statement (which clearly defines what you are going to accomplish and in what timeframe), and a set of organizational values (that are representative of reality). The purpose and values are likely to remain fixed, whereas the Mission and associated strategies are going to shift as both the organization and environment interact. Let's dissect each of these a little further.

Creating Your Purpose Statement

A well-written purpose statement is your guiding light. It is why you and your team show up and suffer through tough moments together. Veterinary medicine has a wonderful purpose baked into its core, to prevent and alleviate the suffering of those who have no voice or ability to do so themselves.

You might be inclined to stop right there. But I encourage you to take a deeper dive. To avoid this step is to align with every other clinic, but I bet you started your clinic for unique reasons. I, for example, operate businesses because I believe deeply that if I create workplaces where people thrive, I can make the world a better place.

It just so happens that I am a vet! So, I do this in the veterinary space. My practice's purpose statement is, "We're a place where pets live well and people thrive."

Another practice with whom I work, Southeast Veterinary Neurology, did this superbly and created the following purpose statement. "We keep families together by giving second chances to pets with neurologic disease and hope to the people who love them."

These statements connect at a deeper emotional level and go beyond the usual trite catchphrases. So, I challenge you to get beyond the surface and peel back the layers of the onion until you get to the very core of why you go to work. That takes time, and it can be a frustrating exercise, but when you get to the very heart of it, I promise you will get goosebumps.

Writing Your Mission Statement

The Mission Statement is all about what you will accomplish as a team. It is the single overarching objective that the business exists to accomplish. As such, a mission statement must meet the criteria of a well-written goal.

You may have seen referenced in other texts the common acronym SMART, used to help create useful objectives. It is used to help us to remember that a well-written objective must be:

Specific
Measurable
Achievable
Relevant
Time Bound

This is a great tool, and I will boldly suggest we modify it slightly to replace Achievable with Audacious. This, of course, is a personal choice. But great people want to do great work, so shooting for the moon can be a great idea. The only caveat is that you must authentically commit to accomplishing your moonshot. Making lofty statements without making the resources available to meet the objective is going to fail. Your people will inevitably see through such fraud.

Audacious missions (eg, to dominate or create a new market), by definition, require large leaps in innovation, scale, and acceptance of risk. They also cost more to accomplish. But the rewards are also potentially very high.

One might think of a company such as Lap of Love, co-founded by Dr Dani McVety and Dr Mary Gardner. Their mission is *"empower every owner to care for their geriatric pets."*

When they started, in-home euthanasia was a back water niche. A decade later, they grew a dominant multimillion dollar, national company with a hundred wannabe startups trailing. That's what I call a moonshot!

Selecting your mission is a highly personal leadership task, so you choose what fits. But be intentional and be authentic. If you want to go big, then go all in. If you are more conservative, then do what feels achievable.

Do not just "career forward" endlessly on the treadmill of veterinary medicine. This endless grinding out of clinical caseload without clarity of purpose and mission is exhausting.

Clear articulation of what you choose to accomplish will have a great bearing on who you retain, who you lose, and who joins your practice. My advice is to aim to create a mission that allows enough time for substantial meaningful work to be accomplished. For my practice, the mission is as follows; "To become a cooperatively owned practice, delivering sustainable, modern care that extends and improves the lives of pets, serving 3000 families each year by 2025." We are well on the way, having upgraded the facility over the first year. Implemented innovative sustainable practices to reduce burnout pressure over the second year. And we have now just launched our employee share scheme to improve rewards for all and introduced a subscription-based payment model for our clients to make access to care easier and less of a burden on family cash flows.

The real beauty and power of a great mission statement, when used as intended, is that things are not happening by accident. There is a plan, and though you might wobble from time to time, the plan will help you stay on track.

Identifying Your Values

The final part of crafting our vision is to define our values. Values matter as they will determine how we do our work and thus complete the "Why, What and How" of a well-written vision.

Edgar Schein[10] provides an excellent definition of organizational values as the fundamental beliefs and principles that guide a company's internal conduct, decision-making processes, and relationships with all its stakeholders, such as employees, customers, partners, and shareholders.

These principles inform the organization's culture, shape its strategic direction, and define its brand identity, influencing behavior and performance within the organization. Perhaps you can see now why a lack of articulated values causes such a giant problem for practices? Like a ship with no compass or rudder, a practice that does not understand and use its values intentionally will be subject to the capricious nature of the winds and currents. Surely, the end result will be a wrecked hull before too long!

Identifying your values is not a terribly complicated task, nor a time-consuming one. There are many ways to do so. But an easy one is simply considering what matters most to you in the workplace. Maybe it is loyalty, honesty, being accountable, acting with integrity, or having fun. The important thing is to take time away from the madness of practice and find the answer to this question. And preferably, have your most trusted and positively influential teammates do the same. Then reconvene, and with some luck, you will have a list of values you can start to group and rank from most important and popular to least. In doing so, you should attempt to arrive at a list of five or six words everyone feels comfortable with. This is a great start, but a word is just a word. What is now required is for you to give that word a real definition. As the entire point of having values is to allow you to navigate the complex and unpredictable world of business in a consistent way that defines who you are as a company, you must give the words deeper and clearer meaning. An example that springs readily to mind is Amazon, a company you will undoubtedly be familiar with. They have a relatively long list of values, which they have expanded on and now describe as "Leadership Principles." I recently experienced how they have shaped their business using at least three.

1. Customer obsession
2. Commitment to operational excellence
3. Long-term thinking

A rather expensive item I had ordered failed to arrive. I contacted the company using a chatbot—usually a loathsome experience. However, within 2 minutes, the bot handled the issue, apologized and reordered the item. No further questions were asked!

I was speechless. They took the hit entirely on the chin without fuss. And, by doing so, deepened my relationship with the brand. Whatever else you might think of Amazon, you cannot fault their operational excellence, customer obsession, and long-term thinking.

Words alone do not accomplish this, especially if they are only drafted for the dusty staff handbook and are never again read or referenced.

Values must be identified, defined, articulated, and used repeatedly to become the standard for "doing things around here." Nothing less will suffice.

So, what does integrity mean to you and your people? How do you expect this to show up? And what do you do when the big (and little) moments arrive, and people live (or violate) the values?

My advice is to use your values when hiring and only hire people who share your values. Use the values when onboarding so new teammates understand what is expected of them. Use the values when you make tough or complex decisions, big or small. Shout people out for living the values both verbally and through rewards. Have a competition to see who lived your values the best each week. Reward people not just for output but also for behaviors consistent with the values. Talk about values when managing performance (more on that below). And, if necessary, fire to the values.

When you have clarity around Purpose, Mission & Values, the entire game of leadership suddenly opens up into a new and insanely fun realm where concrete actions can be taken that allow leadership actions to directly and predictably influence organizational performance.

As such, vision crafting is arguably your most important leadership task.

MANAGING PERFORMANCE

Performance management is a broad category for all activities required to allow individuals to work effectively in their roles and alongside their teammates. It is often confused with Disciplinary Performance Management–the Human Resources equivalent of cardio-pulmonary resuscitation when employee performance or behavior has gone badly askew.

Although this can be effective, it is often a prelude to a parting of ways.

The goal of any performance management process should be to help employees understand the expectations clearly, allow them to see how their work helps the organization accomplish its mission, give them the tools to meet these expectations, and encourage improvement rather than simply punish noncompliance.

Over the past two or three decades, the annual review (or appraisal) has been the dominant performance tool deployed in veterinary practices, large and small. The results have been a dismal failure. Ask for a show of hands from clinicians or managers about the effectiveness (or enjoyment) of the appraisal process, and you will find an overwhelming majority remain statically (or perhaps even painfully) clasped across laps. People hate appraisals and with very good reason.

The broader data support the view that annual reviews are, at best, performative and, at worst, utterly destructive.[11] My suggestion is to terminate this process immediately if you still do this.

The reason why they fail is that they do not meet any of the established criteria for delivering effective feedback! They are usually based on late, deeply flawed opinions on performance delivered awkwardly in a nonpsychologically safe way.

The norm is for new starters in an organization to be tossed in at the deep end with a cursory onboarding process and a poorly defined set of expectations. Behaviors and outputs are largely left unchallenged until the annual review, when a checklist of "problems" is unpacked and delivered from "on high" to the confused or fearful employee.

It is any wonder we have such poor culture scores[12] in veterinary practice?

Setting Expectations and Feedback

The antidote to the status quo is to adopt a system of continuous feedback. Such a system (outlined in **Fig. 1**) starts with clearly defined expectations and moves through a sequence of activities that should, in theory, yield ever-improving results. Although theory rarely survives first contact with reality, in this case, the system works well in the veterinary practice setting when slightly modified as follows.

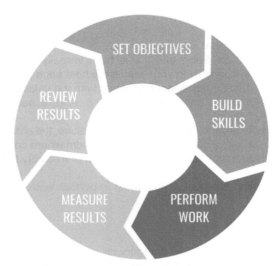

Fig. 1. A continuous feedback model for effective performance management.

Triple-Loop Leadership: Doing Performance Well

The performance management cycle is a continuous process for quality improvement. Done well, it is a respectful process where two humans meet in the middle to understand expectations, needs, and conditions impacting outcomes (good or bad). They then work collaboratively to problem-solve to a point where good performance is established and maintained.

To accomplish this and maximize the chances of good performance outcomes, three types of meetings are essential. Each has a different purpose, duration, and frequency. I created a performance process model I call Triple-Loop Leadership (**Fig. 2**).

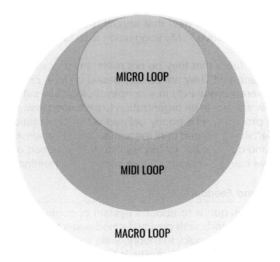

Fig. 2. The Triple-Loop Leadership model.

The Macro Loop: Setting Clear Mutual Expectations

The first loop, or micro loop, is the annual planning meeting (**Fig. 3**). During this meeting, clear expectations for the role over the coming 12 months are discussed and agreed on. This will involve forward-focused discussions of both objectives (what a person must accomplish) and behaviors (how they behave as they perform their role). There will also doubtless be a discussion about what resources, including time, equipment, training, and money, must be allocated to accomplish the objectives.

This conversation should take place with due regard for the organizational mission to ensure the work being discussed helps the team deliver the mission! It is reasonable to allocate 2 hours to such a meeting. With perhaps a maximum of 30 of these minutes allocated to any reverse-looking discussion. All objectives must meet the standard for good objectives previously described in this article (Specific, Measurable, Attainable, Relevant [to the mission], and Time-bound). Each goal must be accompanied by a precise measure of success, so it is easy to recognize to what extent it has been accomplished.

The Midi Loop: How Are Things Progressing?

The next loop exists to help ensure the agreed work is on track. The meeting structure will likely be the same as the annual planning but shorter in duration. The question both parties must seek to answer is, "Are things on track?" (**Fig. 4**)

Preparation is the key to a good meeting and the relevant data should be gathered ahead of time so the meeting can focus on outcomes and collaborative problem-solving to close any gaps between expected and actual performance. Such a meeting should be scheduled frequently enough to allow ample time for course correction. This could vary based on the competency and level of trust that exists between the manager and the employee. A new graduate who has recently joined the practice would benefit from more "face time" with their manager, whereas an experienced practice manager working on a new initiative might not require such hand-holding. It is good practice to hold these meetings every 3 months.

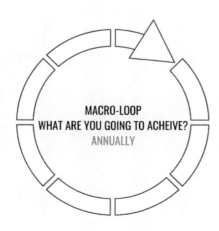

Fig. 3. Macro loop leadership.

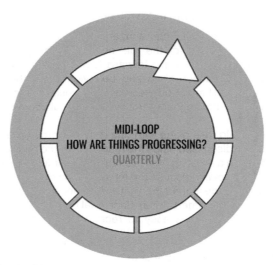

Fig. 4. Midi loop leadership.

Micro Loop: How Can I Help?

The final and most frequent meeting is the third loop, called micro loop leadership (**Fig. 5**).

These meetings are held weekly and for no more than half an hour. I call these BAAM meetings, and there is no meeting I consider more effective when done well. BAAM stand for Bonding, Accomplishments (past focussed), Actions (future focussed), and Mentoring.

Holding a Great BAAM Meeting

The purpose of the BAAM meeting is to connect with the person, understand how things are going with the work, and offer a chance for weekly coaching to occur so objectives

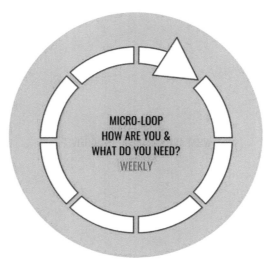

Fig. 5. Micro loop leadership.

are more effectively accomplished. They are a time when the job holder must be accountable for their actions and a time when leaders get to hold them so. (This is the real power of the BAAM meeting.) The leader's responsibility is to make sure these meetings happen. The employee's responsibility is to report on how they have progressed with meeting their weekly objectives and set some expectations for the following week. The structure flows as follows.

Section 1: Bonding (5–10 minutes)

Most people want to know that their manager cares about them. This is readily accomplished by taking a few minute of this meeting to simply chat about the employee's life. "How are you?" is a great question to kick off the meeting! The rest should flow naturally from there but do not rush into talking about the job! If they want to tell you about their kid's recital, then great, listen in and be pleased for them. Just as it is between pet owners and vets, it is also thus between employees and leaders—*people don't care how much you know until they know how much you care*.

Section 2: Accomplishments and Actions (15 minutes)

What has the employee accomplished this week in relation to their objectives? Have they achieved what was expected? If not, what got in the way? It is also important to discuss what they plan to accomplish next week.

Section 3: Mentoring (5–10 minutes)

Is there any advice, tips, or coaching that you can offer to help your employee overcome any challenges? What other ideas do they have for improving performance if they have a challenge? Try not to rob them of the chance to solve their issues with your blessing and support. The meeting closes by checking in on what you have understood and thanking them for contributing to the work and culture.

Ad Hoc Feedback

There is one final piece of the puzzle that does not fit nicely into any fancy framework but is utterly essential. This is the importance of ad hoc, "in-the-moment" feedback. Great feedback happens as close to real time as possible. When you see a team member do something well, take 10 seconds to call out what they did and recognize them for doing so. If something goes wrong, can you help steer people out of trouble without taking over? Far too many managers only bark at people when something has gone wrong. But getting into the habit of catching people in the act of doing things well is a much more effective tactic. Think about the impact of liver treats when it comes to puppy training! A puppy given liver treats right after it goes to poop in the right place will quickly learn that the desired behavior is to poop in the right place (outside), whereas a puppy scolded hours after the accident simply becomes fearful of its owner, with no benefit from a toilet training perspective. Be a "liver treats leader" Doing so will build relationship equity effectively, allowing a safe backdrop for harder conversations that may arise in the future.

SUMMARY

For many reading this, committing so much time to activities such as vision crafting and performance management will be anathema. "Where will I get this time?"

But there is no doubt, Leaders who neglect these activities will inevitably end up stuck on the Hamster Wheel because they have a low-trust culture where the owner or leaders ends up doing the jobs of others alongside their own. They are likely, over the long course, to generate lower rewards as the wider skill set of the team remains limited. Finally, their efforts to accomplish work are hindered by the friction generated by errors and poor behaviors. Regular, intentional performance activities, deployed against the backdrop of a well-crafted vision, are the antidotes to all of these ails.

As we wind up this article, let me again return to my working definition of Leadership as *the process by which a group of people come together and work to accomplish a shared objective sustainably.*

The crafting of a grand vision is a critical step in bringing the right people together to form your group or tribe. One that is likely to work effectively in your practice, and the performance management process allows the required work to be done well.

Veterinary practice ownership has long been a financially rewarding option. High time it was an emotionally rewarding one for all concerned, too. This is the gift that strong leaders bestow on those lucky enough to work on their team. If more of us developed these skills, the course of veterinary medicine would change inevitably for the good.

CLINICS CARE POINTS

- Clarity underpins all aspects of good leadership.
- Creating an inspiring vision is nonnegotiable for those who wish to build effective practices.
- Setting clear performance objectives allows team members to understand what is required of their work.
- Setting clear measures of success allows everyone to understand when a job is being done well.
- Regular accountability meetings allow performance to be reinforced or corrected early, with lower penalties for poor performance as variations can be corrected swiftly.
- Giving valid feedback is an essential skill all leaders must master.

DISCLOSURE

The author has nothing to disclose.

REFERENCES

1. Skogstad A, Einarsen S, Torsheim T, et al. The destructiveness of laissez-faire leadership behavior. J Occup Health Psychol 2007;12(1):80–92.
2. Schyns B, Schilling J. How bad are the effects of bad leaders? a meta-analysis of destructive leadership and its outcomes. The Leadership Quarterly; 2013.
3. McInerney D, Nicol D. Leadership actions and their effects on veteriary practice culture. VetX International; 2021.
4. Northouse PG. Leadership: theory and practice. SAGE Publications; 2016.
5. Judge TA, Piccolo RF. Transformational and transactional leadership: a meta-analytic test of their relative validity. J Appl Psychol 2004.
6. McKinsey. Leading innovation in organizations. McKinsey Quarterly; 2017.
7. Project Management Institute. Success in disruptive times: expanding the value delivery landscape to address the high cost of low performance. PMI's Pulse of the Profession; 2018.

8. Burnout Among Vet Professionals. A literature review. Niamh Farrell. Veterinary Times 2022;52(42):12–6. Available at: https://www.vettimes.co.uk/article/burnout-among-vet-professionals-a-literature-review-part-one/.

9. Beyond Entrepreneurship. *Turning your Business into an Enduring Great.* In: *Company.* Hoboken, NJ: James Collins and William Lazier. Prentice Hall; 1999.

10. Organizational Culture and Leadership. San Francisco, CA: Josey-Bass; 2010.

11. Wigert B, Harter J. Re-engineering performance management. Gallup; 2017. https://www.gallup.com/workplace/238064/re-engineering-performance-management.aspx.

12. McInerney D, Nicol D. Leadership actions and their effects on veterinary practice culture. VetX international; 2021.

Building a Veterinary Practice Team

Monica Dixon Perry, BS, CVPM[a,b]

KEYWORDS

- Team culture • Veterinary teams • Team development champion • Team developer
- Healthy culture • Team collaboration

KEY POINTS

- Building a successful, healthy, and collaborative veterinary team should be approached methodically and with focus. The biggest asset to a veterinary practice is its health care team.
- When building or even rebuilding a veterinary team, focusing on the team dynamics and culture is imperative as this will set the tone and foundation for what will make one's practice a consistent employer of choice.
- Because of labor force challenges, it is more important than ever to incorporate strategies that executive and middle management team members embrace as driving forces and inherently a part of a practice's professional DNA.

Imagine having a team that runs like a new, high-functioning well-oiled machine. Now imagine that this is the norm at your practice, not the exception. Does this sound like a piece of heaven on earth or highly unlikely? Having managed a practice with world-class dynamic team members, this was reality and can be attainable for any DVM owner and management team if so desired. In an industry that is faced with never-ending demands and expectations, building a team that functions at this level does not happen overnight. There is a lot of blood, sweat, and tears that will go into cultivating an environment that allows a team to develop and flourish at this level.

Unfortunately, there is no instruction book, step-by-step manual, or a magical recipe that will make this a reality, but after years of managing a practice and consulting with veterinary practice owners and managers across the globe, it is hopeful that the following recommendations will provide a feasible and digestible blueprint for creating or rebuilding your practice's team to be exemplary on all levels. The beauty of this process is that it will be different for each practice, because protecting and keeping your practice's unique personality is essential.

[a] Burzenski & Co, PC 100 Shore Shore Drive, Mariner's Point, East Haven, CT 06512, USA; [b] 5617 Beargrass Lane, Raleigh, NC 27616, USA
E-mail address: Mdixonperry823@gmail.com

Vet Clin Small Anim 54 (2024) 293–305
https://doi.org/10.1016/j.cvsm.2023.11.002
0195-5616/24/© 2023 Elsevier Inc. All rights reserved.

It goes without saying that a successful veterinary practice strives to consistently meet the needs of its patients and clients, but a successful practice and those who manage and operate it must fundamentally understand that building a phenomenal team is foundational to its success. This may seem like a simple thought and concept, but surprisingly this is a mark that is often missed in the industry. As with building anything, there is a process and although building a veterinary practice team is not rocket science, creating a successful team that will remain victorious when recessions, labor shortages, financial difficulties, negative reviews, a pandemic or a decline or substantial increase in volume takes place should be taken with the same precision and focus as building a rocket. Unfortunately, lots of practice teams have been created and built without truly considering and appreciating the vital role a team plays in a practice's overall success.

To assist practice owners or managers from having to reinvent the wheel when building their practice teams, the following recommendations are simple considerations but will have a great impact on your practice and those who show up every day to help bring your dream to reality. These recommendations are a culmination of more than 3 decades of being in the veterinary management trenches and working exclusively with veterinary practice teams. There is a sincere level of empathy that comes with these recommendations. Although simple in theory, these recommendations should save you time, money, and most importantly lots of headaches in the long run when it comes to developing your team. Keep in mind this process will not take place overnight, but if the commitment is at the forefront, you will be an employer of choice and the envy of others because of low turnover and an awesome culture that resonates within your community.

RECOMMENDATION #1 – IDENTIFY A TEAM DEVELOPMENT CHAMPION
What is a Team Development Champion?

A Team Development Champion is someone who is charged with supporting the practice owner's vision by spear-heading the development, maintenance, and oversight of a world-class, dynamic practice team.

This role can be and should be defined in a way that truly captures what is desired and needed from this position at your practice. Remember, this is your practice and ultimately your dream team. Similar to collegiate and professional sports scouts, your Team Development Champion should be selective and intentional about who they identify as potential candidates for your practice team. Even with the on-going labor shortages and challenges that plague our industry, imagine if those in charge of hiring had the mindset of a sports or talent scout when recruiting team members. How successful would collegiate and professional teams be if their team's scout haphazardly selected individuals for their teams? Scouts are passionate about the process and understand that selecting the best and right talent sets the tone for a successful season and ideally seasons to come. Although sport teams differ on many levels compared with that of veterinary teams, at the end of the day, scouts and veterinary practice owners and managers have a similar goal when it comes to their teams—both want a successful, winning team!

Two simple yet important questions to consider when selecting your practice's Team Development Champion are

1. What type of individual do I want for my practice's Team Development Champion?
2. What are my expectations for this position?

For you to successfully select and decide who will be your practice's Team Development Champion, you must first determine the type of characteristics you would like your team development champion to possess. It is important to think about and establish this expectation from the onset, because doing so will be the catalyst to creating and developing your world-class dynamic team.

Characteristics and traits of a successful team developer (example of characteristics) include

1. The individual must be firm, but fair as he or she interacts and work with the members of your team.
2. The individual must be an influential and positive communicator.
3. The individual must have the ability and wherewithal to create an environment that keeps your practice team motivated and engaged.
4. The individual must be able to inspire your team to not only meet expectations but exceed them on a consistent basis.
5. The individual whole-heartedly supports and fully grasps why this position has been created and is excited about building a team of high-performing individuals.

Writing down the characteristics and traits that you are seeking in this position and person sets you and this process up for success so that when you are considering individuals for this role, you already have a solid vision of what this person needs to bring to the table.

Once you have carefully defined the role, purpose, and characteristics for your practice's Team Development Champion, your work is not done just yet. It is now important to identify at least 5 major duties and responsibilities for this position. Articulating and defining this position's role and purpose come with establishing the major duties and responsibilities in order for ownership to hold the individual and position accountable while simultaneously ensuring that the vision you have for your team is the driving force with each hire and existing team members.

Major duties and responsibilities of a team developer (example duties and responsibilities) include

1. The individual will be responsible for identifying and selecting team members to join the practice who not only come with specific skills and talents to enhance the practice, but a sincere desire to be a part of a world-class dynamic team.
2. The individual will support team members so that they consistently find their positions challenging yet rewarding. This will minimize team members from getting bored and finding what they do mundane.
3. The individual conducts monthly pulse checks to assess each team member's happy factor. Although physical pulse checks are not taken, the power of these check-ins will allow ownership and management to have a better sense of what is working and what is not working for their team.
4. The individual develops personalized professional growth development plans to ensure each team member is consistently growing and evolving in their respective positions.
5. The individual identifies resources that support the overall mental health and well-being of the team. Although this position does not require someone that is professionally trained in mental health, it does require someone who has the ability to research and determine applicable resources to assist team members.

Although some may believe job descriptions have become a thing of the past, it is strongly recommended that providing clear expectations of one's duties and responsibilities be presented. Using a traditional job description is not necessarily a requirement, but taking the approach of presenting expectations in written format will increase the likelihood of a favorable outcome. Being explicitly clear as to what is expected so that there is no room for assumptions or confusion regarding the purpose of this position and who assumes these expectations is critical.

Some of these duties and responsibilities have traditionally fallen under the umbrella of a practice manager, but it is recommended that this position is created with the intent of 1 (a different) individual being designated as the Team Development Champion. Because this concept may be new for many owners and practice managers what should be considered is that senior level management has full plates and hiring someone that assumes this role on a three-quarter to full-time basis would be ideal. Yes, there will be additional costs associated with creating this position, but far too many practices have struggled and continue to struggle with having flawed teams and an unhealthy cycle of turnover. What the industry has done in the past when it comes to building teams simply is not enough in today's workplace. The demands that have evolved in managing teams require more attention and that have become overwhelming for 1 individual to effectively oversee and successfully manage.

When planning and budgeting for a Team Development Champion, the wages for this position would fall under your practice's administrative/managerial expenses, as he or she would be a member of the practice's management team. In addition to the suggested duties and responsibilities, other tasks can be added to the position's scope but keep in mind this person will be the ultimate cheerleader for your team.

In addition to defining the position and identifying major responsibilities with this position, it is recommended that you establish characteristics and traits that you would like for your team developer to possess based on the needs, personality, and team dynamics within your practice.

Once you have defined what a Team Development Champion will be at your practice and the primary responsibilities for your practice team, you have put one of the most essential steps toward building a successful team in motion.

It is imperative that practice owners take time to think long and hard about what they desire for their practice when building their practice team. Most DVM owners are focused on many factors such as honoring their commitment to animal welfare, having a strong, positive reputation in their communities, and creating a financially healthy business all while practicing high-quality medicine. These factors are important, but to achieve a high level of success, selecting someone who enjoys creating, building, and cultivating a healthy, high-performing team will set you and your practice up for a greater level of success.

There are many parallels that take place in a veterinary hospital and our personal lives. Through story time, I will share some personal experiences that have taken place to bring home recommendations that are shared in this article.

STORY #1

As a former hospital administrator, being a team development champion was imbedded into day-to-day operations, but the level of attention required by an effective team development champion cannot be shared with too many other responsibilities. As an administrator, it was difficult to consistently ascertain the needs of the practice health care team. Had I been able to focus on the more immediate needs of 1 individual who comes to mind, I would not have been so taken aback during her exit interview when she made it clear that I had not exceeded her expectations as a leader, but that I was nowhere near even meeting those expectations. The fact that she said I was ineffective as a manager was a hit below the belt. Although I had never been told this, I made sure that this sentiment would never cross one's mind ever again under my leadership. Having a better handle on what was working and not working for each of my employees became a part of my management style, one that I formalized via periodic check-ins (ie, pulse checks) to make sure each employee had one-on-one time with leadership. Everyone wants to have a voice and be heard. What I found out with that exiting employee is that I was ineffective as a leader because I hadn't taken time to meet with my team individually and routinely enough for her to feel valued as a member of the collective team. Sure, being a member of a health care team is similar to being on a sports team, but as talent scouts are charged with doing, they focus on the star, top players to build a phenomenal team. After that employee's exit interview, I better understood that as the hospital administrator, I had assembled my team of top players, and after doing so, it would become a lifeline of sorts to take care and nurture all top players so that they could shine as I had selected them to do. All members of management are expected to play an active role in supporting team members, but a team development champion can take this role to the next level and enhance every aspect of an employee's experience because of the primary purpose they will play by being your team's support system.

RECOMMENDATION #2 – CREATE A HEALTHY AND COLLABORATIVE CULTURE

When an owner and Team Development Champion are focused on building world-class dynamic team members, they are also committed to creating a healthy, collaborative work culture. Culture means different things to different people, so it is important to articulate what a healthy work culture will look like at your practice and the dynamic role it will play for you, your clients, patients, and your biggest asset, your team.

What does a healthy and collaborative team look like to you and your Team Development Champion? In other words, what type of workplace and environment are you all committed to creating for your world-class dynamic team members?

Healthy and collaborative culture (examples needed to create a healthy culture) should include

1. Team members understand and appreciate being supportive of each other and making every effort to work together in a harmonious manner.
2. Team members appreciate a healthy workplace and understand the owner and management will do what is needed to ensure a healthy, collaborative workplace.
3. Team members strive to exhibit positivity toward each other and are intolerant of any type of negativity, especially if it has the potential of derailing a healthy, collaborative work environment and culture.
4. The team, management, and ownership are a unified front working together to keep the practice world-class dynamic team intact and constantly growing and thriving.
5. When the practice's culture is threatened, the team will come together and resolve any issues so that everyone can get back on track and stay focused on the practice's vision for a strong, healthy, and high -performing team.
6. Team members understand and participate in open, healthy communication, because they understand this is needed for a team to work well together.
7. The Team Development Champion will conduct championship sessions that are culture-focused meetings, but not the typical or traditional team meeting. These sessions should not be griping sessions, but sessions that celebrate the team and practice's success over the last 2 to 4 weeks. In other words, these sessions should be conducted every other week or a minimum of once a month. Championship sessions focus solely on the strengths of the practice team and areas of excellence in between sessions. These sessions should be no more than 30 minutes. Although brief, these sessions will positively impact your practice team's

disposition and demeanor as members head back to the trenches of patient care and client service.

There is much more focus on workplace culture with this process. The veterinary industry is one of the best professions on earth, but it is not immune to factors that can easily break and crack a practice team. Ownership and management are ultimately responsible for creating and maintaining a successful practice culture. To achieve success, it is important to eloquently communicate and convey that a healthy, collaborative culture will be a part of the practice's DNA. Depending on your practice team, identify culturally focused activities that will ensure and protect your practice's positive, healthy culture.

Your Team Development Champion should create activities and/or exercises that are a part of your practice's daily operations. This will support the vision of having a healthy, collaborative culture, because these activities will be a daily part of your practice.

Day-to-day activities to enhance your team's culture (daily activity/exercise examples) include

1. Those in leadership roles are expected to and should make a concerted effort to lead by example. If management and ownership expect their team members to speak positively among each other, management and ownership should positively reinforce this behavior when they see their team members exhibiting this expectation and ensure their interactions and conversations are equally positive and demonstrate the level of positivity that is desired for the practice team.
2. Encourage open lines of communication to prepare team members to work through challenges as they come their way. If there are episodes or scenarios that take place where team members feel that their healthy workplace is being challenged, the team member should be encouraged and instructed to locate the Team Development Champion so that he or she assists team members by coming together for a culture protection rally (CPR) session to work through what resulted in any tension or harsh feelings. These CPRs allow for immediate attention, and, ideally immediate resolutions. Most importantly CPRs provide an opportunity for the involved team members to talk and work through any of their frustrations. The goal is that no team member will leave their shift carrying any frustrations, hard feelings, or negativity. Each day should start out on a positive note and end on a positive note. CPRs are an activity to assist with achieving this goal.
3. Celebrate throughout the day. Whether it is getting a pet owner to microchip his or her pet, sign a pet(s) up for pet health insurance, or a technician successfully placing a catheter, celebrate these successes! Although these are common occurrences within a practice, celebrate these routine tasks that your team performs day in and day out, because what they do truly makes a difference in the lives of your patients and clients. Unfortunately, much of what DVMs and veterinary teams show up each day to do is taken for granted. While celebrating these efforts, ensure you are sincere and genuine when deciding to celebrate your team. Do not show favoritism or have your efforts perceived in a way that may cause division within your team. Keep track of who and what is celebrated so that there is an equal display of appreciation and acknowledgment.

These are a few examples, but with your Team Development Champion creativity and your practice's unique personality, ideas for daily activities and exercises will be limitless.

STORY#2

Having a daughter who is currently a member of 2 high school sport teams allows me to see firsthand the importance leadership plays in the overall vibe and feeling she experiences by being a member of those 2 separate teams. She is on the tennis and lacrosse teams. Although she plays these sports at the same school, the teams are led by 2 different coaches. I get to see firsthand the role her coaches and the team captains play in the team's demeanor and how they influence the team's behavior, attitude, and how they interact with each other. On 1 hand, I see what works well together and a team that is passionate about winning because of the team dynamic the coach and leadership created during the season. The players seem happy and motivated during practice and during games. This is evident in how they interact with each other and the energy my daughter exhibits on our rides home after practice and games. On the other end of the spectrum are observations that are polar opposite. To see team members crying because their coach has yelled and used profanity took a toll so much so that instead of trying to make it to the state championships, team members suggested not trying their best so that they could lose and bring the season to an end. Imagine if your health care team showed up to work with an attitude along these lines? Ownership and management, do you have a committed team focused on winning or a team that is only going through motions and therefore not in the fight and subsequently causing your practice to lose in many respects? If you have a high number of client complaints, employee turnover, reoccurring mistakes, and tasks consistently being completed incorrectly, this equates to a losing team or a team that is not committed. An effective Team Development Champion will have the team focused on doing their best individually and collectively.

RECOMMENDATION #3 – ENSURE EACH DEPARTMENT HAS DAY-TO-DAY LEADERSHIP SUPPORT IN ALIGNMENT WITH YOUR VISION

Owners and practice managers cannot effectively oversee and perform all that is needed and expected based on the first 2 recommendations when it comes to building a veterinary team. Therefore, it is recommended that middle management is established when a department has 3 or more individuals. This will not only provide the daily supervision, guidance, and direction needed for your health care team members, but it also provides opportunities for growth and development within your practice. There are few opportunities for team members to grow in a veterinary practice. Creating new roles and positions allows for this growth and development and will also help challenge those individuals who are seeking additional responsibilities.

Traditionally the titles of the individuals who lead and oversee the following departments within a veterinary hospital are called head/lead receptionist (front desk/reception department), head/lead technician (technician/assistant department) and kennel manager (boarding/kennel department). To take a new, innovative approach to building a team that is led by culturally driven and focused middle management, consider renaming your departments leads as follows. For reception, Client Experience Manager (CEM), for your technical department, Patient Experience Manager (PEM), and for the kennel department, Recreation or Resort Experience Manager (REM). The roles of your CPR management team (CEM, PEM and REM) take on a completely different life simply by steering away from the traditional middle management terms used within veterinary medicine. The goal is to engage leadership and ignite excitement within leadership members' respective roles. They will be more effective and productive components of building and sustaining a world-class dynamic team. The term CPR is associated with lifesaving techniques within human and veterinary fields as it relates to patient care, but because of the challenges facing many practices, there is certainly a need for a bit of CPR with many veterinary teams. What has worked in the past may have gotten many practices where they needed to be to build productive teams, but team dynamics have greatly changed for veterinary practices. Therefore, there is a great need for ownership and management to think outside of the box regarding the building or rebuilding of their teams in order to successfully press through these challenges. Unlike in the past, teams need more collaboration and communication so that they have an enhanced sense of purpose. Team building needs reinvigorating, and this process will assist those who are seeking a different approach to lead and direct them. Overhauling your middle management teams' focus can bring life back to existing teams or if building a team from scratch, be the driving force that gives your team an awesome start to being happy and healthy.

STORY #3

It is wonderful to have a management team that works well together and appreciates the role of all employees in their respective positions and departments. When this takes place within a practice, the end result is a well-oiled machine that is led by ownership and middle management, that values the work and efforts of each and every team member, There is an appreciation that every person plays a vital role in the day-to-day success of the practice, When the alternative takes place, there is a lack of structure and focus that allows chaos to reside within the practice. I am reminded of a time when a practice had gotten large enough to have middle management, but the owners elected not to promote and leverage team leads but instead decided to create an environment where all employees were expected to lead. Unfortunately, the result was too many chiefs or cooks in the kitchen. When there is a lack of organization and clarity in who has certain authority and is selected to lead a team or a division, confusion will eventually find its place and creep into your practice. When there is clarity in who is the department decision-maker or leader, there is an understood level of order. As with any department, leadership is needed so there is a go-to person, designated problem-solver, and most important professional cheerleader and supporter for your team members. Middle management offers a level of growth within your practice and under the right leadership, effective order and authority. Do not let your practice be taken over by chaos. Your employees and practice deserve better.

RECOMMENDATION #4 – PROPERLY DEVELOP YOUR TEAM

Developing your team begins with proper training and onboarding. Unfortunately, the veterinary industry has been challenged when it comes to effectively training and onboarding team members. If an approach consistently does not work or produce the successful outcomes, a different approach is needed. When you have identified and selected your middle management team, it is now time to map out an action plan for members to replicate what ownership and management expect from each team member hired to work at your practice. Think lifesaving techniques! What is needed from all team members to ensure that during every shift they are scheduled to work they are supporting and allowing the execution of your practice's vision and mission in each interaction they have with each other as well as your clients and patients? A loaded question, but this is what your middle management team members must understand is their main role in leading and guiding their direct reports.

Charging your middle management team to creating lifesaving techniques that are instilled in your team is a great way to begin.

Create Lifesaving Culture Techniques (Example Techniques)

Create a lifesaving culture techniques list that every team must know and embrace to support team building at this new heightened level recommended. Go beyond your practice's core values and challenge your management team to think over and beyond the practice's existing core values. Get your management team leads thinking about the true value that team members bring to veterinary practices across the globe.

Example #1–Let team members know that at your practice they are seen as a Veterinary HERO!

H–Highly
E–Esteemed
R–Reliably
O–Outstanding

Referring to your team member as a Veterinary HERO provides a level of recognition and appreciation for those in the veterinary field that was never recognized on a global basis like the human health care professionals during the coronavirus disease 2019 (COVID-19) pandemic. There is no question the level of respect and appreciation that is owed to human health care professionals. They were on the front lines caring for and saving lives during an unprecedented time in history. Although many service industries came to a complete halt, veterinary medicine never skipped a beat. What was never publicly acknowledged was the level of commitment veterinarians and their teams demonstrated by being on their respective front lines. Veterinary professionals remained accessible and available to pet owners and their pets on a global level also. It is because of the human-animal bond and the care pets needed and required that veterinary practices could not and did not stop being there for patients. When it comes to building and rebuilding teams, the fact that so many veterinary professionals put their lives at risk and showed up every day is a message that ownership and leadership should use as catalyst and show appreciation for those team members who stayed in the trenches during such a challenging time. And, for those that are new to the industry, referring to team members as Veterinary HEROs will empower them while simultaneously sending a message that the strength, courage, and resilience they bring to the profession are valued and appreciated.

Building a team that is valued and appreciated in an environment that is committed to creating a healthy, collaborative culture becomes much more obtainable when those team members are seen and treated as the most valuable assets your practice has. Once team members are acknowledged as Veterinary HEROs, they will experience what it feels like to be recognized for the extraordinary efforts they bring to the field of veterinary medicine. This experience will be the powerful force that brings the vision of a building a successful team to fruition and reality.

STORY #4

There is a time in most of our lives that someone says something that resonates with us and impacts how we see and conduct ourselves personally and/or professionally. The words of wisdom that my father passed on to me as a young manager that stuck with me and laid the foundation for my communication and management style were – "you can't party with them on Friday night and expect to properly manage them on Saturday morning." What my father unknowingly established for me was the backbone of my understanding and respecting my leadership role so that I could better appreciate the role of my employees and prevent the blurring of any lines. Because of his words of wisdom, I was able to value my role as a leader so that I could provide the support my team desired and deserved. When leaders truly understand the influence and impact they have and the crucial role they play in their practice's success, a sense of pride and empowerment should take place. Leaders can make or break their teams in how they conduct themselves and treat their employees. If leaders get this right and treat their employees as the valuable assets they are, their work becomes much easier and with less headaches and challenges. It goes back to the basics of doing unto others as you would have them do unto you. Everyone wants to be respected, appreciated, and valued. It is that simple, and when leaders and managers grasp this simple concept, the impact they have over their team and the success of their practice is limitless.

RECOMMENDATION #5 COMMIT TO EFFECTIVE COMMUNICATION

Effective communication begins at the recruitment phase but is the center and focus of all that has been recommended. Starting with the owner communicating and articulating his or her vision followed by management wholeheartedly accepting these new approaches to building a successful team.

Recruitment Phase

From the recruitment phase, it is important to express the cornerstone of team building at your practice in your employment advertisement. Your advertisement should illustrate the culture your practice has and the type of team members you desire. Include video testimonials of your existing team members in your advertisement to showcase the culture your practice has to offer. Attempt to differentiate your practice so that you are seen as the preferred employer or employer of choice in your community. Be so effective in your delivery that you not only attract world-class, dynamic applicants, but potentially entice employees of other practices and locations to apply to your practice. When your practice is established as the practice that everyone wants to call their place of employment, you not only have achieved the ability to effectively recruit, but employee retention will also increase. You may think that in the current climate, establishing your practice along these lines seems unattainable. Don't allow this mindset to compromise the vision you have for your practice and practice team. Despite employment challenges, there are employees who are excited to show up for work and are committed to meeting the expectations of their employers. Attracting this caliber of employee so that they can become a Veterinary HERO at your practice ensures your efforts yield the outcomes you desire for your team.

Yes, a healthy, collaborative culture has to be created, but equally, if not more important, is creating an environment where these efforts and recommendations are sustainable.

Hiring Phase

When considering candidates, it does not and should not take long to determine if the candidate is a good fit or not. You have already determined the type of candidate who will transition and acclimate well within your practice, because you have team members who possess the necessary characteristics to excel within your practice's culture. You should document the characteristics that your top Veterinary HERO possesses so that each applicant is assessed comparatively. This does not mean you do not welcome and encourage differences in your team members. You are open and will consider all valid candidates, but there should be a common thread between your applicants and existing team members. How will you know if you should move forward with a particular applicant? You do your due diligence in checking references and asking how they were as an employee when they were at their best. You are trying to determine if they have the capability of being a Veterinary HERO at your practice. Sometimes environments and managers completely demotivate employees. You want to take the feedback you receive when checking references, but include questions that give you an idea of that employee's potential to thrive and contribute to a healthy, collaborative culture.

Onboarding Phase

Although the message of the type of team members you are committed in having at your practice should be vividly clear during the recruitment and hiring phase, it is important that this messaging continues during the onboarding phrase. When onboarding team members, establish basic, but concrete expectations when interacting with team members, your clients, and your patients. Never assume your team members know how you want and expect them to conduct themselves. Verbalize and document your expectations. It is ownership and management's sole responsibility to tell team members everything so that they have no room to assume anything. When you leave the possibility of assumption to sneak into your practice and practice's culture, you open the opportunity of damaging circumstances. Do not allow this to happen within your practice and your team building efforts.

Team Meeting Guidelines

Departmental meetings, all-inclusive team meetings, and pulse checks are all at the core of keeping communication intact at your practice. Having productive, upbeat team meetings is essential to having a practice with effective communication. Team meetings are the oxygen and glue for healthy teams. If these meetings are properly conducted, your team members will leave meetings feeling empowered, leveraged, part of solutions, valued and appreciated.

Departmental meetings

These meetings should be held a minimum of one a month. Your management team leads bring their respective team members together to discuss departmental successes and areas of opportunity. Your associate DVMs should meet with the medical director and if there is not a medical director, they will then meet with the practice owner(s). Leverage your team to resolve issues. When you leverage and encourage them to become problem solvers, they will be more inclined to embrace the solution, because they were allowed to be a part of the decision-making process.

All-inclusive team meetings

These meeting should be held a minimum of once a month. These meetings are led by Team Development Champion and Practice Manager. Executive leadership brings together all team members (this includes part-time employees, associate DVMs, the owner, and groomers). A healthy team does not exclude any team member. Mandating team members is not recommended, because expecting team members to come in when they are off is not fair or realistic. A valued Veterinary HERO deserves time off to relax, regroup and enjoy life outside of your practice. Consider scheduling these meetings on days that most of your team members are already scheduled to be at the practice. Do not schedule meetings that require team members to come to work earlier or stay later than normally scheduled. Conduct these meetings during hours of operation and close the practice for the set amount of time needed to have a productive meeting. The agenda should focus on the successes of the entire practice and bring to attention any solutions that were made during departmental meetings so that all team members are on the same page. If you truly have a world-class, dynamic team, you will have minimal problems to solve.

If it decided that your practice needs more meetings than these 2 meetings, ensure any additional meetings follow the same premise of being productive and positive. Your meetings become the mechanism that is needed to keep your team healthy, collaborative, and functioning like that well-oiled machine you imagined for your practice. Teams that do not meet at least once a month are often plagued with communication woes that invade a practice's culture and potentially cause irreversible or damaging effects. Stay committed to having team meetings, because they are comparable to a lifesaving technique used to save a pet or human's life.

STORY#5

Messaging and communication are everything! There is no doubt that it is important to send a consistent message that aligns with your practice's vision and mission. Having had an opportunity to work for 2 awesome employers over a combined 30 years, luckily there was a consistent message of "people before profits" from both of those employers. They both wanted successful businesses, but grasped the idea that taking care of their employees was the catalyst to their business' success. As an example, my first employer made the statement when I first started that she had 2 goals for me. Professionally she wanted me to become a certified veterinary practice manager (CVPM), and personally she wanted me to own my first home within 3 to 5 years of working for her and she was going to help me achieve both goals. When you have an employer who is looking out for you professionally and personally there is an unspoken level of loyalty and commitment that surfaces. In essence, she had my back, and without question, I had her practice's back. The support that she provided me did not stop with me, she wanted the same for her employees even if it came with an expense. She was one of the few employers in veterinary medicine at the time to offer health insurance, retirement plans and wages that were well above regional and national averages. Because of her stance of putting me and her employees first, she created a practice that ended up being very successful and profitable. Her messaging was clear and consistent. She effectively communicated what she expected from her most senior level manager and in return desired for her team of employees. What do you hope to effectively communicate within your practice? Whatever that may be, make sure the messaging becomes a part of your practice's culture and is a message that motivates your manager and team to be top-notch in all that they do.

SUMMARY

Building a successful veterinary team in today's climate can be easily summed up by acknowledging that building a team is simple in theory. The recommendations outlined in this chapter provide a road map that can be applied to today's challenging workplaces. The goal will remain the same today and tomorrow–create a practice team that is healthy and high-functioning with a solid foundation that can withstand any hurdle that comes its way. Being dedicated to building a team along these lines will be one of the most transformative decisions you make for your practice and practice team. Ready Set Go!

DISCLOSURE

The author has nothing to disclose.

SUGGESTED READING

Cavalea D. Habits of a champion team: the formula to winning big in sports, life, and business. Dana Cavalea Companies 2021.

Habits of a champion team: the formula to winning big in sports, life, and business

Gordon J. The energy bus: 10 rules to fuel your life, work, and team with positive energy. Wiley; 2007.

McChrystal S, Collins T. Team of teams: new rules of engagement for a complex world. Penguin; 2015.

Coyle D. The culture code: the secrets of highly successful groups. Bantam; 2018.

Culture

Building Happier, Healthier Teams and Practices in Veterinary Medicine

Jenni George, BA, CVPM

KEYWORDS

• Culture • Team building • Practice success

KEY POINTS

- Culture must be intentional and worked on constantly to maintain a successful team and practice.
- Culture starts with leadership, and it is important to have the proper leaders in place.
- Psychological safety in the workplace must be in place prior to working on your culture.
- For culture building to be successful, the team must be involved in all aspects of building the culture, values, and action goals.
- Culture is always a work in progress and will never be perfect.

My husband Simon and I started our journey working in 2 private practices before opening our mixed animal practice in Deerfield, New Hampshire, United States in 2007. From our experience, we learned a lot about what makes a successful practice and what makes a toxic practice, how to keep a happy team and how to push employees out the door, how to stay happy in a very difficult profession, and how to burn out. What is the secret? Culture!

Culture is the backbone of your practice. Culture is the values that you choose to live by and the actions that help you to live by those values every day. In the workplace setting, this means that you and your team are living in the same culture day in and day out. Maybe your culture needs some work. Most cultures do, so you are not alone. Maybe your culture just needs a few small changes. If so, you understand that culture is a constant work in progress. Maybe your culture is a raging forest fire. Maybe you want to fire your entire workforce and start over—that is, if they show up for work at all. Maybe your clients berate your staff daily and everyone leaves in tears. Or maybe you do not want to practice in the veterinary field anymore. If this is your truth, know you are also not alone.

Deerfield Veterinary Clinic, 150 South Road, Deerfield, NH 03037, USA
E-mail address: csuvet@yahoo.com

Vet Clin Small Anim 54 (2024) 307–316
https://doi.org/10.1016/j.cvsm.2023.10.015
0195-5616/24/© 2023 Elsevier Inc. All rights reserved.

Think of it like veterinary medicine. First, we must diagnose the problem. Second, we do a little surgery—removing deadly tumors and giving our practice a chance to heal. Finally, we prescribe the medication that our practice needs to stay healthy and continue to progress toward a long and healthy life. You are becoming a doctor of your culture.

CULTURE LESSONS

In the early 2000s, "culture" was a buzzword. I attended many conferences where I learned how to copy the culture of Disney where client satisfaction comes before all else. I could also copy the culture of Starbucks where policies and procedures are the recipe for success. There was 1 thing rarely mentioned in all the talks: the care of team members.

Currently, the veterinary industry is experiencing serious staffing shortages with veterinarians and veterinary professionals leaving the industry in droves. The mental and physical health of our team members is at an all-time low. Hospitals are selling out with little thought to how the culture might change for their team and for their clients and patients because practice owners are burnt out. The veterinary industry is having a serious culture crisis.

Let us visit the lessons we learned from my first veterinary jobs. The first practice I joined was a mixed animal practice in a rural part of the country. The owner/leader was an amazing veterinarian whom we will call Doc. He drew my husband in at the age of 13 when he allowed an eager, young 4-H student to tag along on farm calls—Doc's passion for veterinary medicine and animal care immediately transferred to Simon, who knew early on that he wanted to own his own veterinary clinic one day and be the next James Herriot.

Doc was, indeed, an amazing veterinarian. However, he left a lot to be desired as a business owner. Doc was always humble and lived to serve his clients. He and his team were available at all hours of the day and night, frequently doing emergency colic surgery at 2 AM or caring for a tiny kitten with an upper respiratory infection in the middle of routine appointments. He cared so much for his clients that he did not always make them pay for their care. Doc had a trusted practice manager with whom he rarely checked in. Soon after I joined the practice, I noticed a few key points regarding culture.

First, the employees who were rewarded were *not* the ones who worked the hardest. While he did manage a "Thank you" every now and then, the raises were reserved for those employees who complained the most and the loudest. While I am not sure if this was a "reward system," I am sure that it made those of us who worked hard and kept our mouths shut feel less important. Second, because he was rarely involved in the actual running of the business, his practice manager was able to embezzle funds and leave the practice with no warning, which left Doc in quite a pickle. Suddenly, his practice was further in debt than he realized with back taxes owed and a mess of accounting issues. Between his new bookkeeper and his wife Ione (the new practice manager), the practice became profitable again.

Ione taught me many lessons about being a good practice manager. Laughter and joy can be spread by the leaders and can be infectious to the rest of the team. It is a good idea (and is preferable) to get paid for the work we do. If the practice gets paid, the profits can be spread among the rest of the team and better services can be offered to our clients. Finally, culture can change and sometimes, it takes a catastrophic incident to start that transition.

The second private practice I worked at was also a mixed animal clinic with an exceptionally talented doctor; however the culture at this practice was truly toxic. Doc would pull employees into the examination room to berate them in front of clients, technicians would flip doctors off behind their backs, and team members had to dodge instruments that were thrown across the room. The employees who stayed did so out of respect for Doc's clinical skills, not for his managerial skills. But those employees were very rare compared to the high turnover which included a new hire leaving for lunch and not coming back. Doctors did everything and technicians were glorified animal holders. No employee was trusted fully, and rules were constantly changed when Doc decided they should be. While he was a great mentor for Simon as a veterinarian, we learned a lot about what not to do at a practice.

If either of these situations sounds familiar, there is hope. Culture can be changed, but it takes time and patience. Like any good relationship, it needs to be worked on constantly. And, if you act like Ron Popeil with his "Set it, and forget it" tag line, your culture will fail. Poor culture results in lack of retention for the team and clients, constant tardiness or callouts from the team, low profit margin, poor patient outcomes, and/or an overall toxic work environment.

WHAT IS YOUR WHY?

A good culture is intentional, purposeful, and effectively communicated with all involved. The first step is to know your *why*. Simon Sinek, author of *Start with Why*,[1] speaks to the importance of knowing your why. As he explains, "Every business knows what they do." In veterinary medicine, we care for patients. Our doctors perform surgery, diagnose diseases, and prescribe medications. Our credentialed technicians and veterinary and kennel assistants advocate for our patients and assist our doctors in this care. Our customer service representatives care for our clients so that the rest of the team can care for the patients. This is *what* we do.

In addition, Sinek says, "We normally know how we do it." Our policies and procedures outline how we make sure that each patient gets the care they need. The veterinary school prepares our veterinarians for the gold standard treatment, while real life shows us that there need to be plans B, C, D, and E alongside plan A. We have websites, books, forms, and so much more to assist us in our *how*. The state veterinary licensing boards and the American Veterinary Medical Association also tell us how to meet the basics standard of care.

But what is our *why*? All cultures start with *why*. The first doctor that we worked with owned his own practice so that he could care for clients. While that is admirable, a team needs to be considered as they are part of taking care of those clients. The second doctor we worked with owned his own business because he did not like being told what to do with a "my way or the highway" attitude. Ego leads to a toxic work environment where no one is happy.

When Simon and I started our practice, we knew we wanted to do things differently. Our main goal was to have a fun work environment with a happy and productive team that offered the best in customer service and excellent patient care. It was a lofty goal and is still progressing after many, many years. We know that if we take care of our team, they will take care of our clients and patients.

I challenge you to really think about what is your *why*. Why do you work in veterinary medicine? Why do you want to lead? Why are you reading this article on culture? Knowing your *why* can lead you to either a great culture or a disastrous one. If your *why* sounds like "to make more money" or "because I want to do things my way," your practice will *not* have a positive culture. Selfish reasons will not lead to productive results. Sinek's companion book, *Find Your Why*,[2] is a great resource to work your way through discovering your *why*. This workbook can also be used with your leaders and your team.

UNICORN LEADERSHIP

The question of *why* needs to be asked of all leaders in your practice because your leaders are the enforcers of your culture. Culture starts with leadership. Who are your leaders? Leaders can be at every level of the practice, and you can find and mentor them if you look.

There are 7 key components to a unicorn leader:

1. A focus on progress, not perfection
   - Perfection is unattainable and, therefore is the lowest possible standard to hold someone to. They will always fail.
   - Progress is far more important; learning from mistakes and failures is the only way to grow. We do not grow from a place of comfort but from a place of challenge.
2. Compassion
   - Compassion means to empathize with someone who is suffering and to feel compelled to relieve the suffering. This is a very common practice in veterinary medicine because we live to ease suffering in clients and patients.
   - This does not mean to take others' suffering home with us. We must be able to separate ourselves from problems that are not ours after we have attempted to help in whatever way we can.
3. Solutions-based thinking
   - This is the ability to not only see problems, but to see solutions to those problems. This can come from learning from past or present failures or from looking at a problem with fresh eyes.
   - Solutions could be new or something tried before with a new approach.
4. Courage
   - A leader must be willing to do things that others do not wish to do. They must be willing and able to have difficult conversations while being open enough to connect with others. Brené Brown says, "Daring leaders who live into their values are never silent about hard things."[3]
   - A leader cannot be afraid of change or new situations.
5. Good communication
   - Active listening skills and the ability to read body language are a very important part of communication. Emotional intelligence is a must for good leaders.
   - It is important for leaders to know and adapt to different communication styles.
6. Self-awareness
   - We must be aware of our own strengths and weaknesses. Seeing ourselves clearly can help us succeed in communicating with ourselves and others.
   - Knowing how we affect those around us helps leaders be better communicators.
7. Grit
   - Angela Duckworth, the author of *"Grit,"*[4] defines grit as "focused persistence that is more valuable than natural talent."
   - Focusing on the effort put forth and never giving up makes for a tenacious leader.

Remember that unicorns do not exist. Your leaders will not have every one of these attributes. You may have someone who is very compassionate and an excellent communicator but who lacks courage. You may have someone who has amazing grit and solutions-based thinking but who struggles with perfectionism. Choose leaders with intent and do not just promote due to longevity. Ask your leaders if they want to be leaders. If they do want to be leaders, ask them for their *why* (this is an excellent opportunity for you to purchase them a copy of *Find Your Why* and work through it together). Leaders are helpful in getting the team to buy-in to your new and improved culture. You may have some great leaders in place already, while other leaders may show up as you work toward a healthier culture. Be mindful in choosing leaders and your culture will improve automatically.

PSYCHOLOGICAL SAFETY

Before moving forward, you need to be sure your practice has psychological safety for team members. If you are a perfectionist and your team is constantly belittled when mistakes are made, there is no psychological safety. If team members or clients do not feel accepted for who they are (sexual orientation, gender identity, ethnicity, religion, appearance, and so forth), you do not have psychological safety. If team members are afraid to speak up, question leadership, or advocate for the patients and clients because they have been reprimanded in the past, you do not have psychological safety.

Psychological safety means that your practice is a safe place for risk-taking. Brown defines psychological safety as "team members feeling safe to take risks and be vulnerable in front of each other."[3] It is giving people the benefit of the doubt and assuming good intent and they do the same with you as a leader. If your team members do not feel safe taking risks and making mistakes, they will not speak up to help create a positive culture. There are many opportunities to learn how to make your workplace psychologically safe. This must be done prior to any work on your culture. You must learn how to be inclusive and allow team members the opportunity to learn, contribute, and challenge you in safe and meaningful ways.

Another part of psychological safety is owning up to past mistakes. Perhaps your culture has not been great. Perhaps you have not been great at rewarding your hard workers or utilizing your team to the best of their abilities. You need to recognize your past mistakes and plan to fix those mistakes. If you are not able or willing to do this, the rest will be a waste of time. As leaders, we must take responsibility for our part in the failures of our culture. Remember, culture starts with leadership. If the practice owner or practice manager does not lead with integrity, honesty, and hard work, the team will know and act accordingly. Failures can be learned from and not repeated in the future. Your team needs to know you are focused on improving and what your expectations are for yourself moving forward. You can ask trusted team members to help hold you accountable so that you do not fall into past habits. Dwelling on past mistakes without changing behavior to avoid them in the future is insanity. Remember progress, not perfection.

CULTURE BUILDING

Now that you know your *why* and your leaders know their *why*, share this *why* with the rest of the team. Ask them what their *why* is for working at your practice and for being in the veterinary industry. Again, this is a great opportunity to work on a workbook or book group together as a team such as Sinek's or Brown's books mentioned earlier. Your team needs to be involved in all aspects of making and growing your culture. Therefore, they need to understand your *why*. If your reasons do not align with their integrity, be prepared for them to leave, and find a practice that better fits their *why*. Please know that it is better to have team members who fit your culture than to have warm bodies who are there to punch in, mindlessly do their job, and punch out while waiting for a better opportunity.

Culture is an individual sport as well as a team sport. You and your leaders will continually promote your culture. But your team must be actively involved in making the culture. If you do not involve your team and you simply tell them what your culture is, you may lose more people. You will have better retention and more patience from team members who contribute and who feel involved and heard.

Step 1: Goals

Your culture should have specific goals. It should answer the question "What does my practice stand for?" This is for the team to help you decide and can come from finding your team's *why*. If we go back to our *why*, it may sound like, "I got into the veterinary industry so that I could ease the suffering of pets and help them get healthy," "I want to help clients when they are stressed about their pet," or "I want to work in a practice where I feel like I am part of a team and I make a difference." These *whys* are the beginnings of your culture. Work together to list what your key culture points might be.

Your culture points might be practice high-quality medicine, offer excellent customer service, work with a happy and productive team, and have a safe and healthy work environment. They should be the big-picture ideas of what you, as a practice, stand for. This may take a few meetings to hash out as everyone may have opinions. It is important to take everyone's opinions into consideration so that your team is involved and feels heard. This is why we must have a psychologically safe workplace. Without support and the ability to take risks, your team will not participate.

Step 2: Values

Next, ask your team to list values that they feel define the practice. Brown has a list of values on her website, brenebrown.com. Be prepared that your team may pick other values than your own. For example, you might pick "efficiency," "legacy," and "learning" as key values to your practice. Your team might pick "making a difference," "trust," and "teamwork" as their values. All are exceptionally good values to have, and you should choose to focus on the values the team picks, as those would be the best for them to represent in their daily work. You could have your own individual values that you stand up for while the team has values that you, as a practice, can live daily.

After producing your values, define what those values mean to each of the members. For example, teamwork has different meanings for each of us. Some see teamwork as working together toward a common goal, some see teamwork as helping each other overcome weaknesses, and some see teamwork as picking up the slack when other team members are having a bad day. Teamwork can include your work team as well as your clients. Defining each value is a long and tedious process.

Have each team member write their own definitions on sticky notes. The notes can be put up for all to see. Then have a team discussion to pick what they like and do not like to make your own definition. (This is why psychological safety is so important to getting full participation.) This may take multiple team meetings over a period of weeks or months. It is worth the time and energy put into developing the culture.

Step 3: Actions

After defining values, each team member must define the actions they choose to hold themselves and each other accountable for living by these values. Brown has a wonderful list of behaviors to adopt on her website. You can also produce your own. Sticking with the value of teamwork, behaviors could include

- I will bring a positive attitude to work each day.
- I will do my own dishes and not expect others to clean up after me. (Our practice cannot be the only one with this issue, can it?)
- I will help wherever needed and not say "That's not my job."

- I will not gossip about other team members. If I have a question or issue, I will go directly to that person.
- I will communicate my expectations clearly and concisely.
- I will show up before my shift starts and be ready to work at the time expected of me.

You can go on and on with ideas on how to commit to behaviors that will better your team. Each team member should make a list of what they commit to so they can live by these values. Practice managers should meet with team members one-on-one to discuss their lists within a few weeks of this team exercise. Ask how they plan to overcome past challenges themselves. For example, you could have a team member who says they will be ready to work on time. But this team member is consistently late for various reasons. Ask what their action plan is to overcome this in the future. Help them see solutions for past problems. These are truly courageous conversations and give you insight as to what team members are willing and able to do to make the practice the best it can be.

SMART goals
You can help team members produce SMART goals. SMART goals are Specific, Measurable, Attainable, Relevant, and Timely goals. Your consistently late team member could have a goal to show up on time to work for an entire month. Their actions to make this possible could be to charge their phone outside of their bedroom and use an alarm clock. This helps them to avoid scrolling all night which leads them to going to bed late and makes them late in the morning. They could also make their coffee at home or purchase it the night before and leave it in the refrigerator to avoid long coffee lines in the morning. Find the problems and help produce solutions. This shows your team you care and creates a culture of growth.

After everyone has their one-on-one conversations and you know what they are willing to work toward to help live the values your team defined, you need to define your culture. If you go back to your *why*, it may sound like, "I got into the veterinary industry so that I could ease the suffering of pets and help them get healthy." You now need to tie in your values to this idea.

Build your forest
Think of culture as a forest. You have been working on all the small things that build your forest. Your *why* is the root system that gives life to the trees. Your leadership and psychological safety are the trunks and branches that give strength to the trees. Your values and behaviors are the leaves that collect the sunlight and rain to help the forest grow. Your culture is your forest—your big picture. All of it ties together.

One of your culture points might be excellent patient care. Your values of trust, teamwork, and making a difference can be the trees to your forest of excellent patient care. You build trust with your patients by practicing fear-free techniques. Your team can anticipate each other's needs to better care for emergent situations that arise. You make a difference by advocating for our patients so that they have better outcomes.

The final step to creating a positive culture is to list behaviors that align with your values and culture points. In this case, you would give examples of what excellent patient care looks like. It might be simple things like making sure your patients are always warm and clean, playing music in your kennel areas to help keep patients calm, or offering many, many options for treats. It could be a more costly option like installing sound-reducing panels so that the barking is absorbed and not as disturbing to patients. It should always be continuing to learn and grow with the latest procedures and practices for pain management and anesthesia. The team can get highly creative with ways to make the best possible patient experience. Because the team feels like this practice and culture belongs to them, they are more likely to try new ideas and take risks. Seeing team members express their creativity can be a lot of fun!

Once your behaviors and actions for your culture are listed, you should pick 2 or 3 from each category and produce SMART goals for them. For example, your goal is to offer multiple treats to each patient and keep track of their favorite. That is specific and attainable. Your action can be to keep notes on each patient that is seen within the clinic for a month. This can be measured by auditing the appointments seen each day to see if they have a treat note in their record. At the end of the month, if 80% of patients have notes, you can have the team choose their reward.

TEAM BUILDING

Rewarding your team for successes can build a positive culture and lead to a more satisfied team with better retention. Rewards do not have to be expensive (but could be if you have the funds). No matter what, rewards should be chosen by the team. When hiring team members, you could ask them how they like to be recognized (publicly vs privately, in-person vs in writing). You should also ask for ideas for little rewards like favorite junk food, favorite healthy food, favorite place to get gas, favorite place to buy coffee, and so forth. Having a pile of favorite candy bars in a drawer and a stack of blank "thank-you" notes can go a long way to building trust and comfort among leadership and a team.

As for bigger rewards, let the team pick what they would like to do. Maybe a pizza party or an ice cream party for smaller goals. Maybe go-kart racing or a paint night for bigger goals. Remember, what you like may not be what the team wants. If you love cake and bring cake in for every celebration but you have a team that is doing a health challenge, your reward will not mean much and could be seen as sabotage in their eyes. Including your team in all conversations, from culture and values to rewards and recognition, will create a team that cannot be beaten.

Another way to build an unbeatable team is to hire for your culture and values. In a time of employee scarcity, you might frequently be tempted to hire a warm body to fill a position. Sometimes the only requirements are breathing and reliable transportation. To build a successful team, you must do better. You must ask questions during the hiring process that align with your values and your goals. There is a clinic in Tennessee that requires applicants to read *The Energy Bus* by Jon Gordon prior to interviewing. The practice manager has many copies and gives them out. Some come back and some do not. But those that come back know what the practice is all about and it is one step closer to finding a great fit for the team. While this is an excellent book that should be read by everyone, I do not recommend making applicants read a book necessarily. But asking questions that align with your beliefs can help.

If your focus is on client service, invite applicants to share a time when they had to solve a problem with an upset customer or a time when they made a customer's day. If someone is applying from another clinic, invite them to share stories about a difficult case they saw through to the end or what their interest is in fear-free techniques. By inviting applicants to tell stories, you will find out if their personalities align with your culture points. Waiting for the right fit is worth the wait. Hiring warm bodies just invites good team members to jump ship.

SUMMARY

Like any relationship, a culture and team must be worked on. Once or twice a year, practice owners and managers should meet to discuss their *whys* and be sure that their values still align. Practice managers should meet with leads 2 to 4 times a month to avoid any mole hills from becoming mountains. Team leads should meet with their teams monthly. This may seem like a lot of meetings, but communication is key to a successful and positive culture. Think of it as preventative medicine. It is easier to heal diseases if diagnosed early as opposed to when it is too late. Problems are the same way. A proactive approach leads to success and happiness.

- Your culture is always a work in progress and will never be perfect. There may be small fires, but the goal of a great culture is to keep your forest from burning.
- Building up and supporting leaders is necessary to building a good team and a great culture.
- Creating a psychologically safe workplace will allow your team to participate in the creation of your culture.
- Involving your team in defining culture and values keeps them engaged and feeling valued.
- Caring for your team can lead to a happier work environment for everyone involved.
- Your culture can make or break a practice. You must choose to work on your culture with intent to keep your practice, your team, your patients, and your clients for a long, long time to come.

CLINICS CARE POINTS

- A positive culture is important to team retention and a successful business.
- Team leadership must be courageous and open to communication.
- The practice must be a psychologically safe workplace that encourages the team to learn from mistakes and take risks.
- The team needs to be involved in building and maintaining a great culture.
- Building a culture is not a fast process, but it is worth the hard work and time.

DISCLOSURE

The author has nothing to disclose.

REFERENCES

1. Sinek S. Start with why: how great leaders inspire everyone to take action. Penguin Books; 2009. p. 33–51.
2. Sinek S, Mead D, Docker P. Find your why: a practical guide for discovering purpose for you and your team. Penguin Random House; 2017.
3. Brown B. Dare to lead; brave work. Tough conversations. Whole heart. Vermillion; 2018. p. 36–8.
4. Duckworth AG. The power of passion and perseverance. Scribner 2016;3-14: 243–68.

FURTHER READINGS

Gordon. Jon the energy bus: 10 rules to fuel your life, work, and team with positive energy. John Wiley &Sons, Inc; 2007.

Brown. Brené workbook for dare to lead: brave work. Tough conversations. Whole hearts. Cosmic Publications; 2022.

Sinek. Simon leaders eat last: why some teams pull together and others don't penguin random house 2014.

Gordon. Jon the power of a positive team: proven principles and practices that make great teams great. John Wiley & Sons; 2018.

Optimal Veterinary Team Utilization Leads to Team Retention

Heather Prendergast, RVT, CVPM, SPHR

KEYWORDS

- Veterinary team utilization • Veterinary team retention • Culture • Trust
- Credentialed veterinary technician • Optimal utilization • Change management
- Veterinary Practice Act

KEY POINTS

- For veterinary practices to effectively reduce the loss of team members, whole team utilization must be implemented.
- Veterinarians should be diagnosing, prescribing, prognosing, and performing surgery. Everything else should be leveraged to a well-trained team, thereby increasing daily patient capacity.
- Veterinary hospitals that embody optimal whole team utilization, a strong culture, and great leadership have higher revenue, profitability, client compliance, and reduced employee turnover.

THE IMPORTANCE OF TEAM UTILIZATION

There is no doubt that the pandemic has had a vast impact on the veterinary industry. The workforce has changed, not only in the availability to attract talent but also in the dedication and loyalty team members have for their practices. Personal views on job satisfaction have changed because they look for a career that they can be happy and fulfilled in, not just a job. Non-Doctor of veterinary medicine (DVM) team members that are *fully utilized* in their positions are more likely to stay in their roles when they have a positive, healthy culture that they thrive in (not just survive).

The average turnover for credentialed veterinary technicians (CrVTs) is 7 years.[1] Upon graduating from an American Veterinary Medical Association (AVMA) accredited program (either associate or bachelor's program) and passing the National Veterinary Technician Exam (VTNE), they enter the veterinary workforce as either Registered Veterinary Technicians (RVTs), Certified Veterinary Technician (CVT), Licensed Veterinary Technician (LVT), or a Licensed Veterinary Medical Technician (LVMT), all of which depends on the state in which they choose to practice in. For ease of reference, the collective term

Synergie Consulting, Las Cruces, NM 88011, USA
E-mail address: H.Prendergast@synergie-llc.com

Vet Clin Small Anim 54 (2024) 317–335
https://doi.org/10.1016/j.cvsm.2023.10.010
0195-5616/24/

vetsmall.theclinics.com

CrVT is used to refer to RVTs, CVTs, LVTs, or LVMTs. The main reasons cited for CrVTs leaving the profession are lack of utilization, low wages, lack of title protection, and lack of work–life balance.[1]

If the scope of practice in the state Veterinary Practice Act (VPA) or Rules and Regulations (R&R) are not defined to split the 2 roles, veterinary assistants (VAs) will frequently perform the same tasks as CrVTs. However, VAs are usually on the job trained (OJT) and although they may have advanced skills, they do not possess the formal training of a CrVT. In many cases, the skills of a CrVT are *not* fully used because practices have allowed VAs to perform similar tasks thus setting the expectations for both positions as similar but with VAs being hired at a lower wage. The expectations for VAs are elevated, whereas those of the CrVT are diminished, which saves money for the practice while severely affecting the value of the CrVTs. This has created a barrier to entry into the field because the average debt load of a CrVT is nearly US$30,000.[1] VAs do not see the need to seek formal education when the wage is the same and without the debt load.

The DVM role is in jeopardy as well because nearly 3000 veterinarians chose *not* to return to the profession after COVID 2019.[2] Additionally, nearly 40% of younger DVMs are considering leaving the profession in the near future.[3] To further the gap in the veterinary industry, nearly 41,000 DVMs will be needed to serve the estimated 75 million pets in 2030. Veterinary schools estimate that there will be approximately 15,000 graduates by 2030, leaving a gap of 15,000 veterinarians in addition to those looking to retire after serving 40+ years in the industry.[4] Similar to the DVM shortage, it is estimated to take 30 years of CrVT graduates to meet the demand of 2030.[4]

Finally, the Customer Service Representatives (CSRs)/Receptionist Team have one of the hardest jobs in the practice, receive the least training, and receive the least amount of respect from both the veterinary team and the clients. They are the first and last impression clients have of the practice, and if they are used well, they will serve very important roles. They too, must be used to their fullest potential to decrease the rate of turnover.

For practices to reduce turnover of all roles, practice leaders must understand why team members are leaving, challenge the way things have always been done, and implement changes to keep them.

THE BASICS OF A SUCCESSFUL WHOLE TEAM UTILIZATION AND IMPLEMENTATION

Although practice owners and leaders may understand the need for team utilization, many try to implement changes (such as immediate, full utilization) without having basic principles in place. Without a thriving culture that embodies psychological safety and team trust, any change has a high chance of failing. Team members must understand the "why" to buy into any change and believe that leadership will continue with the change (versus reverting to the way it has always been done when it gets difficult). Additionally, team members need to have ongoing educational opportunities to continue bringing collaborative ideas to the team, which also contributes to an individual's ability to become, and sustain internal motivation.

Culture is discussed in article eight, and because a positive culture is the basis for successful change, it is worth highlighting here. Culture is defined as the social order of the practice that shapes attitudes and behaviors that when done well, achieve the goals of the practice.[5] It is driven by leadership and is like a garden; it takes continuous care. One must plant seeds, fertilize, water, and weed the garden for its success. A leader's work on culture must never stop.

Culture is driven by sharing the goals of the practice, including how every role contributes to the achievement of those goals. When *each* team member understands what they bring to the goal(s) and how to positively accomplish daily skills, they become emotionally invested (vs financial investment) in the success of the business. This starts the process of finding their sense of purpose in their role, ultimately leading to long-term, invested team members.

For context, practice goals are defined as the vision, purpose, core values, and achievement of the practice's strategic plan. The vision describes the future of the practice (where will the practice be in the next 2–5 years?). The purpose defines the fundamental reason the practice exists and is also commonly known as the mission statement. The word "purpose" is more relational and resonates better with team members. The purpose is a statement that when practiced enables the practice to achieve the vision. Core values are specific words that describe the desired behaviors that each team member should demonstrate daily in the practice; they serve as guiding principles of the practice that should not be compromised. Collectively, the vision, purpose, and values should lead to the achievement of the practice's long-term strategic plan.

If team members do not know what these goals are, they simply show up to a "job" every day, complete tasks, and go home. Their own sense of purpose is not filled. However, when the CSR team (as an example) understands that their role is to:

- Provide value for clients through education and a frictionless client experience,
- Control the chaos of the day through strategic scheduling, and
- Ensure patients are triaged and seen according to need, they can become emotionally invested in their role.
- By serving clients and patients to achieve the practice's vision and purpose, they too can find their own sense of purpose.

Psychological safety is defined as a shared belief that the team is safe for interpersonal risk-taking.[5] It establishes a culture of safety that allows a space for people to speak up and share ideas without fear of retribution. When psychological safety is present, it enhances employee engagement, inspiration, and creativity. When team members are comfortable, they are more likely to collaborate, critically think, and problem-solve and, thus, improve their mental health and well-being, which allows them to perform at optimal levels. Implementing optimal team utilization requires psychological safety and trust.

Team trust can take years to build and minutes to break down. When implementing optimal utilization, the DVMs must trust the skills of the CrVT, and the CrVTs must display behaviors and skills that allow the DVM to trust them. Similarly, CrVTs must trust the VAs, and the VAs must display the skills and behaviors needed that allow both DVMs and CrVTs to trust them. When a thriving practice culture exists with defined goals and psychological safety, trust comes easier; adding continuous training and education puts the icing on the cake.

Education must be provided to all team members, regardless of role. Although the CSR and VA teams are not required by state regulations to have CE, the practice *should* require it. For team members to achieve self-fulfillment, they must understand why, what, when, and how to deliver exceptional client and patient service. Learning outside of the practice stimulates excitement, especially when they are allowed to implement what they have learned in the practice when they return. If they have not had the opportunity to attend continuing education (CE) outside of the practice or implement what they have learned during a previous CE experience, leadership must set expectations before the event, encouraging them to learn and return to the practice to implement the ideas that were presented.

To further enhance trust between the DVMs and the team (CrVT, VA, and CSR), the DVM team should partake in the development and training of the team on medical procedures that are specific to the practice. Standard operating protocols (SOPs) and standard of care (SOC) should be developed with a collective agreement of the DVM team, allowing the team to deliver exceptional care every time, not dependent on which doctor sees the patient. SOPs and SOCs keep the team aligned and allow them to educate clients with the same consistent message and care (often, clients need to hear a recommendation at least 3 times to accept). SOPs and SOCs, when delivered in a positive environment, allow the team to deliver a frictionless client experience for every client (while driving trust within the practice team).

The DVMs license is on the line, and every team member must understand and respect that. Therefore, if the DVMs train the skills that are expected and team members deliver the skills and behaviors consistently, optimal team utilization will occur without the micromanagement of cases.

Internal motivation can best be described using Maslow's Hierarchy. People are not self-motivated when they work in an environment that has a negative culture that lacks safety, trust, and clarity of practice goal achievement. Therefore, it is the responsibility of the practice to create an environment that encourages collaboration and emotional ownership, both of which contribute to each team member finding and fulfilling their own sense of purpose.

Maslow's breaks down the motivation of team members into 3 categories of basic, psychological well-being, and self-fulfillment needs (**Fig. 1**). Food, shelter, and sleep are factors outside of the practice while working conditions and wages are factors from within and make up the first category. Although shelter and sleep are factors outside of the scope of responsibility of the practice, leadership must understand if anyone on their team is struggling with this basic level because it will inhibit motivational progression. The practice has 100% responsibility for creating safe working conditions and adequate wages for team members. The 2022 NAVTA demographic study cites that 33% of CrVTs work more than one job to sustain livable conditions. Team members of this state are less likely to progress to the next level because they consistently worry about providing for their families. Food, shelter, sleep, safe working conditions, and wages must be met before advancing to the second category.

Category 2, psychological well-being, includes the practice culture, purpose, inclusion, self-confidence, and self-esteem. When the practice culture is strong, clear expectations are communicated, and goals are implemented into daily activities, inclusion and a sense of purpose naturally occur, thereby resulting in self-confidence and esteem for

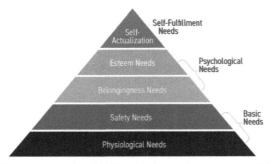

Fig. 1. Maslow's Hierarchy; reprinted with permission from Practice Management for the Veterinary Team, 4th ed; Elsevier 2023.

their roles. When category 2 is achieved, self-fulfillment (category 3) naturally occurs because team members are highly motivated to obtain practice goals and seek additional growth opportunities within the practice.

Leadership must understand Maslow's and ensure ample opportunities are provided to help team members achieve their sense of purpose while cultivating a culture that creates a psychologically safe environment rich with team trust, and the ability to take risks and try new things that result from continuous education.

WHY OPTIMAL UTILIZATION DRIVES TEAM MEMBER RETENTION

When the basics above are implemented into daily routines, the practice is on the way to implementing and maintaining optimal utilization with loyal and dedicated team members that have a desirable work–life balance. When all team members are used for their maximal skill, their sense of purpose is fulfilled.

However, maximal skill does not stop with the knowledge team members graduated from school with (CrVTs and DVMs); that is simply the beginning. New graduates need a mentorship program during the onboarding phase to help them apply the skills obtained in school (DVMs and CrVTs alike) resulting in increased confidence and loyalty to the practice in the first 90 days of employment. To continue fulfilling a person's sense of purpose, team members must be allowed to grow through advanced education and be allowed to implement what they have learned through that experience. For example, if a CrVT attends CE in which they learn advanced cardiopulmonary resuscitation (CPR) or catheterization skills, they must be allowed to bring back the knowledge to the practice, have the opportunity to teach the team, and implement into daily protocols as necessary. If a DVM attends a hands-on tibial plateau levelling osteotomy (TPLO) course, they must be allowed to provide that service to their clients (potentially attracting new clients).

VA and CSR teams also need outside education to maintain their sense of purpose as well as have the knowledge and skill to be able to contribute inventive and unique ideas to practice growth. Stagnant team members that depend on knowledge only provided within the practice are at a higher risk of disengagement and decreased loyalty, ultimately leaving the practice. Educational budgets must be implemented, allowing every team member to equally contribute to the growth of the practice through maximal utilization while also achieving a sense of fulfillment and pride. Historically, 0.5% to 0.9% of gross revenue has been allocated to continuing education expenses and reserved for DVMs and CrVTs that were required to have annual CE. However, this low amount does not support whole team growth and utilization. In the author's experience, 2% to 3% of gross revenue (yearly) should be allocated to CE that supports the practice's vision and strategic goals.

When the whole team can provide patient and client care at their maximal skill level without micromanagement, the burnout and compassion fatigue rate dramatically reduce because responsibility is equally shared, everyone embodies emotional ownership, and everyone is accountable for their actions and the success of the practice.

OPTIMAL TEAM UTILIZATION BY ROLE

It is critical to understand the state VPA and/or R&R because it applies to CrVTs and OJT VAs. VPAs and R&Rs vary by state, some of which define the title of a CrVT and reserve the title for those that have graduated from an AVMA-approved school, passed the VTNE, and the state licensing examination. Additionally, some states define the scope of duties allowed to be carried out by that role.

Some states do not define the difference of in the scope of duties in the 2 roles and is therefore a driving factor for CrVTs to look for positions in practices that voluntarily split the duties that allow optimal utilization by formal training and advanced skills. Recall one of the top reasons CrVTs leave a practice (or the field completely) is lack of utilization and overall competition for VAs that are paid at lower wage rates.

Regardless of the role or title, all team members must have respect for one another and the strengths they bring to the team. Common behaviors include the senior tech that treats lower level team members with little to no respect, the VA that has been at the practice for 20 years that refuses to help a recent CrVT graduate, and/or all medical team members that fully disrespect the CSR team. Practice must establish "one team" that is aligned, has each other's back, has respect and trust for one another, and empowers others to carry out skills based on training and the demonstration of such skills.

Leveling up

Practices will have different levels of skill sets of team members within the same role. Although the goal will likely be to bring everyone up to the highest level of skill, not all team members can do so, nor have the drive to achieve that higher level. It is normal to have these levels within the team and that is acceptable; it allows the team members to achieve greatness within their level and allows improved utilization of those with higher skills. A lower level team member can carry out the base level skills, while a higher level carries out advanced duties (instead of the advanced level doing all things). For example, a level 1 VA may have tasks associated with cleaning cages, feeding patients, retrieving patients for treatments and diagnostics, and restraint of patients. A level 3 VA will likely carry out a higher level of nursing care, client education, and so forth (based on state VPAs and R&R). This splits the duties, sets clear expectations of what role/level does what, and encourages the team to work smarter and more efficiently in a collaborative manner.

Leveling also provides team members with an understanding of how to grow in their role, can accommodate wage ranges for transparency, and have training protocols built in to ensure that everyone has been trained as they grow within the practice. Examples of leveling by role that leads to optimal utilization can be found in **Table 1**.

The CSR team is the first and last impression for clients, and it is important that they are knowledgeable on veterinary procedures, and can communicate positively, confidently, and clearly, ultimately creating value for clients from the first interaction (and thus setting the medical team up for success). They should not have to defer recommendations for the top services and products sold within the practice to the medical team but instead have the knowledge to make the same, consistent recommendations (often, clients need to hear a message 3 times before accepting recommendations). They should be able to understand and communicate the SOPs and SOCs developed by the medical team and have the autonomy to address and fix client concerns and complaints immediately (not defer to the manager at a later time).

Having CrVT-specific appointments can offset the workload of the doctor team by allowing the CrVTs to manage vaccine booster appointments, specific rechecks (incisions, dental rechecks, dermatology, wound/bandage care, and so forth), diagnostics, treatment plans, and client education. Additionally, CrVTs should be able to carry out advanced nursing care and case management of hospitalized patients when a treatment plan has been established. VAs increase the efficiency of the CrVT team by obtaining patient history, vitals, loading rooms with patients, obtaining basic diagnostic samples, and providing basic patient care and client education. When telehealth is used by the practice, the CrVT can obtain advanced vitals and examination findings

Table 1
Leveling by role that leads to optimization utilization

CSR Level 1	CSR Level 2	CSR Level 3	VA Level 1	VA Level 2	VA Level 3	CrVT Level 1	CrVT Level 2	CrVT Level 3	Veterinarians
Greeting clients	Medial record preparation	Client complaints	Complete a medical record audit and identify all reasons for the visit	Basic client education	Basic blood sample collection	Drug therapy calculations familiar with potential drug interactions	Apply splints or casts	Advanced level diagnostic sample collection	Diagnose
Client check-in and check-out	Medical record audits	Accounts receivable	Check client in	Run samples on in house blood machines	Fecal analysis	IV fluid therapy calculation	Advanced Imaging, Anesthesia support for CT, MRI, PET procedures	Advanced level diagnostic completion	Prognose
Invoicing clients	Reminder reviews and corrections	CSR work schedules	Obtain history and TPR/HR	Prepare reference lab samples	Collect free catch urine	Administer vaccines	Suture (closing existing skin incisions)	Advanced imaging (MRI, computed tomography, PET)	Prescribe medications
Reviewing invoices with clients	Maintain email communication	Onboarding and training new CSRs	Patient restraint	Administer PO, SQ injections, SQ fluids, and topical medications	Complete basic diagnostic labs (UA, CBC/Chem, PCV/TP)	Bandaging	Advanced level radiographs (Shoulder, OFA, spinal series, and so forth)	Advanced level nursing care	Perform surgical procedures
Process payments	Maintain third party client communication dashboards		Patient care and husbandry (food, water, and walk)	Nail trims	Obtain basic level radiographs	Urinary catheter care	Urinary Catheter placement	Nasogastric tube placement	

(continued on next page)

Table 1
(continued)

CSR Level 1	CSR Level 2	CSR Level 3	VA Level 1	VA Level 2	VA Level 3	CrVT Level 1	CrVT Level 2	CrVT Level 3	Veterinarians
Discuss payment options with clients (Care Credit, and so forth)	Communicate with clients regarding normal basic labwork results		Cleaning examination rooms, treatment areas, and surgery	Manage prescription and appointment requests	Obtain patient vitals	Anesthesia induction and monitoring (III–IV)	Advanced level client education	Telehealth/follow up appointments	
Answer phones	Basic client education		Clean and sterilize surgical instruments, gowns, and towels	Admit surgical patients	Administer SQ injections	Tracheal intubation	Dermatological testing	Central line placement	
Schedule appointments	Pet insurance education			Admit hospitalized patients	IV Catheter placement and fluid administration	Advanced level/complicated anal gland expressions	Esophagostomy tube maintenance	Arterial blood pressure monitoring	
End of day reconciliation				Complete client call backs and address client queries	Basic level, uncomplicated anal glad expression	Perform intake physical examination/assessments	Perform euthanasia	Gastric intubation	
Process new client cards				Mediate client concerns	Ear cleanings	Perform initial triage/tele triage	Perform chest compressions	Chest tube placement	
Be familiar with patient emergencies and schedule appropriately					Basic anesthesia monitoring (ASA I–II)	Perform pain assessment	Advanced surgical patient discharge	Chest/tracheal tube maintenance	

Fill prescriptions	Calculate constant rate infusions	Advanced inpatient discharge	Ultrasounds
Mediate client concerns			
Attach patient records from previous hospital to medical record and update reminders			
Suture removal	Dental prophy, charting, and radiographs	Cytology	Ultrasound-guided nerve blocks
Microchip insertion	Dental blocks	Blood transfusion and cross matching	Blocked cat catheter placement
Neonatal care and resuscitation	Cystocentesis	Critical care assessments	Epidural catheter care
Recover postop/sedated patients	Gastric intubation	Physical rehabilitation treatments (laser, shockwave, ultrasound, TENS, and so forth)	Leading code (RECOVER)
Onboarding and training/mentoring new VA's	Blood typing	Regenerative medicine preparations (PRP, stem cell processing, HA injections)	Place IV catheter and administer drugs during cardiopulmonary arrest
Treatment plan/estimate plan development and delivery	Controlled substance handling and monitoring	Emergency triage	Establish airway in cardiopulmonary arrest

(continued on next page)

Table 1
(continued)

CSR Level 1	CSR Level 2	CSR Level 3	VA Level 1	VA Level 2	VA Level 3	CrVT Level 1	CrVT Level 2	CrVT Level 3	Veterinarians
					Surgical prep	Ophthalmological testing (Schirmer tear, fluorescein stain, tonometry)	Multimodal analgesia and interventional prescriptions (vasopressors, gastrointestinal, and so forth)	Onboarding and training/mentoring new CrVTs	
					Obtain EKG		Intraosseous catheter placement		
							Fine needle aspirates		

Abbreviations: CBC, complete blood count; EKG, electrocardiogram; OFA, orthopedic foundation for animals; PCV/TP, pack cell volume/total protein; SQ, subcutaneous; TPR/HR, temperature, pulse, respiratory, heart rate; TENS, transcutaneous electrical nerve stimulation.

and provide a remote doctor with the information needed to make a recommendation for the diagnostics and treatment plan.

The DVM team can then focus on diagnosing, prognosing, prescribing, and performing surgeries with the ability to see (and "fit in") critical cases that need their attention, resulting in optimal work–life balance and mental wellness.

GETTING FROM LOW UTILIZATION TO OPTIMAL UTILIZATION

When looking at the overall picutre of optimal utilization, the implementation process may seem daunting. A "gap analysis" will help identify specific objectives that must be achieved to achieve the greater goal. Set objectives will prevent steps from being missed that will slow the progress of the goal, or worse, set the team up for failure to achieve the goal.

A gap analysis defines the starting and end points of a goal. *What does utilization look like in the veterinary practice today, by role? Who does what?* Be specific and detailed during this part of the exercise to ensure all inefficiencies are uncovered.

Next, dream of what ideal utilization should look like in the future, again by role. Do not associate who can do what in this step, rather focus on what the role should accomplish. Details are critical in this step as well as it sets the stage for a complete gap analysis.

The third step identifies what needs to occur to get from today to the ideal. This step may include training, advanced education, role-playing, enhanced interteam communication systems, technology to enhance the client experience, and so forth. See **Fig. 2** for an example of a gap analysis.

A gap analysis is then followed with SMART goals that include specific objectives to make sure that optimal utilization is achieved. Goals and objectives (measurable steps taken to achieve a goal) must be specific and measurable, and the person responsible for carrying out the goal must be motivated and empowered to use resources outside of the practice to achieve success. Objectives can be assigned to different team members, resulting in greater goal achievement and team buy-in.

An SMART goal sheet helps define the needed elements to successfully implement goals.

S—Specific defines the specific goal that is to be achieved.

M—Measurable identifies how the success of the goal will be measured.

A—Action items identify what tasks will need to be completed to achieve the goal.

R—Resources identify what resources will be needed to achieve and implement the goal successfully.

T—Timeline and accountability identify when the goal will be achieved by and establish check-in points with the responsible individuals.

Goals and objectives will often hit snags that were not previously identified in the gap analysis, and this is normal. By critically thinking and being creative, team members can overcome hurdles together and still achieve the goal. Expect there to be continual assessments and change as needed to yield successful implementation. See **Fig. 3** for a completed SMART goal sheet.

CHANGE MANAGEMENT

Implementing change is difficult. It is easy to stay with what is comfortable, and when challenging the status quo, a sense of chaos and discomfort is created. Many times, team members will use their energy voicing resistance to change, versus critically thinking, problem-solving, and creating solutions. This is a common scenario and leadership must be able to positively influence change to take the practice to the

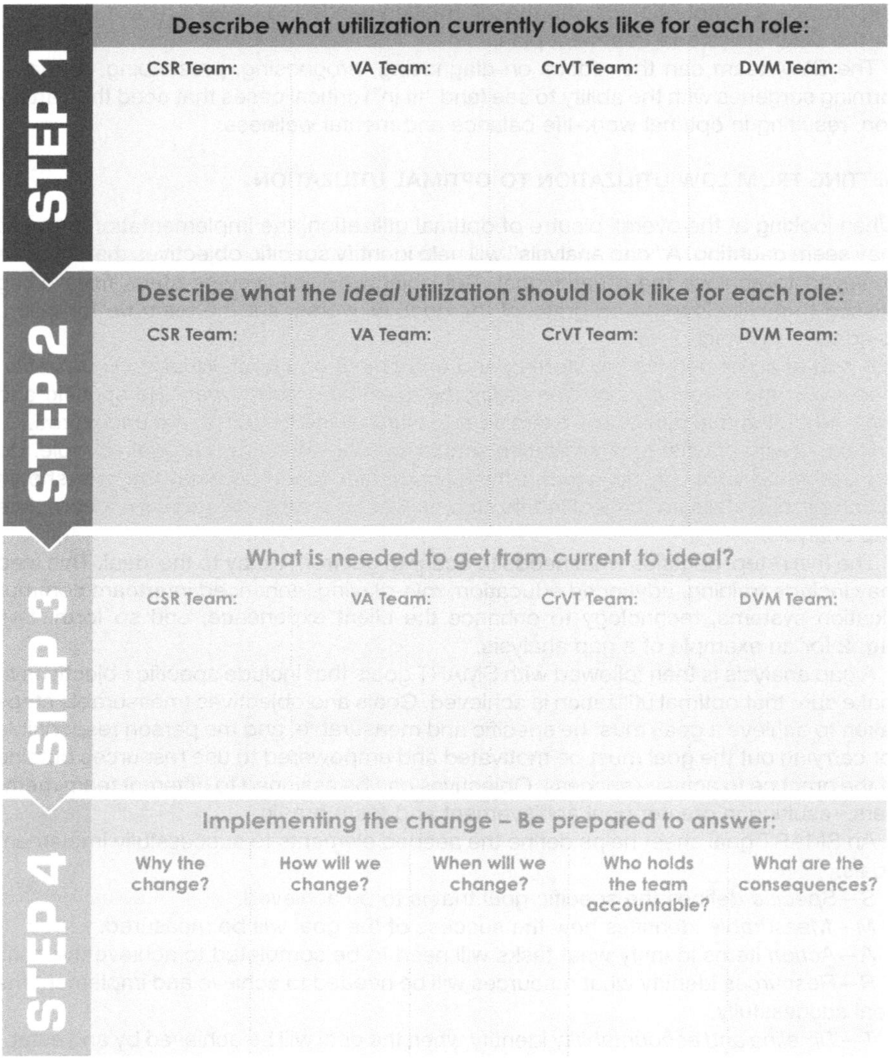

STEP 1	**Describe what utilization currently looks like for each role:**			
	CSR Team:	VA Team:	CrVT Team:	DVM Team:

STEP 2	**Describe what the *ideal* utilization should look like for each role:**			
	CSR Team:	VA Team:	CrVT Team:	DVM Team:

STEP 3	**What is needed to get from current to ideal?**			
	CSR Team:	VA Team:	CrVT Team:	DVM Team:

STEP 4	**Implementing the change – Be prepared to answer:**				
	Why the change?	How will we change?	When will we change?	Who holds the team accountable?	What are the consequences?

Fig. 2. Example of a gap analysis.

next level. Understanding the most common reasons for change resistance will help leaders plan and overcome patterns of resistance.

"*Informational resistance*" is defined as team members not knowing why a problem exists, how it affects the practice, and where potential change could occur. Although most team members will understand the need for optimal team utilization, some may resist full optimization without having all the information needed as to how and when the change will occur. It is important that leaders be prepared to answer and support.

- Why the change?
- What is the goal?
- How will we change and achieve the goal?
- When will we change?

PROJECT: CrVT Utilization	
GOAL: Our practice has determined that we do not utilize our team to maximal efficiency, resulting in the loss of team members, decreased revenue, and burnout. As practice leaders, we must reverse these results to improve revenue, reward the team, decrease turnover, and improve client retention and satisfaction.	
Specific	Implement CrVT utilization to the maximal capacity allowed by state regulation through team development, a gap analysis, and an understanding of maximal capacity as defined by state regulation.
Measurable	1. Less than 10% team member turnover year over year. 2. Increase revenue by 10% through organic growth (not just price increases). 3. Increase wage ranges based on the scope of duties. 4. Increase client satisfaction (as measured through surveys) from an average of 3 to 4.8.
Action Items/ Accountability	1. Create a Utilization Team with representation from all practice roles (veterinarian, CrVT, veterinary assistant, customer service representative, and kennel team) to contribute to and participate in all decisions and activities of the team utilization plan. ASSIGNED TO _____. 2. Complete a gap analysis to assess the current situation by evaluating the team's daily duties and tasks. Identify which tasks are routinely performed by veterinarians that could be performed by CrVTs, as well as future growth opportunities if tasks are not a current duty (Table 5.3). ASSIGNED TO _____. 3. Review the state practice act, rules, and regulations for a scope of duties that can be delegated to CrVTs and other team members with Immediate Supervision, Direct Supervision, and Indirect Supervision. ASSIGNED TO _____. 4. Review the scope of practice as outlined by AAVSB. ASSIGNED TO _____. 5. Create a foundation of transparency with the team; present the findings of the gap analysis and seek input for successful goal implementation.
Resources	State Veterinary Practice Act/Rules and Regulations found on the state Board of Veterinary Medicine Webpage AAVSB Model Regulations – Scope of Practice for Veterinary Technicians and Veterinary

Fig. 3. Example of a complete SMART goal sheet.

- Who will hold the team accountable?
- What are the consequences of failure?

"*Personal resistance*" is a result of the loss of familiar patterns or relationships with fellow team members. This is likely the second largest hurdle a practice faces when implementing optimal utilization as years of patterns and behaviors must be broken. New patterns and behaviors can take 30 days to become a habit, so it is easy to revert to the status quo quickly, as new patterns can cause chaos, confusion, and loss of confidence. Psychological safety, trust, collaboration, and emotional ownership are critical to overcoming personal resistance. Leaders need to be prepared to answer and support:

- DVMs that wish to protect their license.
- Not having skilled staff
- Not having enough staff

"*Cultural resistance*" is the opinion that change is not possible within the organization, or leadership is not capable of carrying out the change. This is the largest factor that inhibits change in veterinary practices. A 100% of leadership (owner, practice manager, associate DVMs, lead techs, and lead CSRs) must be onboard with goals, how the team will get there, maintaining leadership alignment (being on the same page at all times), changing their own habits and behaviors, and holding each other accountable

	Technologists	
Timeline	1. Action item #1 due: _____ . Checkpoint date #1 _____ ; Checkpoint date #2 _____ .	
	2. Item #2 due: _____ Checkpoint date #1 _____ ; Checkpoint date #2 _____ .	
	3. Action item #3 due: _____ Checkpoint date #1 _____ ; Checkpoint date #2 _____	
	4. Action item #4 due: _____ Checkpoint date #1 _____ ; Checkpoint date #2 _____ .	
	5. Action item #5 due: _____ Checkpoint date #1 _____ ; Checkpoint date #2 _____ .	
	6. Begin implementation: _____ and adapt as needed to continue improvement.	
Projected Outcome	Whole team utilization	

Fig. 3. (continued)

for the optimization of team utilization. Leaders need to be prepared to overcome being too busy to train, have team meetings, or openly communicate goals.

ADAPTABILITY

During this critical time of change management, there must be the opportunity to pivot and adapt if the goal that the team is working toward is not progressing. Although it is important to allow time for the team to adapt to changes and establish new behaviors, leadership may see that the team needs additional resources (or other tools) to continue achieving the long-term goal. There will likely be some things that are working well, some things that need slight adaptation, and others that may need to be completely rebuilt. These are normal processes a practice goes through as they work to find the most efficient methods to achieve optimal utilization. The goal during the gap analysis is to identify a majority of these hurdles during the planning process but the adaptability quotient must be considered.

OPTIMAL WORKFLOW PATTERNS

Although optimal workflow will be slightly different in each practice due to building layout, space restrictions, and team member skill limitations, finding optimal patterns is critical to both efficiency and utilization. **Table 1**, **Table 2**, and **Figs. 2** and **3**, **Fig. 4** provide examples of leveling and optimal utilization, and **Fig. 4** demonstrates a gap analysis to identify hurdles. A practice should also consider time and motion studies and identify what bottlenecks halt efficient, optimal processes. **Table 2** provides examples of optimal workflow patterns for various types of cases seen in all practices.

Once levels, optimal workflow patterns, and role expectations have been created for the practice, leaders need to update job descriptions, onboarding and phase training programs, rewards programs, and performance feedback mechanisms. This ensures new employees are hired with clear expectations and have appropriate training and support in place to succeed long-term in the practice (a career, not just a job).

THE IMPACT OF OPTIMAL UTILIZATION

Optimal utilization in the veterinary practice has both tangible and intangible impacts, with the latter being harder to measure in revenue production.

Table 2
Examples of optimal workflow for a variety of case types

Category	Steps by Role →					
	CSR:	CrVT (with VA):	Veterinarian and CrVT:	CrVT (with VA):	Veterinarian:	CrVT and team:
Appointment/ Initial Assessments (General Practice)	• Obtain initial information, reason for visit, previous medical records	• Data collection • Obtain the relevant history • Initial triage • Note problems identified • Create a preliminary diagnostic plan (ie, if the patient is pale, order CBC), • Basic level of care or initial diagnostics started (ie, collect ear swab samples for cytology) • Present case to the veterinarian	• Agreement/ prioritization of problem list— patient assessment → Veterinarian • Therapy plan recommendation • Case management check ins with CrVT are predetermined • Presumptive or working diagnosis given	• Diagnostics/ therapy planned carried out	• Prescriptions written or surgery performed	• CrVT creates and facilitates nursing plan • CrVT develops and facilitates/delegates to go home information/keys to clinical outcome success • CrVT sets and performs follow-up and recheck appointments
Initial Assessments/ Emergency situations (ER)	• Obtains initial information, reason for visit, previous medical records	• Data collection • Obtain the relevant history • Initial patient assessment • Initial Triage and assessment • Note problems identified	• Agreement/ prioritization of problem list— patient assessment → Veterinarian • Therapy plan recommendation	• Diagnostics/ therapy planned carried out	• Prescriptions written or surgery performed	• CrVT creates and facilitates nursing plan • CrVT develops and facilitates/delegates to go home information/keys to clinical outcome success

(continued on next page)

Table 2
(continued)

Category	Steps by Role →				
	• Create therapy plan *based on agreed protocolized medicine* (algorithm) (defined as standard operating procedures, ie, if/then steps) • Order diagnostics (ie, if patient is pale, order CBC), • Basic level of care (ie, if patient is blue, start oxygen) • Initial therapies, to-go-home information gathered • Present case to veterinarian	→	• Case management check ins with CrVT are predetermined • Presumptive or working diagnosis given	→	• CrVT sets and performs follow up and recheck appointments

Surgical Utilization—Veterinarian diagnosis	CrVT:
	• Patient assessment
	• Pain score
	• Anesthesia/Analgesia protocol and preparation (as per protocol(algorithm)/ Veterinarian direction)
	• Create surgical plan
	  ○ Equipment
	  ○ Preop
	  ○ Monitoring
		Veterinarian:
		• Performs surgery
			CrVT:
			• Anesthesia/pain monitoring,
			• Incision documentation, surgical record keeping
			• Postop pain score
			• Facilitate nursing care with team
			• Communicate patient updates with clients
					CrVT:
					• Prepare, communicate, and discharge instructions
					• Create follow-up and recheck appt plan

	All Team Members / CSR	CSR/bot	CrVT	Veterinarian	CrVT
Triage and Teletriage (assumption VCPR is already established) VVCA Sample Vet Tech Flowchart Asynchronous1 - http://vvca.org/virtual-care-guides/	**All Team Members:** Clear understanding of definitions for telehealth/triage/ VCPR AAVSB RECOMMENDED GUIDELINES	**CSR/bot:** • Initial response (signalment and historical information collection • Automated information collection for what can be collected (no need for CrVT)	**CrVT:** Performs teletriage: • Asks questions to collect more clinical information, photos/video. • Uses critical thinking skills to ask differentiating questions • Synthesizes generalized problem list • Makes recommendation on action: ER, see doctor, home care/education, and/or builds plans from SOPs previously approved by a doctor and patients already having VCPR	**Veterinarian:** • Diagnoses problem remote or in person visit or review tests • Prescribe treatment	**CrVT:** • Schedules necessary tests, communicates with client/patient, performs treatments, prepares discharge and educational info for client. • Prepares follow-up plan

Telehealth - follow up appointments and check ins, rechecks VVCA Sample Vet Tech Flowchart Hybrid Curbside 1 - http://vvca.org/virtual-care-guides/	**CSR:**
	• Schedule telehealth appointment with CrVT based on treatment or discharge plans
		CSR:
		• Schedule telehealth appointment with CrVT based on treatment or discharge plans
			CrVT:
			Performing telehealth appts remotely can include the following:
			• Postop rechecks (such as incision checks)
			• Post-Dx discussions
			  ○ Check-in visits regarding Cushing's/Diabetes/DJD/senior pet care
			    ▪ Restating disease pathophysiology
			    ▪ Restating outcome/prognosis discussions
			    ▪ Refreshing timing of repeating laboratories and reasoning for continued monitoring
			    ▪ Scheduling of CrVT appointments for sample collection when deemed necessary.
			  ○ Restates medication expectation/compliance
			    ▪ Challenges of compliance
			    ▪ Lifestyle changes
			    ▪ Exercise routines
			    ▪ Nutrition discussions		

Abbreviations: Appt, Appointment; CrVT, credentialed veterinary technician; CSR, client service representative; DJD, degenerative joint disease; VA, veterinary assistant; VCPR, veterinary client patient relationship.

Adapted with permission from the 2023 AAHA Technician Utilization Guidelines. Copyright © 2023 American Animal Hospital Association (aaha.org/technician-utilization).

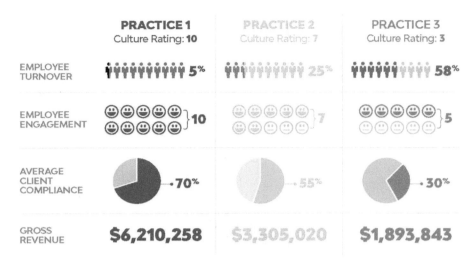

Fig. 4. Summary of a study looking at the impact of culture and whole team utilization (among other factors) from 3 practices each with 4 full time equivalent (FTE) DVMs. Practice #1 had a dramatically higher revenue-producing team resulting in happy team members and clients, whereas practice #3 struggled with team member engagement and client compliance. (Graphic courtesy of Synergie Consulting.)

Team member retention increases when employees feel valued and are used to the optimal potential. When a practice is willing to invest in the team to build their skills and provides a culture that is a great place to work, employees will not want to leave. In fact, when a strong employer brand is built (that team members brag about), it attracts highly skilled and talented team members to further help the practice achieve long-term strategic goals.

On average, for every team member lost, it costs the practice up to 1.5 times the annual salary of the individual leaving to recruit, interview, hire, and train a replacement.[6] This does not include lost revenue that results from decreased client compliance because of strained team members or reduced customer service during the time of team member shortage. The average turnover rate of CrVTs and DVMs is currently 25%, an increase from 13% prepandemic.[7]

Healthy team members that love their job and maintain a work–life balance perform at a higher level during working hours than those experiencing burnout and fatigue. Optimal utilization leads to increased job satisfaction and a fulfilled sense of purpose. Ensuring they maintain that healthy balance is an important key performance indicator (KPI) that should be tracked through hours worked, overtime hours, lunch breaks, when the team leaves at the end of the day, paid time off (PTO) taken, and leadership check-ins with each individual team member.

When looking at the revenue generated from 2 different studies in North America, one with data from 2007 (Fanning and Shepherd, 2010) and the other with data from 2020 (Shock and colleagues), fully using a CrVT for their education, licensure, and training accrues a revenue benefit of approximately US$104,976 to US$137,240 per CrVT, per veterinarian.[8] Additionally, if an full time equivalent (FTE) DVM spends 15 minutes per hour per day doing non-DVM skills (prepping/reading a U/A, placing a catheter, client education, and so forth), the practice has the potential to lose more than US$350,000 (in revenue) per DVM per year because additional patients could not be seen due to the inefficient workflow process.[9]

Data from a third study looked at the impact of a positive culture, team member engagement, whole team utilization, and leveraging in 3 comparative practices. Each practice had 4 FTE DVMs, whereas the number of team members varied to support the higher utilized team. Practice 1 in **Fig. 4** had the highest culture rating, employee engagement, and client compliance, with the lowest employee turnover, resulting in the highest revenue (and ultimately profitability). When a veterinarian makes an initial recommendation to a client and a CrVT or level 3 VA provides additional clarification and education that supports the initial recommendation, client compliance and satisfaction increase dramatically.[9] Optimal utilization is a team sport. When done well, everyone benefits, including clients and patients.

CLINICS CARE POINTS

- Optimal team utilization helps retain staff members of all roles, including DVMs.
- Culture, trust, and psychological safety are required for successful optimization implementation.
- CrVTs leave the profession (on average) within 7 years of graduation due to lack of utilization and leveraging.

DISCLOSURE

The author has nothing to disclose.

REFERENCES

1. 2022 NAVTA Demographic Study. Available at: https://navta.net/news/navta-survey-reveals-veterinary-technician-pay-and-education-have-increased-but-burnout-debt-are-still-issues-2/. Accessed May 2023.
2. AVMA 2022 State of the Veterinary Profession. American Veterinary Medical Association. Available at: https://www.avma.org/resources-tools/reports-statistics. Accessed August 2022.
3. Salois M, Weathering the Next Storm, VHMA Webinar presented Aug 2022. Available at: www.vhma.org.
4. Welser J, We Must Unite as an Industry. Today's Veterinary Business. June 1, 2022. Available at: https://todaysveterinarybusiness.com/workforce-shortage-innovation-station/. Accessed: October 2022.
5. Prendergast H. Leadership. In: Practice management for the veterinary team. 4th edition. St. Loius, MO: Elsevier; 2023. p. 11–30.
6. Whitfield B, The True Costs of Employee Turnover. Built in. Available at: https://builtin.com/recruiting/cost-of-turnover. Accessed June 2023.
7. Rose R, Smith C. Career choices for veterinary technicians. Denver, CO: AAHA Press; 2013.
8. Fanning J, Shepherd AJ. Contribution of veterinary technicians to veterinary business revenue, 2007. J Am Vet Med Assoc 2010;236(8):846.
9. Data on file with Synergie Consulting; http://www.synergie-llc.com/.

Practice (In)Efficiency in Veterinary Medicine
Moving from Chaos to Control

Peter Weinstein, DVM, MBA

KEYWORDS

- Efficiency • Effectiveness • Teamwork • Profitability • Delegation • Systems
- Processes

KEY POINTS

- The veterinary business model needs to improve its efficiency.
- Improving efficiency means focusing on place, products, people, and processes.
- You can measure improvements in efficiency.
- Profitability and practice enjoyment will increase with improved efficiency.

INTRODUCTION

At the time of this article, the veterinary profession is 3 years into its response to the initial coronavirus disease 2019 (COVID-19) pandemic. In some ways, this period was very revealing for the veterinary profession. At its earliest stages, the companion animal practice delivery model was forced, by the threat of disease and death, to change. The biggest change was from the classic 'over the stainless steel table in a cozy examination room' model to a 'curbside' model. This required using cars as waiting rooms and staff members as 'runners' to bring patients into the hospital *without* their owners—probably the most dramatic update in the veterinary profession in millennia. Among other things, this showed that the veterinary profession can change and it truly revealed how inefficient the veterinary delivery model was and is. As clients had to wait in their cars for hours, hospital staff were overwhelmed with calls and clients, appointment books were overfilled, surgeries were deferred, cases (that previously would have been handled) were referred to specialists, and appointment books were filled for 2 weeks or more, preventing even some of the best clients from being seen.

Over the last few years, the American Veterinary Medical Association (AVMA) Economics Division has focused on the efficiency of the small animal veterinary delivery model and using the variables that they measure, they have determined that there

PAW Consulting, 3972 Barranca Parkway, Suite J-137, Irvine, CA 92606, USA
E-mail address: peterweinsteindvmmba@gmail.com

Vet Clin Small Anim 54 (2024) 337–353
https://doi.org/10.1016/j.cvsm.2023.10.012   **vetsmall.theclinics.com**
0195-5616/24/© 2023 Elsevier Inc. All rights reserved.

are a percentage of highly efficient practices. On the other hand, AVMA's calculations show most practices have efficiency ratings below 50%, meaning that most of the practices have lots of room for improvement.

The AVMA studies indicate an underlying problem of chronic inefficiencies with the delivery of veterinary services. In this case, efficiency is defined as how well resources are used, to differentiate it from productivity (output per unit of input). The studies in 2021 measured efficiency on a scale of 1 (highly efficient) to 0 (highly inefficient). Only 1% received a 1; 34% were 0.3 or less; 59% were 0.4 or less; and 73% were 0.5 or less. The study covering 2017 to 2021 found 60% of practices to have severe inefficiency problems.[1]

According to the AVMA, veterinarians' average productivity decreased by nearly 25% from 2019 to 2020.[2] All of these factors have resulted in veterinary professionals experiencing greater stress and anxiety, which lead to a higher risk of burnout[3]

At the 2022 AVMA Veterinary Business and Economic Forum, Dr. Fred Ouedraogo was quoted as saying, "I am convinced that increased efficiency and value innovation is the key at this point to cope with change."[4]

GETTING STARTED

"Efficiency is doing things right; effectiveness is doing the right things."

"There is nothing so useless as doing efficiently something that should not have been done at all."

—Peter Drucker

Let us start with some definitions of terms that are frequently misinterpreted or misused.

Efficient most often describes what is capable of producing desired results without wasting materials, time, or energy. While the word can be applied to both people and things, it is far more commonly applied to things, such as machines, systems, processes, and organizations. The focus of the word is on how little is wasted or lost while the desired results are produced.[5]

Effective typically describes things—such as policies, treatments, arguments, and techniques—that do what they are intended to do. People can also be described as effective when they accomplish what they set out to accomplish, but the word is far more often applied to things.[5]

Operational Efficiency is the ability of an organization to reduce waste in time, effort, and materials as much as possible, while still producing a high-quality service or product. Financially, operational efficiency can be defined as the ratio between the input required to keep the organization going and the output it provides. Input refers to what is put into a business to operate properly, such as costs, employees, and time while output refers to what is put out or gained, such as rapid development times, quality, revenue, customer acquisition, and customer retention.[6]

Using the term "inefficient" to describe the delivery of companion animal veterinary services reflects on the fact that the current delivery model routinely wastes time, energy, and resources to get to its desired outcome.

A very direct outcome of an inefficient operational model is exhaustion, a feeling of overwork, and burnout. Thus, anything that can be done to improve operational efficiency will relieve these sequelae while concurrently improving profitability.

The optimal goal is to develop a plan to be both effective and efficient. Being efficient is only worthwhile if it leads directly to achieving your purpose. And after you identify what you need to do (effectiveness), you can work on improving your skills to master the ultimate outcome (efficiency). Metaphorically, winning a race (outcome) requires knowing where the finish line is (goal); knowing how to run the race (pacing); and practice to master the skill (training). Do not just be busy. Make sure you are busy with the right things. Efficiency is getting a lot of things done, while effectiveness is choosing and getting the right things done.

Both efficiency and effectiveness are critical for business success, but when should you focus on which, and how do you achieve them?

The next sections will focus on identifying areas to improve efficiency and strategies to achieve goals and identify focus areas to help practices decrease costs and increase revenues through appropriate allocation of resources such as time, space, supplies, and effort.

ISSUES: WHERE IS THE DELIVERY MODEL MOST INEFFICIENT

There are 4 areas that can be readily highlighted. Each of these impacts both profitability and people—2 of the variables that determine long-term success. The 4 areas are

- Place/Physical plant
- Products
- Processes
- People

PLACE

Place refers to the physical location such as the brick-and-mortar building, the car, the truck, or whatever 'unit' houses the veterinary business. As a business, the place is reflected as rent, mortgage, loan, or so forth. To be most effective in using the physical plant, you must optimize every square foot. At any time, you are routinely paying for 100% of the building or vehicle. As a result, if you are not using any portion of the place that portion is being paid for while *not* generating revenue. Thus, it is an expense without a return on your investment.

With 1 doctor, when the doctor is seeing patients in the examination room, there may be no income generated in the treatment area, surgery suite, radiology room, or laboratory area, although they are being paid for as a part of the rent or mortgage. Similarly, when the doctor is in surgery, the examination rooms are not generating income unless there are technicians generating income from technician-based procedures.

Are there components of your practice that are collecting dust instead of printing money? Of course, we do not expect our bathroom to generate revenue, but we do expect our radiology room to. The staff lounge does not directly add to profitability but indirectly helps your team clear their heads for the next onslaught. Optimizing physical plant space means making sure every square foot is generating as much income as possible.

As there are more and more doctors (full-time equivalents [FTEs]) added to a veterinary team, and with effective scheduling, the entire practice can generate income concurrently. Envision, 1 doctor seeing patients in 2 examination rooms; 1 doctor in surgery; 1 doctor handling hospitalized patients, treatment area procedures (dental care), walk-ins, and emergencies; and so forth. It is suggested to always have at least 1 examination room more than doctors seeing patients in the outpatient area.

With effective scheduling, surgery could be started at 800 AM and handled by the surgery doctor. Outpatient consultation could start at 800 AM and be handled by the examination room doctor. And drop offs, hospitalized patients, and dental procedures can start as early as 800 AM as well. This also allows for more effective utilization of time for the doctors because when they are torn in multiple directions, their efficiency and efficacy both decline. It also builds teams that work together more efficiently. Add high density or block scheduling and you can increase client visits by 50% to 100%.[7,8]

Inventory, which we will address, is an inefficient area when you think about space utilization and profitability for pet food; toys, leashes, and other pet accessories; and pharmacy.

Other areas of the physical plant that need to be assessed for efficiency would be boarding and grooming. These areas require significant labor and square footage and do not always have high occupancy and thus might be productive for weeks at a time and then totally nonproductive. However, the staff is still paid. The rent or mortgage on the square footage is still paid.[9]

Space—The Final Frontier

Let us add one more variable to physical space efficiency—*workflow*. Are there ways to optimize the workflows, patient flow, and client flow to maximize outcomes and minimize steps?

As you move about the building, are there extra steps that you must take to get from point A to point B and how often are your navigating those steps? There is a reason that the pharmacy is placed just outside the examination rooms!! On the other hand, how far from the treatment area is your surgery suite? Where are the supplies that you need for a dental prophylaxis relative to where you perform the procedure? Take a walk on the wild side through your kennels and get a feeling for how many steps per day are wasted. 10,000 steps are readily achievable by lunch in many veterinary hospitals. Are there workflow changes that can mollify that number?

Can a practice be built without a 'waiting/reception/lobby' area? Could more examinations room be built to replace chairs? Think about the client going from the car directly into the examination room. No waiting!! Waiting does not generate income and frequently generates ill will. Keep the assembly line moving: car to examination room to car. We did it during COVID; the only difference now is that the client comes along.

Would having a smaller physical plant be more profitable? Would not inventorying food allow for more profit from a larger treatment area or more examination rooms? Would not doing boarding and grooming cut overhead without sacrificing profitability?

Think about the benefits from a simpler physical plant toward efficiency and profitability.

PRODUCTS

In addition to veterinary services, virtually every veterinary practice also uses and sells products. From cotton balls to euthanasia solutions; from antifungal medications to dog or cat food; and from flea and tick preventives to shampoos, there is a huge inventory housed in a veterinary hospital. For any business that sells or uses inventory, turns drive earns. Inventory sitting on a shelf unused is an expense waiting for an income to happen. Of course, some of the products are not resold to clients but are used in the delivery of medical care, for example, catheters, laboratory reagents, paper towels, and cage cleaners, while others are specifically purchased for resale value.

In the world of inventory, there so many moving parts that include people, ordering, inventorying, data entry, counting, packaging, shrinkage (theft), wastage, human error, and so forth. And let us not forget that the physical plant that houses inventory should be included in its cost. This is routinely reflected in the markup and margin at which a product is sold. But what about the product that sits on the shelf? Or a product that is back-ordered? Or even the process of refilling prescription requests? The cost of human capital is rarely considered when it comes to products.

When it comes to food, the physical plant, staff time for inventory, staff time for invoicing, shrinkage, wastage, and so forth are just some of the costs. How much margin do you have to charge to make food profitable? And if you moved food to a home delivery model, how much more efficiencies could there be from a physical plant standpoint as well as a greater use of human capital for higher margin income generation—examination rooms, treatment area, and client service?

The same thoughts on food can be extrapolated to nonfood, nondrug, and over-the-counter (OTC) product sales.

One of the greatest areas of income (and expense and profit) is prescription medications. With increasing competition from online pharmacies that are not affiliated with your veterinary practice, this margin is shrinking. With the increasing numbers of requests from online pharmacies into your practice, this also decreases your staff efficiencies. As noted for food, there are a great number of unaccounted for expenses beyond the hard costs for the prescription medications. Would there be a benefit to having a smaller in-hospital pharmacy and an online pharmacy you control? Could a smaller pharmacy allow you to have another higher margin extra examination room? Would a smaller pharmacy increase staff efficiency and profitability since rather than counting pills and putting labels on bottles your staff can increase the client value proposition?

Inventory is both a boon and a bane and should seriously be assessed for ways to improve how practices can effectively and efficiently provide these offerings to clients. From online pharmacies to practice information management system (PIMS) software and inventory managers to best pricing, there are several ways that must be considered to optimize effective and efficient outcomes for our practice's products.

PROCESSES

"If you don't have time to do it right, when will you have time to do it over"
—John Wooden

In my experience with veterinary practices, the only thing consistent about how we do things is its inconsistency. From answering the phone to putting together surgical packs; from invoicing a client to cleaning a cage; from paying payroll to taking thoracic radiographs; and the list goes on—there is limited consistency in the way services are provided or tasks are performed. With practices ranging in size from 1 or 2 employees to 100s of employees, it is paramount to create the systems and processes that are repeatable, predictable, and perfected to deliver the ultimate desired outcome.

Why are processes so vital to efficiency? By creating a consistent way of doing things that is documented, you are defining the optimal way of doing something. Through trial and error, practice, and repeated practice, you have optimized a process so that anybody can learn it and perform it without error. And by doing it right each time, you do not have to repeat it, say I am sorry, or fix something because it was not right. Processes allow for the entire team to do things the same way consistently. And consistency improves efficiency.

Doing it correctly each time, every time, without fail comes from having systems, processes, and checklists.

System—"A system is a repeated course of action, a way of doing things that brings about a result." Systems produce predictability, sustainability, and consistency. As

Michael Gerber stated in his book *The E-Myth Revisited*, "The best systems allow you to devote your mental capacity to work on your business, such as improving your system's efficiency. Unpredictability is the enemy of profitability."[10]

Process—A business process is an activity or set of activities that accomplish a specific organizational goal. Business processes should have purposeful goals, be as specific as possible, and produce consistent outcomes.[11]

Checklists—Atul Gawande, Checklist Manifesto,[12] is quoted: "Experts need checklists–literally–written guides that walk them through the key steps in any complex procedure. The volume and complexity of knowledge today has exceeded our ability as individuals to properly deliver it to people—consistently, correctly, safely. We train longer, specialize more, use ever-advancing technologies, and still we fail." Gawande suggests that well-honed checklists can be applied to prevent the most uncertain of possible errors. He suggests that checklists provide order.

Only a small amount of what is performed daily should be improvisation. On the other hand, the vast majority of what we do depends on systems, processes, and checklists. It makes complete sense to create structured workflows and processes for the vast majority of what we do repetitively every day to ultimately improve efficiency and consistency. By doing away with disorganization, you will do away with stress.

Think through the steps of the client experience, the patient experience, the hiring experience, and any other system within the practice. Identify and perfect all the touchpoints for these. The scripts, the handoffs, the training, and the standard operating procedures can be delineated in such small detail that anybody can pick up the standard operating procedure and do it.

Do the same for the most common things you do every day. Create your systems, create your processes, create your checklists, and then organize them in operations manuals.

Operations Manuals

The goal of systems, processes, and checklists is not to create robots as much as to create consistency. Documenting your systems and processes in a digital or analog operations manual tells everybody on your team that this is how you do things at your practice until you find a better way. It creates a consistent manner for doing everything that anybody on your team can pick up and, using the defined process, perform.

Additionally, operations manuals become training manuals so that new hires will perform the same way as everybody on the team.

A huge issue seen in veterinary practices is inconsistency in everything from answering the phone and making an appointment to cleaning a cage. This inconsistency leads to mistakes, having to do things twice, and costs the practice both in time and money. It is easy to extrapolate that inconsistency leads to inefficiency.

One of the more common causes for inefficiency is not optimizing the processes that you use to deliver an outcome. The workflows that are associated with a client visit, cat spay, dog thoracic radiograph, cleaning a cage, and virtually everything that we do should have systems and processes to ensure a consistent delivery each time, every time, without fail.

In no way, shape, or form is the author suggesting we dehumanize what we do to the point of being robotic. What the author is suggesting is that if everybody on the team knows how to do something the right way and the best way, you will increase effectiveness and efficiency.

PEOPLE

"You will never get a second chance to make a first impression."
—Will Rogers

The effective and efficient utilization of the veterinary team is a HUGE component of the efficiency and inefficiency measures noted in the AVMA research. The final and probably greatest challenge to move from inefficient to efficient or from chaos to control is to optimize the outcomes of your team. Teamwork makes the dreamwork.

Effective use of people starts with hiring correctly. Then it is a question of orientation, onboarding, and training. The skills, knowledge, and attributes needed to be a successful veterinary hospital employee vary from position to position. The better trained an individual is, the more that they can contribute. The more that an employee can work within their job description, the more effective they are in contributing to the efficiency of the hospital. When employees must work 'below' their job description, efficiency ratings will decrease. When employees can move up within their job description, the more valuable they can become. For example, when a credentialed technician is restraining animals, they are not using their credentials, that is working down. When a credentialed technician is doing a dental prophylaxis, that is within their job description. When a credentialed technician legally (within their state's practice act) induces anesthesia, they are working at the top of their job description and thus allowing a doctor to work within their own job description and not below it.

To improve efficiency, we need to think about hiring for careers by investing in people from day 1. Efficiency goes up with longevity as people learn their roles and determine how they can grow and contribute. Constantly replacing people drops your efficiency level. Look at your staff retention rates and your efficiency ratings concurrently, the longer a team stays together and plays together, the more they can metaphorically think like the other person, finish the other person's sentences, and be prepared for the next task without even being asked.

"Train people well enough so they can leave, treat them well enough so they don't want to."
—Richard Branson

How do we invest in people? Start training them for careers on day one. Investing in training as a long-term return on investment pays off as people get to grow, get more responsibility, and thus contribute more. Training leads to retaining which leads to efficiency. On the other hand, the higher the turnover, the more inefficient you will find yourself as you must continually train new people.

Additionally, consider job descriptions with different growth levels and with higher pay scales as people move up the ladder. Job descriptions are a must for efficiency so that team members know what their expectations are *and* what their opportunities could be. Clearly define what each role entails, provide the resources and training to be successful, and acknowledge that productivity and efficiency can lead to promotions. Job descriptions leave no questions as to what is expected to be completed in a highly efficient business model.

"When a cynic asks, "what if we train people and they leave?" Winning organizations respond: "what if we don't train them and they stay?"
—Peter F Drucker

So, to optimize return on a team member, you combine personality, talent, training, and engagement. The concept is to encourage people to work to the top of their skills and then provide additional training so that they continue to grow and contribute. Working at any level below optimal would be considered inefficient. However, this is commonplace in veterinary practices.

Training

"Failing to prepare is preparing to fail."

—John Wooden

For licensed professionals, veterinarians, and technicians, education does not stop with attaining a degree and a license, but it just begins. Professionals who only operate at the level that they graduate are not working effectively or efficiently in a profession where change is so rapid. For all team members, after onboarding, orientation, and initial training periods, education should be a mandatory aspect of employment. The author might even suggest that employers use goal setting rather than performance reviews to determine the commitment of team members. And to add to that, goals must include further development of skills and talent. Training can be soft skills–based—communication, leadership, compassion. Training can be hard skills–based—next-level dentistry, ultrasound, Microsoft Excel, QuickBooks, PIMS software, nutrition, and so forth.

Training for the entire team should be scheduled, measured, and monitored. Training should be to a level of accomplishment that the individual can be trusted to perform a task or skill. As people are trained and grow, they are pushing peak performance higher and higher and the closer they come to the ideal performer. And the more skills they have, the greater value and the more efficient the practice becomes.

One final thought on training, by growing people's skills and value (responsibility), by acknowledging the growth that they have shown (recognition), and by letting them know how much you appreciate their development (respect), you will help to retain employees. And, as in any successful team, the more people stay together and work together, the tighter the team becomes and the more efficient the team becomes.

Delegation and Team-Based Health Care Delivery

Delegation is one of the weaknesses in many small businesses and veterinary medicine is no different.[13] Veterinarians (and doctors in general) have seen themselves as sole healers. Entrepreneurs have often been 'solopreneurs' doing everything by themselves. Veterinarian entrepreneurs have been experts at doing everything by themselves because of their role models (think James Herriot). It is a proven fact that small business owners that learn to delegate are more successful.[14] Why?

Delegation and associated leveraging are part of delivering health care in a team fashion. It is time to move from a classic doctor-centric business model to a team-based health care delivery model. What is a team-based health care delivery model? It is when each member of the team knows their role, their skills, has the systems and processes, and delivers the vision of the practice at its optimal performance. The model is all about coordinated efforts featuring all team members pulling together. The potential of this model is to improve the coordination, efficiency, effectiveness, and ultimately the value of the service and thus the satisfaction of the team *and* the clients.[15]

One of the best places to improve on efficiency through delegation is the client experience.

The Examination Room Experience

One of the areas of greatest inefficiency in veterinary practice is the examination room experience. For many, the client visit is all doctor driven. From greeting the client in the waiting room to walking the client to the reception desk at the end of the visit, the doctor does everything. This terribly limits how many patients per day a practice can see. In a team-based health care model, the right people with the right training can be leveraged to buy time for the doctor and allow for a much more efficient client and patient experience. And an increase the number of patients can be seen, sometimes from 50% to 100% per day. This is the role of an examination room advocate (ERA).

Examination Room Advocate

This has also been called a room tech, examination room nurse, loader (loading the room), and so forth. The role of this person is to handle all things that are not necessarily doctor dependent during the client visit.

If the examination room experience is driven by the ERA, the doctor can see between 50% and 100% more clients/patients per day.

So, what can the ERA do to help the process be more efficient?

- Call the client the night before or e-mail and get a scripted history
- Have the client text upon arrival
- Greet the client and engage
- New client, review the welcome form (focus: how they found the practice)
- Guide to the examination room
- Review a previously collected history and any updated history (scripted and visit-specific)
- Ask also about any other pets in the household
- Get the pet's weight
- Review wellness parameters
- Perform a temperature, pulse, and respiration
- Grade body condition
- Grade dental status
- Review nutrition/diet
- Collect samples as appropriate
- Enter all of the aforementioned details into the medical record

---

Upon the entry of the doctor, the ERA will.
- Review the aforementioned details
- Remain in the room to help restrain, as needed
- Become a medical record scribe (see the following section)
- Create estimates

Upon departure of the Doctor of Veterinary Medicine (DVM).
- Fill prescriptions
- Get food, shampoos, and so forth
- Review estimates
- Provide educational handouts

- Admit patients for testing, hospitalization, and so forth
- Collect deposits
- Collect payments
- Call the client back with information as appropriate
- Follow-up on test results as appropriate

One client, 1 patient, 1 doctor, 1 ERA, 1 room

With the aforementioned handled by an ERA, the doctor is free to go to the next room and see another patient. And if this is done with 10 minutes of doctor time instead of 30 minutes, think about how many more patients per day a doctor can take care of.[16]

The Scribe

Most veterinarians do not leave their practice late because of emergencies; they leave late because they still have medical records to write up from earlier in the day. In human health care, an examination room scribe was shown to save doctors 2 to 3 hours per day while not impacting the quality of their records *and* while positively enhancing the patient experience.[17]

If the veterinarian can effectively and efficiently use a scribe, the same can be expected. There is some teaching, training, and roleplaying needed, but a doctor can completely change their work dynamic by developing the trust in a staff member and empowering them to be their medical record scribe.

Whether digital or paper medical records are being used, the scribe and the ERA will undeniably improve veterinarian efficiency and thus practice efficiency.

If not a scribe in the room, consider any of the other options using voice recognition or online scribe resources.

Medical records are without a doubt a *huge* source for inefficiency.

Think about the concept of delegation and leveraging and team-based health care in the treatment room, the surgery suite, imaging, and management. What can the team take on and improve efficiency and effectiveness?[18]

TECHNOLOGY

Veterinary medicine is best and most optimally delivered via a team-based health care system where everybody contributes and optimizes the time that they are working doing what they are best at and what is clearly defined within a job description. Any technological advance should not replace people but allow for better utilization of people in the high-touch aspects of the practice.

Technology has been a huge boon to efficiency when you think about computerized medical records, e-mail communications, digital radiographs, in-house laboratory equipment, and short message service (SMS) communication. As much as these have become second nature to practices, there was a learning curve until they were part of the norm. That learning curve hampered efficiencies at times as staff were frequently slowed down to learn and trust the technology.

There is a rapid growth of technological options that when fully integrated can be a huge asset to time saving, cost saving, and income generation and expense control. As practices look to bring on more technology, remember that the onboarding will negatively impact efficiencies at first. It is imperative to look at the outcome as the process can be painful.

Some examples of high-tech options

- Phone call management systems
- Online appointment books
- Online hospital controlled pharmacy
- Online food ordering and delivery
- Online store
- Automated texts or e-mails
- Automated reminder systems
- Two-way SMS from the computer desktop with clients
- Voice recognition software
- Automated social media posting
- Online payment options or app-based payment options
- Artificial intelligence and imaging interpretation (tele-radiology)
- Inventory tools within the PIMS
- Tele-health (See Veterinary Clinics of North America)
- Medical record templates
- Virtual cytology (tele-cytology)
- E-prescribing
- Better utilization and more useful electronic medical record
- Employee scheduling
- Employee internal communications

And others that are being released as this is being written.

Anything that can take a task from a person and automate it *without* compromising the high-touch nature of the profession is worth considering. Understand what problem a technology will solve; which efficiencies it will improve; what the cost benefit ratio is; and, how easy or difficult it is to integrate into your workflows.

To help gauge the aforementioned, let the end users (*your team*) have a voice in choosing the new technologies. Make sure they try them out. Call other practices using them. Time invested up front will hopefully be rewarded with decisions that improve your bottom line of time and money. Investing in the right technology can help boost your productivity, while helping you cut down on unnecessary costs. When implemented correctly, technology can also help your staff up their game, while making their life easier. This in turn may improve employee satisfaction and retention.

More and more technologies are being integrated into the veterinary business workflows. Each of these technologies should be considered if they save time, save money, decrease errors, and improve efficiency by allowing people to be used for their highest skills. And of course, the technology should never, ever substitute for touch-logy.

MEASURE IT TO MONITOR IT

"Don't mistake activity with achievement."

—John Wooden

When it comes to judging your (in)-efficiencies, there are some numbers that you should collect and monitor. The author suggest initially tracking *production* (totals) and then using time-stamped measures, you can measure and track *productivity* (a better measure of efficiency).

Operational Production:	Operational Productivity:
Revenue change year over year • Total practice revenue per FTE doctor • Total medical revenue per FTE doctor • Total practice transactions per FTE doctor • Total medical transactions per FTE doctor • Total practice ATC • Doctor ATC • Active clients per FTE DVM (12 mo) • Active patients per FTE DVM (12 mo) New clients per FTE DVM • New patients per FTE DVM • Transactions per client • Annual revenue per active patient	• Total practice revenue per doctor per hour worked • Total medical revenue per doctor per hour worked • Total practice transactions per FTE doctor per hour worked • Total medical transactions per FTE doctor per hour worked Many numbers you can collect can be converted to productivity numbers by using a time stamp—minutes, hours, day, or other units of time.

Abbreviations: ATC, average transaction charge; DVM, Doctor of Veterinary Medicine; FTE, full-time equivalent.

From your PIMS software:
Revenue by category.
From your accounting software:
Expense by category.
What is your margin/profitability per category?

Categories may include but are not limited to
• Examinations and consultations
• Immunizations
• Professional services
• Laboratory services
• Diagnostic imaging
• Anesthesia
• Surgery
• Dentistry
• Hospitalization
• Pharmacy
• Diets

- OTC sales
- Boarding
- Bathing/grooming
- Discounts

PERSONNEL RATIOS:

- FTE non-vet staff per FTE doctor
- FTE administrative staff per FTE doctor
- FTE credentialed technicians per FTE doctor
- FTE veterinary assistants per FTE doctor
- FTE receptionists per FTE doctor
- FTE kennel staff per FTE doctor
- FTE groomer per FTE doctor
- Revenue per FTE non-veterinarian employee

Consider also converting these into staff hours and doctor hours, for example, Hours of non-vet staff worked per DVM hours worked.

Determine *your optimal* staff to DVM ratio depending upon the services provided and standards of care. Studies do indicate that the most productive doctors have more staff to support them.[19]

Track how your staff are contributing individually by giving each staff member a line item linked to what services they provided:

- Your technician today was
- Your customer service representative today was
- Your groomer today was
- XX and YY took care of your pet while here
- Your prescription was filled by
- Start to link $$ to line items associated with staff to give them a value

---

Physical plant and inventory

- Revenue per examination room
- Revenue per square foot
- Revenue per hour of operation
- Average cost of inventory on hand at any given time
- Know how many square feet are dedicated to each of the earlier mentioned categories
- What is your cost per square foot overall (expenses/square feet)
- What is your cost for your surgery suite per square foot per year; imaging area; pharmacy; and so forth

Anything that you measure on an annual basis can be calculated to a daily basis or a per shift basis. For example, average number of patients seen by FTE per day. By converting to a per shift or per day basis, efficiency can be more readily tracked.

The American Animal Hospital Association (AAHA)/Veterinary Management Groups Chart of Accounts[20] is a useful resource for the categorization of income and expenses. Benchmarks for these may be found in resources such as

- Well-Managed Practice Benchmarks study[21]
- AAHA Financial and Productivity Pulsepoints[22]
- Veterinary Industry Tracker[23]
- AVMA Economic State of the Profession[24]

Even without specific benchmarks, you can create key performance indicator for your practice and monitor change over time, but to quote Peter Drucker, "You can't manage what you don't measure," or Seth Godin, "If you measure it, it will improve."

Calculations For Pharmacy

Work toward improving profit not just gross. There are lots of unaccounted for expenses with inventory management, think of this not all-inclusive list:

Time: to order, inventory, update price in software
People: phone calls, counting pills, printing labels, faxes
Supplies: cotton balls, pill vials
Shrinkage
Expired drugs
Returns
Online competition
Physical space

This is why we have always added a significant margin to our prescription medications. If you have charged $15 in the past and garnered a $7 margin, did that margin consider all the aforementioned. On the other hand, what can you net with your own online pharmacy? And, with competition being what it is, if you net $0 from clients that go to an online behemoth and can have a real net of $1 from 'your' online pharmacy and maintain the relationship, could you increase the effectiveness and efficiency of your pharmacy by having an online option?

SUMMARY

With manpower issues being front and center, improving efficiency and outcomes from those currently in the industry could put off needs at least temporarily while other solutions are developed.

If practices were efficient in their use of their physical plants, there could be an increase in profitability which *might* allow for higher salaries. By sacrificing certain highly people-dependent service areas, there might be a need for fewer people as well. Ask yourself, could you give up boarding and grooming/bathing and still net as much financially with fewer people? Could you convert those areas to higher margin income areas? Could you downsize your physical plant and earn more per square foot with medical services only?

If practices were efficient in their inventory control, there could be an increase in profitability *and* more time for staff to focus on greater income generating areas or even a need for fewer staff do the labor-intensive component of inventory. Can you develop an online pharmacy to compete with others that provides the same *profit* (not revenue!) for the practice and free up people and room for other income-generating opportunities that are medically based?

If practices were efficient by having systems, processes, and checklists, could they do it right the first time and not have to apologize, repeat things, and overall be inconsistent? By performing tasks correctly one time and each time, efficiency escalates, the number of people needed decreases, and profitability soars! Can you build your systems, processes, and checklists so you do things the same way, each time, every time, without fail?

If practices were efficient by using people to the top of their job descriptions, could they leverage people to greater outcomes from a time-savings and income-generating standpoint? The AVMA notes that more efficient practices are more likely to utilize their veterinary technicians'[4] entire skill sets than less efficient practices. By changing the delivery model to a team-based health care model, can we increase the value of our para-professional team in the eyes of the pet owners and in the bottom line of the practice? Can you build an examination room system that leverages an ERA to handle most of the experience thus allowing the doctor to work to the top of *their* job description and thus free up time to see more people, do more procedures, and allow for everybody to get home on time at the end of the day? Using your technicians to their full ability will not only improve efficiency but increase their job satisfaction as well. Give nonmedical tasks such as cleaning examination rooms, scheduling appointments, answering phones, and other office work to nonclinical staff. This frees up your clinical staff to focus on the work they are trained to do.[25,26]

And with all of this, could the feeling of running in quicksand, swimming upstream against the current, or being pulled down into a vortex be replaced with job satisfaction and a happier, healthier workplace? Can burnout and fatigue be replaced with laughter and enjoyment? Improving efficiency has so many subjective and objective benefits that it must be considered an ongoing focus for the veterinary profession.

Things you can do immediately to improve efficiency
1. Train to trust and delegate so you can work to the top of your job description.
2. Develop systems, processes, and checklists to ensure a consistent way of doing everything.
3. Identify low-profit areas in your practice and remove them from your service offering.
4. Add technology in areas such as appointment book scheduling, social media scheduling, client follow-up, texting, online pharmacy, and so forth.
5. Either using a scribe or voice recognition software improves the efficiency of medical recordkeeping.
6. Rethink appointment book scheduling for most effective use of time and space.
7. Add credentialed technicians and practice managers and empower them to work to the top of their job description and skills.

DISCLOSURE

The author has no conflicts to disclose.

REFERENCES

1. Practice inefficiencies compound veterinary stress. Available at: https://www.avma.org/javma-news/2021-12-01/practice-inefficiencies-compound-veterinary-stress, Accessed June 1, 2023.
2. Are we in a veterinary workforce crisis? Available at: https://www.avma.org/javma-news/2021-09-15/are-we-veterinary-workforce-crisis, Accessed May 23, 2023.

3. How veterinarians can manage burnout and support well-being. Available at: https://www.mwiah.com/our-insights/how-veterinarians-can-manage-burnout-and-support-well-being, Accessed June 5, 2023.
4. Study explores secrets of highly efficient veterinary practices Available at: https://www.avma.org/news/study-explores-secrets-highly-efficient-veterinary-practices, Accessed June 5, 2023.
5. https://www.merriam-webster.com Accessed May 15, 2023.
6. Operational Efficiency. Available at: https://www.techtarget.com/searchbusinessanalytics/definition/operational-efficiency, Accessed May 15, 2023.
7. High Density Scheduling = Effective Time Management. Available at: https://www.vin.com/apputil/content/defaultadv1.aspx?id=3844094&pid=11131, Accessed June 10, 2023.
8. Block Scheduling: Understanding the Benefits for Your Practice and Team. Available at: https://www.practicelife.com/en/latest/block-scheduling-understanding-the-benefits-for-your-practice-and-team/, Accessed June 10, 2023.
9. The Business of Boarding. Available at: https://todaysveterinarybusiness.com/animal-boarding-1222/, Accessed June 10, 2023.
10. The E-Myth Revisited- Michael E. Gerber
11. Business Process. Available at: https://www.techtarget.com/searchcio/definition/business-process, Accessed May 15, 2023.
12. The Checklist Manifesto, Atul Gawande
13. Cost Benefits of Delegation for Your Small Business. Available at: https://finance.yahoo.com/news/cost-benefits-delegation-small-business-130014093.html, Accessed June 15, 2023.
14. To Be a Great Leader, You Have to Learn How to Delegate Well. Available at: https://hbr.org/2017/10/to-be-a-great-leader-you-have-to-learn-how-to-delegate-well, Accessed June 15, 2023.
15. Creating Teams and Team-based Care. Available at:https://www.ahrq.gov/ncepcr/tools/transform-qi/create-teams.html, Accessed June 15, 2023.
16. The Outpatient Nurse Technician. Available at:https://www.vin.com/apputil/content/defaultadv1.aspx?pId=11227&catId=31635&id=3862728, Accessed June 5, 2023.
17. Impact of Scribes on Physician Satisfaction, Patient Satisfaction, and Charting Efficiency: A Randomized Controlled Trial. Available at:https://www.ncbi.nlm.nih.gov/pmc/articles/PMC5593725/, Accessed June 5, 2023.
18. Non-DVM staff: Doing more with more. Available at:https://www.ncbi.nlm.nih.gov/pmc/articles/PMC1624915/Accessed June 10, 2023
19. Nonveterinarian staff increase revenue and improve veterinarian productivity in mixed and companion animal veterinary practices in the United States. Available at:https://avmajournals.avma.org/view/journals/javma/260/8/javma.21.11.0482.xml Accessed June 10, 2023.
20. Chart Of Accounts. Available at:https://www.aaha.org/practice-resources/running-your-practice/chart-of-accounts/Accessed June 10, 2023.
21. Well-Managed Practice Benchmarks Study. Available at:https://www.wmpb.vet/ Accessed June 10, 2023.
22. Financial and Productivity Pulsepoints, Tenth Edition. Available at:https://ams.aaha.org/eweb/DynamicPage.aspx?site=store&Action=Add&ObjectKeyFrom=1A83491A-9853-4C87-86A4-F7D95601C2E2&WebCode=ProdDetailAdd&DoNotSave=yes&ParentObject=CentralizedOrderEntry&ParentDataObject=Invoice%20Detail&ivd_formkey=69202792-63d7-4ba2-bf4e-a0da41270555&ivd_cst_key=00000000-0000-0000-0000-000000000000&ivd_cst_ship_key=00000000-000

0-0000-0000-000000000000&ivd_prc_prd_key=DCD2A161-F778-498B-A097-3
D107E993FE2 Accessed June 10, 2023.

23. Monitor veterinary industry trends. Available at:https://vetsource.com/resources/
veterinary-industry-tracker/# Accessed June 10, 2023

24. AVMA 2023 Economic State of the Profession. Available at:https://ebusiness.
avma.org/ProductCatalog/product.aspx?ID=2094 Accessed June 10, 2023.

25. A Recipe for Success. Available at:https://todaysveterinarybusiness.com/
veterinary-technicians-success/Accessed June 10, 2023

26. How empowering veterinary technicians supports practice success Available
at:https://www.avma.org/resources-tools/how-empowering-veterinary-
technicians-supports-practice-success Accessed June 10, 2023.

The Magic of Customer Service in Veterinary Practice

Adam Christman, DVM, MBA*

KEYWORDS

- Practice management • Disney • Customer service • Client service • Culture
- Mission statement • Vision statement

KEY POINTS

- Both Disney and the veterinary profession place a strong emphasis on creating positive experiences they share common principles in delivering exceptional service.
- Your internal customer service is just as crucial as your external customer service for strong culture and quality service.
- The physical setting creates the stage for exceptional client service. If the setting is not right, then client service will fail.
- Creating a strong team allows for better efficiency and increased client satisfaction.

When thinking about client service in veterinary medicine, there are many business models outside of the profession to find synergy and best practices from. Perhaps one of the strongest examples of exceeding client service is the Walt Disney Company (Disney). The Disney customer service model and health care's business model might seem like unrelated concepts at first glance, but on closer examination, there are several valuable connections between the two. Both industries place a strong emphasis on creating positive experiences for their customers and patients, and they share common principles in delivering exceptional service and care.

1. *Customer/Patient Experience*: Both Disney and health care providers strive to create memorable experiences for their customers and patients. In Disney's case, this involves providing outstanding entertainment, exceptional hospitality, and attention to detail in every aspect of their theme parks. Similarly, health care organizations focus on delivering compassionate, patient-centered care that addresses not only medical needs but also emotional and psychological well-being.

dvm360® & Fetch Conferences
* www.dradamchristman.com
E-mail address: docchico@gmail.com

Vet Clin Small Anim 54 (2024) 355–367
https://doi.org/10.1016/j.cvsm.2023.10.009
0195-5616/24/© 2023 Elsevier Inc. All rights reserved.

2. *Personalization*: Disney excels at tailoring experiences to meet individual preferences. Whether it is personalized greetings or customizing vacation packages, they understand the importance of making customers feel special. Health care providers are increasingly adopting a personalized approach as well. With the rise of precision medicine, individualized care is crucial as we will discuss shortly.
3. *Employee Training and Engagement*: Disney's commitment to training its "cast members" is renowned. They invest heavily in equipping their staff with the necessary skills to deliver exceptional service. Similarly, health care organizations are realizing the significance of employee engagement and training in improving patient care. Well-trained and engaged veterinary professionals are more likely to provide better service and foster positive patient experiences. Ultimately, this leads toward greater retention.
4. *Emphasis on Safety*: Disney theme parks prioritize the safety of their visitors through rigorous safety measures and protocols. In health care, safety is also paramount. Veterinary professionals follow strict guidelines and procedures to ensure patient safety, minimize errors, and reduce the risk of injury.
5. *Brand Loyalty and Reputation*: Disney has mastered the art of building strong brand loyalty, with many visitors returning for repeat experiences. Likewise, health care providers aim to cultivate patient loyalty by delivering high-quality care and earning a positive reputation. Satisfied patients are more likely to return for future veterinary needs and recommend your hospital to others.
6. *Guest/Patient Feedback*: Disney actively seeks guest feedback to improve its services continually. In health care, patient feedback is increasingly sought after and valued. Client satisfaction surveys and feedback mechanisms help veterinary leadership identify areas for improvement and enhance the overall patient experience.
7. *Innovation and Technology*: Both industries embrace technological advancements to enhance their services. Disney constantly introduces cutting-edge attractions and experiences, whereas health care leverages technology (virtual care, artificial intelligence [AI], and digital platforms) to improve better workflows for hospitals.
8. *Accessibility and Inclusivity*: Disney endeavors to make its parks accessible and inclusive for all visitors. Similarly, health care organizations are striving to provide equitable access to health care services, address health disparities, and ensure that everyone receives the care they need.

WHAT'S SO "MAGICAL" ABOUT CLIENT SERVICE?

I want you to imagine a time in your life when you experienced or consumed a Disney product. Have you vacationed at any of the theme parks or watched a Disney movie? If you went out and asked people to describe Disney, they would most likely say nostalgia, happiness, expensive, family memories, and/or customer service. When you stop and think about that, it takes people to make, deliver, and execute an incredible product or service to you so that you feel fulfilled, satisfied, and wanting or even yearning to come back and indulge in another product in the Disney portfolio. Walt Disney understood innately that the long-term success of his company depended on his ability to motivate people, one day and one innovation at a time. He understood that the secret behind his theme parks would be the ways and experiences guests feel from the setting and its employees, commonly referred to as "cast members."

What are some words when your team, clients, and you think of your veterinary practice? Are they words that evoke emotion, credibility, and brand loyalty? When asking veterinary professionals around the country, I often hear family, knowledgeable, compassionate, friendly, and expensive. This is a good question to ask your team during a huddle or team meeting.

Where do you think the very first client interaction occurs at your practice? I hope that when a client calls into your clinic, this is the very first client experience they have with your clinic. For this reason, applying these basic Disney principles into the veterinary space is so crucial for client satisfaction.

I remember sharing an interaction with a top management cast member one day when visiting Walt Disney World in Orlando, Florida. We had a profound conversation about our professions, and she leaned into me and said quietly, "You know, Adam. You and I are in competition for the same commodity in this world." I looked at her with disbelief, not knowing what veterinarians could possibly be in competition with Disney for. I replied, "I honestly have no idea what you mean."

"Disposable income. Our guests save up for these magical vacations. Your clients save up for bettering their pets," she explained to me. After she said that, I completely understood, and she was correct. Both of our professions have us under the microscope with people wanting us to exceed their expectations because their perception of the dollar is that of high value than those of other commodities in this world. Let's dive in and look at some concepts on how we can enhance the client experience even further.

THE SETTING
Physical Hospital Structure

One of the many things Disney is known for is their attention to detail. It successfully creates a setting that is warm, inviting, and inclusive that allows greater service to happen. Have you ever walked into a booth at a restaurant where they forgot to clean the table before you sat down? How did that make you feel? Being able to create a healthy work environment both culturally and structurally are crucial for any organization's success.

Did you know that none of the Disney parks have 90° turns? When was the last time you arrived at a sidewalk intersection and made a precise 90° turn? No one does it! Not even our animals. That's why you will notice curves and flowy walk patterns throughout the parks for guests to meander which creates a better flow. Think about what that does for our workflow and client flow? I am sure you have jammed your hip on some corner of an examination table. The future of workflow efficiency has significantly changed the landscape in which we practice medicine today. Hospitals are busier than ever, and we want to make sure we provide a workplace that allows for better client, animal, and employee flow.

For example, some hospitals are now eliminating reception areas as many animals start their fear, anxiety, and stress at that point. We are now realizing that curbside or simply taking the animals from car to examination room may be a better workflow for everyone. Your clients will also have greater piece of mind knowing the safety of their pet is top priority.

Below are some selected components of setting that Disney Parks use to exceed guest's expectations.

- Architectural design
- Color
- Directional design on carpet
- Focal points and directional signs
- Internal/external detail
- Landscaping

- Lighting
- Music/ambient noise
- Signage
- Smell
- Taste
- Texture of floor surface
- Touch/tactile experiences

Do you work in a run-down building? The plumbing is sub-par, and your machines are starting to go. Have any of your clients asked, "What did I just pay $200 for? Certainly not for this building!" Well, it happened to me and the practice I worked at. It was embarrassing. It almost felt like the building we practiced in was a poor reflection of the great medicine we practiced. Sound familiar?

In fact, did you know that veterinary hospitals are shifting to a more concierge style vibe? But simple adjustments go a long way to achieve successful client service. I hope that by now you are providing refreshments to clients. For example, diffusing a neutral odor such as coffee into veterinary clinics is equally important as sights and texture. You should do a walkthrough of your clinic through the eyes of a client and patient. As you walk through, do you feel like you are in a safe, welcoming, and clean environment? As a client, would you feel comfortable bringing your pet here? I hope so but if not, make note of what feels off or wrong to you and work on creating a better space.

The Front and Back Stage

Disney Parks are noted and touted for their legendary terms of performance. Let's face it, it is not so in veterinary medicine. Being in front of the guests is referred to as onstage and anything where there is not a guest interaction is referred to as backstage. Signs are strategically placed that read "Cast Members Only" so that there is a clear differentiation between the front and backstage because no guest wants to hear how Cinderella had a rough weekend. Creating an experience that has consistency where guests can receive the highest level of quality service is important to the Disney Parks and it keeps guests coming back.

Have you ever had a client tell you that they overheard a team member oversharing through the door? This scenario is a very common in our field as the walls are thin and we often have a difficult time differentiating the front stage from the backstage. It is absolutely crucial to have an employee lounge and/or offices where team members can decompress away from clients. However, it is equally paramount to know that all team members are on stage the moment they walk in the door. Every single interaction may be scrutinized by a client or another team member. If team members have had a difficult client, end-of-life case, or any other challenge, it is so crucial to allow team members to be human and have their time to collect their thoughts. A few ideas to help team members cope and work through challenges are to encourage them to go outside, meditate, and talk to management.

THE KEYS FOR SUCC-YASSS!

Disney strives and lives by its four keys of quality standards in the order of most significance.

1. Safety
2. Courtesy
3. Show

4. Efficiency

Think how these standards work into your veterinary practice. Would the order of significance change? Let's find out.

Safety

Policies and procedures are put into place to ensure the safety of both cast members and guests. Training programs, design considerations, and workflow patterns are studied and executed in a way that provides a safe work environment. Think about this for a moment. If you have ever traveled to a Disney Park and rode The Haunted Mansion, there is a likely chance that the ride had slowed down or even come to a halt. This omnimover is consistently moving but occasionally will slow down or come to a stop to accommodate those individuals that may require extra time to board the ride. Is efficiency compromised? Absolutely. Did this affect the show and your experience? Potentially.

Think how safety affects the veterinary practice. Every day we experience situations where safety is a top priority, and this should equally be our number 1 quality standard.

Courtesy

Everyone deserves to be treated as a very important person (VIP) and in new era of customer service, the "I" stands for individualized. Not every family vacation is the same way, and Disney provides many options through their hotels, theme parks, and extra add-ons that truly make a customizable vacation while adding personal touches such as celebrating birthdays, anniversaries, graduations and they are done with a smile on each cast members face.

Think how far our profession has come in terms of individualized patient care. We are talking more than ever on spectrum of care as well because our clients have individual concerns regarding their pets. Not every cat receives the same vaccine protocol and not every dachshund may receive the same recommendations as the golden retriever who was in the room before them. DNA testing, liquid biopsy, pet insurance, vaccine and wellness protocols, feline-friendly hours, and more are just several ways we can provide exceptional service. I will never forget how nice it was to have my name on a billboard themed sign in my orthodontist's office for my first visit. It made me feel welcomed, seen, and I knew I was going to receive the right care that met my needs. This quality standard cannot be emphasized enough; we are in a profession full of compassion, passion, and empathy.

Because the very first interaction with a client typically occurs on the phone, if the clinics voice on the phone does not meet a client with courtesy, respect, and active listening, chances are you lost the client. Courtesy is like an aroma diffuser; it must permeate throughout the entire hospital, and it starts with your team. If the diffuser starts to go stale and not work, then it is time to get a new diffuser.

I have one very simple motto to live by in veterinary medicine: HIRE ATTITUDE. TRAIN APTITUDE! Have you ever walked into a store and had an incredible interaction with an employee and wished they worked for you? Well, you can easily make that wish a reality. Oftentimes, I find fellow veterinary professionals are hiring for experience and overlook candidates that may have had a rocking interview and previous work experience in high touch points of customer service. Do NOT overlook them! I have hired quite a few rock star employees just from interactions at restaurants and malls whom all went on to achieve veterinary success and continue to be customer-centric employees. They can and will be the bedrock to your quality standard of courtesy. As long as you have a great courtesy standard in place that provides training, education, and mentorship, your eagle of an employee will soar.

Show

Cast member appearance, costumes, and standards manuals are all major player for the "show" to commence. They wear visible name tags with the hometown of the cast members, allowing for connection and commonality to occur with guests. In the world of veterinary medicine, think about scrubs, business casual wear, and appearance. We want our "show" to reflect our medicine and quality of care. An unkempt appearance may be perceived by clients as poor attention to patient and pet parent detail.

Now, various hospitals throughout the country have stickers of the employee's languages they can speak with their country of origin. This can help foster an inclusive show because it is crucial for the power of representation to be seen and heard.

Efficiency

Efficiency is defined as the degree to which organizational resources contribute to productivity. In other words, doing things right. Oftentimes, this gets confused with the term effectiveness—the degree to which managers attain organizational objectives. In other words, doing the right things. I like to think of efficiency being an umbrella for three buckets—speed, quality, and cost. By no means is this referring to being a speedy doctor in an effort to turn an examination room over quicker at the expense of sacrificing poor medicine. Think how speed, quality, and cost affect your day-to-day practice.

Now, think of how Disney is successful and not successful in their guest flow patterns. They have realized that waiting in long lines for hours is not the best use of a guest's time while in the parks. So how did they fix this issue? They created virtual queues that provide guests with a window of an estimated time to arrive for their ride. As they wait, guests can walk the parks and make additional purchases on merchandise or food and beverages while still creating a magical experience.

Disney even maximizes its space to its fullest potential through new themed lands which are continuously being added while maintaining a healthy footprint for guest flow patterns.

Efficiency is quality standard that many veterinary practices struggle. Many have adapted and continue to use curbside as a means of better space utilization for the examination rooms because it became a necessity during the pandemic. Some practices reserve curbside appointments for technician visits and recheck appointments, whereas wellness, new client, and sick visits are used in the examination rooms. Efficiency is all about making the best possible use of available resources. Efficient companies maximize outputs from given inputs, thus minimizing their costs. When a company's efficiency improves, its costs are reduced and its competitiveness enhanced, if the focus is also on productivity.

In fact, Disney provides Seven Service Guidelines (tied to the Seven Dwarf of course!) that can easily be implemented into the veterinary sector.

1. Be *Happy*...make eye contact and smile! This is something that I strongly encourage your team to role play with.
2. Be like *Sneezy*...greet and welcome every guest. Spread the spirit of Hospitality...It is contagious!
3. Don't be *Bashful*...seek out guest contact by asking clients questions such as have I answered of all of your questions today or can I provide you or Max with a drink of water?

4. Be like *Doc*…provide immediate service recovery. If a pet vomits in the waiting area, clean it up right away. When you have to call someone else in, it looks like you are not part of the team and the clients will notice this immediately.
5. Don't be *Grumpy*…always, always display appropriate body language. As you know, pets read body language very well.
6. Be like *Sleepy*…create DREAMS and preserve the magical guest experience. How can you find one "mini-magical moment" in the office visit? Maybe taking a picture of the pet for social media?
7. Don't be *Dopey*…thank everyone! Remember they are the ones responsible for our salaries. We need to make sure we provide an environment of mutual trust and respect for our clientele.

Guestology:Clientology

How well do you know your clients? Disney defines "guestology" as the art and science of knowing and understanding customers because this is how the company moves forward. This is also referred to as the customer compass. Guestology puts Disney's service strategies in context because it answers two critical questions: Who are we doing this for and why are we doing it this way? Have you ever completed a data analysis to see what your demographic audience is and then address their needs and wants? Perhaps you realize that you may not need reminders mailed to client homes as they prefer text messages and automated phone call reminders instead. Understanding your customer compass will allow your hospital to achieve better client service.

There are two kinds of information developed through guest research. There's demographic: Factual or quantitative data—physical attributes, such as where guests come from or how much money they spend. Demographic information provides a team data to meet goals and create target points. It can often reveal marketplace insights like who else they can market to, why, and how to best accomplish it. For example, certain schools in the United States have early spring break in February versus March. As a result, Disney will geotarget and market to that demographic knowing that people within these school districts may consider a Disney vacation at that time. Most veterinary practices have a high millennial population with social media competencies. As a result, practices now have social media campaigns dedicated to this segment of pet owners in recommending or marketing a particular initiative or campaign for their pets.

THE CUSTOMER COMPASS

The second kind of guest research information is psychographic. The customer compass, imagine it to be like a directional compass, is a way of Disney understanding the psychology of their guests. This compass is a useful tool in understanding the guest's strengths and reason as to why they attend a Disney theme park. Let's look at this further as we see how crucial this is in our profession of veterinary medicine.

Needs (North) and Wants (West)

Psychographic data are different with the customer compass. This captures the mental and emotional states of guests. What are the guests needs and wants? Guests may need park maps, sunscreen, strollers, and then want souvenirs and cotton candy to help keep the magic going when they leave the park. Their needs tend to be obvious, usually corresponding to the products and services you offer. Consider what the client needs from you, but their wants are less obvious and can suggest a client's deeper purpose. Although needs meet a predetermined service or product need, wants can be defined as the desired outcome. In other words, why do your clients come to see you?

Stereotypes (South)

The preconceived notions, also known as stereotypes, are ones that your clients may have when they do business with you. As you identify client stereotypes, you obtain valuable clues about their expectations. These clues help us fill in the features of the client portrait. I know you have heard clients say all veterinarians are the same or veterinarians are overpriced and just want to take my money. This notion is a common barrier we, as veterinary professionals, face and help paint a portrait of us learning to be incredibly specific and detailed when delivering price, value, and treatment plans.

Emotions (East)

Arguably the most important compass tool for the veterinary profession is connecting with your clients and their pets on an emotional level to help give differentiation. Pet owners have a deep and wide range of emotions when it comes to the decisions for their pets. When striving to understand your clients on a holistic scale, you must recognize and be sensitive to the different emotional levels they are experiencing. That's why emotional intelligence and training with your team is very important. Role playing various situations are crucial for the emotional well-being of your team. Think of the emotion that is invoked when you just hear the word Disney let alone see Cinderella's Castle on Main Street, USA! It is as if nothing else matters and the credit card has no limit.

Having this crucial data helps organizations build better understanding of their clients/guests that enable leadership to make informed decisions about how to enhance the experience and Disney customer service. For example, building a new attraction that does not get used or meet expectation is not just a waste of money; it affects the guests' impression of their trip and could impact future sales. Whatever the organization does always circles back to their common purpose (*create happiness by providing the finest entertainment for people of all ages, everywhere*) and their four compass points.

FROM THE INSIDE OUT

There is a famous phrase: "Employees don't leave their job; they leave their bosses." It certainly holds true in the veterinary profession. We know that we enter this field with compassion, a calling, and an understanding of elevating the human–animal bond. Yet, we sometimes lose our way when the team, culture, or hospital is not aligned with your mission, vision, and values.

Throughout my career as a veterinarian, I had found that most employees want to be involved in something greater than just being paid for a job like staying later to assist with a surgery. They fill in when employees are sick because they truly care about the animals, clients, and team. I wanted the team to feel they are more important than cleaning the kennel, walking the dog, or removing sutures. They are creating healthy pets to live longer and thus create happiness for clients. Let's face it; nothing brings us greater joy in this profession than seeing happy clients with healthy pets and Disney is no different with its customers! They work very hard as a team, collectively around the world, in creating happiness for everyone. This obviously does not happen overnight, but how do they have everyone aligned with the same mission? It is not easy but it starts with words.

Imagine seeing a Disney cast member walk into work unkempt, no name badge, and a dirty uniform. What would their manager do? They would of course rectify the situation right away before the cast member appeared on stage. At Disney.

- They don't have customers—they have Guests.
- They don't have employees—they are hosts, hostesses or cast members.
- They don't wear uniforms—they wear costumes.
- They don't have a crowd—they have an audience.

These words are so crucial for the organization as every task is centered around being on stage. Work is their performance, and nothing gives the cast members greater joy than delivering happiness. I challenge you to start changing your mindset in practice to terminology such as this.

In veterinary medicine.

- We don't have clients—we have pet parents.
- We don't have patients—we have guests.
- We don't wear scrubs—we wear costumes.
- We don't ask for signatures—we ask for an autograph.
- We don't have cranky pet parents—we have disenchanted ones
- We don't have overworked cast members—we have pixie-dust deprived ones

You're probably thinking, "This all fine, but at the end of the day, work is work and it's hard for a team to stay motivated." Well, it is time to chat about our actions.

ACTIONS SPEAK LOUDER THAN WORDS

When Walt Disney researched his competitors before building Disneyland, he found that they were filthy. Nothing was updated, litter was everywhere, and the employees did not take any pride in their work. It was from that day forward he knew that Disneyland, as well as the cast members who worked there, would be a model for cleanliness and motivation. It is known that every single cast member from the CEO down to the first-year intern is responsible for trash in the theme parks. If a wrapper or napkin is on the ground, it is the responsibility of everyone to clean it up because no one is above a dirty work environment at the Disney Parks. This is a true testament of teamwork by constantly reinforcing its core beliefs of creating a good show. Cast members from foods and merchandise assist the operations during peak evenings of fireworks and parades. This makes all cast members feel part of a team with equal recognition and responsibility.

Have you ever walked past a urine or fecal deposit in the reception area? Maybe you were too busy or maybe someone on your team thinks it is above their pay grade. Actions speak volumes especially when it comes to your internal customer service and your team. A general rule veterinary professionals need to adapt from the Disney model is "no one is above any rule when it comes to client service." In other words, cleanliness, courtesy, respect, and teamwork all play a vital role, regardless of the position you are in or how many years you have been at your practice. Your internal customer service is just as crucial as your external customer service. Clients notice when teams are broken, disenchanted, and devalued and there is a good chance that at least one of your employees will leave your practice, hopefully on good terms. Perhaps they are moving, going to veterinary school, or changing a career. Whatever it is, these former employees have quite an influence on the way in which your internal customer service has been established. Here are five questions you should be asking yourself to ensure that your internal customer service is just as strong as your external customer service?

1. Do you treat your employees' pets well and allocate the time you need to work up the cases?
2. Does your team provide nonmonetary motivational recognition to your team daily?
3. Do you recognize, listen, and act on constructive feedback from your team?
4. Do you routinely revisit your hospital's mission and vision to make sure all team members, including the recently onboarded ones, are aligned?
5. What signs and symbols do your hospital have that reflect your culture, mission, and vision?

TEAMWORK DOES MAKE THE DREAM WORK!

Imagine the enormous number of teams that are involved in working just at the Disney Parks alone! There are hundreds of them, and they all serve by one guided principle— creating happiness. Let's chat about the various types of teams that can exist in a hospital as many veterinary hospitals are different. Some are specialty hospitals, mixed animal hospitals, urgent care facilities and clinics.

The terms group and team are not synonymous. A group consists of any number of people who engage with one another, are psychologically aware of one another, and think of themselves as a group. A team is a group whose members influence on another toward the accomplishment of a hospital's objectives. What does your team(s) look like? Believe it or not, there are three types of teams in today's hospitals: problem-solving teams, self-managed teams, and cross-functional teams.

Problem-Solving Teams

Your hospital confronts many problems daily. The typical problem-solving team consists of 5 to 12 employees who discuss ways to improve quality in all phases of the hospital. Perhaps client service is inefficient or maybe doctors are speaking with clients on the phone too long. These kinds of teams help to improve the overall work environment. Instead of a team, some clinics choose a task force or committee where employees work with other teams to reach their goals.

Self-Managed Teams

These teams are also referred to as self-directed teams. These teams plan, organize, control, and influence its own work situation with only minimal intervention and direction from management. These teams take care of common tasks such as.

- Establishing work breaks
- Developing vacation schedules
- Performance evaluations
- Hospital ordering

Larger hospitals will take the team lead from each department and create these self-managed teams. To ensure the success of a self-managed team, the manager or owner should carefully select and properly train its members for success. These teams tend to be popular because today's hospital environment requires such teams to solve complex problems independently. You know that common phrase, "Don't come to me with a problem without a solution?" Self-managed teams work to correct those bottleneck issues.

Cross-Functional Teams

A cross-functional team is a work team composed of people from different functional areas of the hospital. They may or may not be self-managed but has the expertise to coordinate each department's activities within the organization that affect its own work. My hospital had "techceptionists" and it really was a great team of employees that knew each other's roles, responsibilities, and skill sets. Not every team member was a "techceptionist," but those who were truly embraced the mission and values the hospital represented and successfully (and efficiently) performed them well.

NO SUCH THING AS A FREE LUNCH...OR IS THERE?

I will close this article by mentioning the importance of employee autonomy. You or someone you know hired your doctors and support staff because they are knowledgeable, friendly, and trustworthy. Imagine the following scenario on "Peter Pan's Flight." Sarah, a custodial cast member is cleaning around the guests in line when she suddenly hears a little boy have a melt down in tears, having a full-on crying hysteria—enough for other guests to stop and see what is wrong. He accidently dropped his Peter Pan popcorn bucket, spilling the contents of the popcorn. Within nanoseconds, Sarah, the cast member knew exactly what she needed to do. Without question, she rushed to the popcorn kiosk and instantly replaced the bucket turning the boy's tears of sadness into a happy smile and giving his parents some relief. Sarah leaned down to the little boy and said to him "Peter Pan told me you accidently dropped your popcorn, so me and Tinkerbell went back and got you some more!" Mission accomplished. That boy and his family will remember that day long after their stay.

Did you notice that Sarah did not ask her manager if she could receive authorization to provide a complementary popcorn bucket filled with popcorn to the boy? She just sprang into action and did the right thing. Hospitals that undermine its employees trust, morale, creativity, and effectiveness up and down the veterinary leadership chain with restrictive policies are destined to create disenchanted employees. Our profession is FULL of incredibly talented, creative, and innovative employees. It is part of the customer experience to make sure managers and leaders' harness and embrace that creativity. Clinics handing out free stuff is obviously not the answer to every problem, but think about what a complementary chew toy, squeaky toy, or even a selfie can do for your hospital. Think of how nice is it to receive a complementary appetizer at a restaurant? You're obviously going to have a great entrée but knowing the appetizer was free makes you want to do additional business there, right?

Giving your team the autonomy to make individual decisions without repercussions is powerful. "I'll have to ask my supervisor" reflects the terrible state of hospital health and their very disgruntled clients. In other words, from a Disney perspective, allow your team to go off script and then celebrate the positive outcomes it can create. Employees will feel that VIP experience (remember, the "I" stands for individualized) and that will reflect on the patient's VIP experience! I strongly implore you to role-play situations during your staff meetings to better provide leverage and lead way to your employees. The cost of a box of popcorn from Disney is simply pennies to Disney compared with the message it conveyed to its guest and family during that difficult moment. In my eyes, it was pure gold! I encourage you to think about a situation where a client is concerned about pilling her dog. You send the pet parent home with a complementary bag of some pill masking treat. Why? Because actions speak louder than words. This pill story is telling, we really do care about your human–animal bond.

Employee empowerment encompasses your hospital's culture and intentionally keeps them engaged and part of the show. Remaining true to your core values internally will be a strong reflection on how your team provides organizational success, externally. Putting people first over profit will allow a more natural flow of profit. Walt Disney once said, "You can dream, create, design, and build the most wonderful place in the world, but it requires people to make the dream a reality." Magic just does not happen with some fairy princess (though that would be ah-mazing). Magic comes from the people who are bought in to your core values, find alignment in your quality standards, and believe in the culture that provides the best patient care for people and animals. THAT is what I would call magic in a bottle.

In conclusion, the Disney customer service model and health care's business model share common values such as customer/client experience, personalization, employee training, safety, brand loyalty, feedback, innovation, and accessibility. By adopting and adapting these principles from Disney's successful model, you and your fellow veterinary professionals can further improve their services and create a more positive and patient-centric experience for those they serve. Although the two ideologies may appear emotionally different because one focuses on creating happiness and making dreams come true while the other is full of mixed emotions, species differentiation, and of course, health care.

CLINICS CARE POINTS

- Disney strives and lives by its four keys of quality standards in the order of most significance: safety, courtesy, show, and efficiency.
- The client compass refers to needs, wants, stereotypes, and emotions.
- Hire attitude and train for aptitude. Building a strong culture requires a positive attitude with proper training and mentorship along the way.
- There are three types of teams in veterinary medicine: problem-solving teams, self-managed teams, and cross-functional teams.

DISCLOSURE

The author has nothing to disclose.

SUGGESTED READINGS

Certo C, Certo S Trevis. Modern Management: Concepts & Skills. 11th Ed. Prentice Hall; 2009.

Disney Institute (2019). Disney Customer Experience Summit. Available at: https://www.disneyinstitute.com/.

Lee F. If Disney Ran Your Hospital. 9 ½ Things You Would Do Differently. 1st Ed. Second River Healthcare; 2004.

Lipp D. Disney U. How Disney University Develops the World's Most Engaged, Loyal and Customer-Centric Employees. McGraw Hill Education; 2013.

Smith D. The Quotable Walt Disney. Disney Enterprises, Inc./Disney Editions; 2001.

Lee F. If Disney Ran Your Hospital: 9 1/2 Things You Would Do Differently. Second River Healthcare Press; 2005.

Kinni T. Disney's Approach to Quality Service: When You Wish Upon a Star. Disney Editions; 2007.

Bearden WO, Rose RL. Attention to social comparison information: An individual difference factor affecting consumer conformity. Journal of Consumer Research 1990;16(4):461–71.

Schneider B, Bowen DE. The service organization: Human resources management is crucial. Organizational Dynamics 1993;21(4):39–52.

Heskett JL, Jones TO, Loveman GW, Sasser WE, Schlesinger LA. Putting the service-profit chain to work. Harvard Business Review 1994;72(2):164–74.

Parasuraman A, Zeithaml VA, Berry LL. A conceptual model of service quality and its implications for future research. Journal of Marketing 1985;49(4):41–50.

Traditional Marketing Is Not Dead in Veterinary Practice

Robin Brogdon, MA

KEYWORDS

- Traditional marketing • Digital marketing • Target audience • Clients
- Marketing plan • Branding

KEY POINTS

- No marketing, traditional or digital, can succeed without first defining your brand and the promise you make to clients.
- Only then can you create strategies and tactics mostly likely to inspire potential clients to choose your practice and for current clients to remain loyal.
- Delivering an experience that is consistent with your brand will earn the trust needed to gain satisfied clients and team members.

With the proliferation of the Internet and an ever-connected world, it would be easy to assume that traditional marketing has lost favor. In fact, traditional marketing is very much alive and experiencing a resurgence in popularity.

WHAT EXACTLY IS TRADITIONAL MARKETING?

Traditional marketing is any form of marketing that uses offline media to reach an audience. Examples include things like newspaper ads and other print ads, billboards, direct mail advertisements, television, and radio advertisements. Although most of these tactics are not widely used in veterinary medicine, traditional tactics also include participation in a community event, sponsorship of your local shelter or rescue organization, support for the local high school athletics program, or a Q and A column by the practice owner in the community paper. In today's world, we might see traditional marketing as any marketing technique that was used before digital options.

You may be saying to yourself, "why would I consider traditional marketing tactics when I can quickly reach a targeted audience online?" Well, not so fast. Traditional marketing allows a business to reach people in ways not afforded to them by digital. Although digital tactics allow specific targeting, it can only reach people while they are at a device. Whether it is a billboard that sits on the side of a major road, an advertisement in the pages of a widely read newspaper, a booth at a pet expo, or an ad during a favorite TV show, traditional marketing allows people to be reached in places that digital just cannot touch.

BluePrints Veterinary Marketing Group, Huntington Beach, CA, USA
E-mail address: robin@blueprintsvmg.com

Vet Clin Small Anim 54 (2024) 369–379
https://doi.org/10.1016/j.cvsm.2023.10.004
0195-5616/24/© 2023 Elsevier Inc. All rights reserved.

vetsmall.theclinics.com

There are many benefits of traditional marketing as well as some downsides.

1. People simply trust traditional marketing more. A survey by MarketingSherpa[1] showed that the top five most trusted methods of advertising are printed material, television, direct mail, radio, and publicly displayed posters/billboards.
2. Surprisingly, traditional marketing is more well-received than most online marketing. A Hubspot[2] survey found that most of the consumers find online advertising to be bothersome. Many people tune it out or even block online ads.
3. Digital marketing has its issues and is ever-changing. Google and Apple are phasing out third-party cookies in 2023. This means that tracking user behavior and collecting data will get more difficult. As a result, many companies are increasing their traditional marketing budgets to try to make up the difference.

There are also some big downsides to traditional marketing.

1. Measurement is a challenge. We have gotten accustomed to easy access to digital analytics that help us evaluate and manage our marketing campaigns. We can then adjust them based on what the numbers tell us, further improving performance. With traditional marketing, data are much more difficult to collect and are less accurate.
2. It is more expensive. In general, traditional marketing is more expensive. It is easy to understand the cost of a TV spot, but even printed material (think distribution) is not inexpensive.
3. It takes time. Executing a digital campaign can be as fast as a few clicks, whereas traditional avenues take much longer. Producing a print ad, buying media, or simply securing space for placement all take time. Furthermore, anyone can launch a digital campaign, but many traditional channels require knowledge of "how-to" and "who" to work with to create the best product that will appeal to an audience.
4. It seems old school. At a glance, yes, traditional marketing can seem like a bore because digital tactics are viewed to be the more modern approach to marketing. This can diminish any "cool factor" the product or service hopes to attract, simply by the medium used to reach consumers.

Be careful not to overlook the perhaps less obvious benefits of traditional marketing. It allows businesses to reach consumers they might not otherwise be able to, such as less technology savvy individuals. This is important for veterinary practices because baby boomers are widely considered the second largest group of pet owners. Although many seniors are active online, they may also be more comfortable with some of the more traditional and familiar marketing tactics. A fascinating potential upside is that although traditional marketing is typically less targeted than digital marketing, it can unveil unpredictable interest by groups that the product or service is not expected to appeal to. We can learn a lot about how consumers view our offerings simply by listening and watching their behavior, and this can reveal untapped markets. Last, back to upside #1, the physical presence of traditional marketing has a psychological effect establishing credibility. It is obvious to the consumer that time and money have been invested in reaching a specified audience and that creates legitimacy. Conversely, anyone can spam your social media feed with scam ads and unscrupulous "deals." This, alone, makes some people tune them all out.

TRADITIONAL MARKETING IS MAKING A COMEBACK

Although digital marketing has been the rising go-to tactic for over a decade, consumers are causing a bit of a shift in preferences. According to data from the 28th

Edition of The Chief Marketing Officer (CMO) Survey,[3] consumer-facing companies, in particular those who provide a service, will make the greatest leap in traditional marketing spending. So why exactly is traditional marketing on the upswing?

1. Too much digital noise. The more time one spends online, the more they become desensitized to the glut of ads, particularly those that are of no interest to them. Furthermore, many people get frustrated with the bombardment of ads that prevent them from reading an article or having to watch a video first before proceeding to the desired content. Thus, marketers are trying to find more creative ways to cut through the clutter to actually reach and engage their intended audience. Because of this, traditional ads are experiencing increased engagement. According to MarketingSherpa,[4] more than half of consumers often or always watch TV ads and read print ads they receive in the mail from companies they are satisfied with. Furthermore, digital advertising costs are rising, whereas traditional have declined. This encourages marketers to rebalance their advertising portfolio if you will, based on consumer behavior. You may be saying to yourself, I am a veterinary practice owner of a small business and I do not advertise on TV, but you might consider a small cable spot, sponsorship of a community event, a column in a local newspaper (digital and/or print), participation in a charitable organization's newsletter, all forms of traditional marketing. Do not get lost in the digital frenzy and miss an opportunity to creatively appeal to prospective clients in traditional ways too.
2. Trust is a virtue, and traditional marketing is viewed as simply more trustworthy. Another survey by MarketingSherpa[1] found that the top five most trusted advertising formats are traditional including print ads, television, direct mail, and radio to make purchasing decisions. Just look at the growing distrust of social media or brand influencers (One need look no further than the recent Bud Light blowback). A survey commissioned by Emplifi, a UK company, and conducted by Google Surveys[5] in 2022 found that consumers rarely trust the products and services being promoted to them by social media influencers, especially those with more than 1 million followers. This flies in the face of what we are witnessing in the veterinary industry. More and more veterinarians are building personal brands online and subsequently being hired to represent and promote specific companies and their products. Furthermore, influencer marketing budgets are skyrocketing. After all, people relate to people and consumers can more easily be persuaded to make a purchasing decision if someone they like or admire recommends it. The takeaway here is that brands must select influencers who demonstrate authenticity, believability, and are relatable to better convert buyers. Consumers can spot a fake recommendation and respond more positively when they believe the influencer is genuinely enamored with the product.
3. Return on investment (ROI) is getting more difficult to track with digital marketing. This may seem strange, but the digital powerhouses are under pressure to consider user privacy and pull back on data collection. Thus, we continue to see the decline of third-party cookies. Cookies are simply text files set by a website on a user's browser to collect data for better targeting in the future. Things like shopping preferences, buying habits, location, search history, and general interests help create consumer profiles beneficial to the advertiser and make for a more personalized ad experience. Google is phasing out the third-party cookie on Chrome browsers in 2023, and Apple already implemented changes to its iOS14 operating systems so the writing is on the wall. It only makes sense then that some reshuffling of marketing dollars goes back to more traditional methods. Without specific data-driven tools, marketers will need to refine how they reach consumers.

4. Podcasting, the new traditional media. Yes, podcasts are a form of digital media, but they use an on-demand approach, like radio, which is one reason they are quite popular. In fact, more than 100 million listeners tune into podcasts each month resulting in a rapidly growing audience who tend to believe their hosts use the brands they endorse on their shows. According to Edison Research's Super Listeners 2020[6] study, almost half of podcast listeners pay more attention to podcast ads than those of any other format. Because podcast content is specifically sought out by listeners, they have proven to be an effective way to get a company's brand in front of a relevant audience.
5. Leveraging digital media makes traditional marketing more effective. A perfect example of this is the shift back to direct mail because a strategically placed QR code can be an effective call to action. A practice can use a unique tracking code (URL, phone number, landing page) to gather data from interested consumers which provides more opportunities to not only retarget these individuals but also to analyze which marketing approach is performing the best.
6. It is a brand builder. Traditional marketing vehicles are great for generating awareness and establishing the company where it wants to be positioned in the mind of consumers. This is brand building 101 and is the first step every business needs to invest in to capture attention. Then, it can communicate what it is all about and how they can benefit consumers. If done well, the consumer will take the next step in the sales journey to learn more. Other marketing channels are best for conversion or inspiring consumers to act (buy, click, call, form fill, and so forth). These would most likely be digital tactics although not always. Because marketing is both an art and science, traditional marketing will be a perfect fit for some brands, but not all, so do not miss an opportunity to reach your ideal pet parent where they are and via a delivery mechanism that satisfies how they like to absorb media. As an aside, it is a good practice to ask clients how they wish to receive information (phone, fax, email, text) so you can customize communication as much as possible.
7. Concerns about digital analytics. With all the ongoing changes to Google, tracking cookies, and digital advertising platforms, it is no wonder companies are suspect about the ROI they are receiving. This of course makes buyers of digital advertising less than confident that the analytics they are seeing are in fact, true. Because these platforms control both the advertising inventory and the analytics, it can sometimes be seen as though the wolf is protecting the hen house—a clear indication of transparency issues. Because most advertisers are not experts at executing and analyzing marketing campaigns, they often do not know better. This lack of expertise adds to the tentative acceptance of the data and can drive consumers to revert to what is familiar—traditional tactics.

THE BRAND COMES FIRST

Building a sustainable business requires an investment in building a brand. A brand is a psychological, emotional relationship between your business and your clients. Simply put, your brand is your promise to your current and prospective customers. It is your purpose for being in business and the "why" you are doing what you do. It is what you stand for and plays a pivotal role in the culture and personality of the practice. It is instrumental in who you attract (and keep) as team members, and how you are perceived by pet owners and the community at large. Good branding creates an experiential differentiation in the mind of the consumer, even if there truly is no difference. Bad branding creates no differentiation in the mind of the consumer, even when there is a difference. Many think of a brand in terms of a logo, or typeface used in the design of the logo, even the color combinations in these visual elements of the brand. However, a brand is much more than a name, tagline, or logo. This is where marketing and investing in the brand comes in. To fully actualize a brand and communicate its values to an intended audience, it must be strategically brought to life over time. It requires nurturing with intention and an emphasis on building a relationship based on trust, respect, consistency, and authenticity. Time and patience are essential as well as buy-in from the team. Ideally, the business has a brand champion to lead the charge. Typically, this falls to senior leadership, but a brand champion can be anybody at the company and should be a role that many volunteer to embrace. To bring a brand to life, a business needs a strategic marketing plan. Branding is about creating an experience for the customer. It is an intuitive, natural expression of the culture. It is a subconscious, emotional tool, whereas marketing is about the promotion of that experience. It is an intentional, strategic, publicizing of your organization. It is a conscious, intellectual tool.

THE BUILDING OF A STRATEGIC MARKETING PLAN

Deciding which tools to use to market your veterinary practice is very similar to how to approach treating a patient. You begin with an examination, progress to diagnostics, then create a treatment plan, and monitor the outcome. In marketing terms, the examination equates to developing the brand, values, differentiators, attributes, and benefits of the business. Diagnostics in this case refers to identifying the obstacles or challenges the business faces as well as the goals desired to achieve its mission. Once step one and two are complete, you have the information needed to create the strategies and tactics or the treatment/marketing plan. At defined intervals, you can then assess the performance of the marketing efforts, adjust based on the results, and reengage with a refined plan. This is exactly what you would do when caring for a patient. Although it is tempting to want to go right to the treatment plan, skipping the first two steps puts you at a significant disadvantage and greatly lowers your chance of success. Working in a prescribed order is not only more efficient but also much more cost-effective.

There is a concept in marketing referred to as the "Four Ps." The 4 Ps were first formally conceptualized in 1960 by E Jerome McCarthy in the highly influential text, Basic Marketing: A Managerial Approach.[7] It was developed to help businesses succeed at marketing. The four Ps are a marketing mix composed of four key elements.

Product–Price–Place–Promotion

A thriving business typically considers the four Ps when creating marketing plans and strategies to productively market to their target audience. The goal of course is to develop the right product (or service), at the right place, with the right promotion, at the right price, to appeal to a specific group of consumers and meet the objectives of the business. The four Ps have a dynamic relationship with one another with each being equally important to the plan.

1. Product–no surprises here. This is the actual product or service being marketed to a specific audience. The best products fulfill a need in the marketplace. An example would be a low cost, high volume spay/neuter clinic in an underserved area where demographics indicate most pet parents have limited disposable income. As you plan to market your practice, it is essential to consider your target audience and their unique needs. Ask yourself the following questions:
   a. What are you selling?
   b. What does your product or service do? Does it meet an unmet need?

    c. Who is your product or service's target audience, specifically?

    d. How is your product or service different than what others offer?

2. Price—simply put, the cost of a product or service to the consumer. Pricing can and will have a significant impact on the overall success of a product or service. It is important to price your product or service commensurate with the expectations of your desired audience while simultaneously meeting the goals of the business. The chosen price plays a key role in how the brand is perceived. If you are priced on the higher end of the market, you will need to demonstrate value for the additional cost. If, on the other hand, you sell at the lower end of the market, some may simply pass because they are concerned about the quality of care. To determine the right price, you must understand your target pet parent and their willingness to pay for the product or service. Consider:

    a. What do your competitors charge for the same service?

    b. What price range is acceptable to your target audience?

    c. What price would be too high or too low for your target audience?

3. Place—where you set up shop and sell your product or service, as well as your distribution channels to reach the consumer. Choosing the right location to open a practice or buying one for that matter is equally important to what you are selling and for how much. The right location is one where there is an unmet need, the target audience is willing to pay for the product or service, and you can sell it at a price that allows for a healthy profit. Of course, this will be different for every type of veterinary practice model and community. A mobile wellness practice will have to choose the geography that they are able to cover and still operate in the black, whereas a fixed location practice will have other considerations to think about such as what type of visibility does the location have, will prominent signage be allowed, what is the parking situation, and so forth.

4. Promotion—how you market your product or service. With so many ways to get the word out about your product or service, what resonates with your target audience is all that matters. Traditional methods include word-of-mouth, print advertisements, sponsorships, TV, radio, billboard, and the like. Our toolbox of marketing tactics continues to grow with so many ways to connect digitally: Website, social media, digital ads, email marketing, QR codes, and many, many more. The key is to go where your target audience is and with messaging that is relevant and deemed to be beneficial to compel a desired action (call, download, schedule, learn more, and so forth). When it comes to promotion of your product or service, keep in mind:

    a. What is the best time to reach your target audience? Digital ads for an emergency hospital, for instance, are great in the hours after most primary care clinics close.

    b. What marketing channels are most likely to reach your target audience? Where do they spend their time?

    c. What advertising approaches are most persuasive to your target audience? How do they like to consume media?

I have always suggested that there really are "six Ps," with the fifth being People and the sixth, Personality. It is the people that work at your practice that are unique and cannot be replicated. All other factors essentially can be duplicated in some fashion. Likewise, the personality or culture you have created can be your biggest differentiator. Long-tenured employees who know the names and faces of clients for generations can create such loyalty among both staff and pet parents that it pays to invest in a healthy environment built around quality individuals who genuinely enjoy caring for animals and each other.

Marketing = Sales? NOT!

Is not marketing just sales cloaked in a more palatable word? Well, if a product or service can truly benefit someone with a need, I'd say, not. Frankly, if a business can communicate how a product or service can be of value to a consumer, I call that education. The consumer then gets to choose if or when they take advantage of that product or service. In veterinary medicine, we are in the business of educating pet owners on how best to care for their animals. If we believe that we are sharing the best ways to keep Fluffy and Tigger healthy, then we have done part of our job. Developing trust and encouraging acceptance is another thing all together. However, we have got to start with "why" and explain in ways pet parents understand what the consequences of not following our guidance are, or better yet, the potential upside if they do.

Let's talk about the sales funnel or how you acquire clients and put all the pieces together. A sales funnel is essentially the consumer's path to becoming a client. It is a visual (literal or figurative) representation of the steps in the purchasing journey, and it illustrates how consumers move through the steps from first exposure to repeat buyer. The process is known as a funnel because the path narrows as interest grows, such as the shape of a funnel. The top of the funnel is broad, to expose many people to the company. As people express interest and engage with a company's marketing activities, the funnel narrows, indicating growing interest in becoming a potential customer. The goal, of course, is for the prospect to complete a purchase and become a client.

Every business has its own sales funnel, but for the purposes of how we reach pet owners in veterinary medicine (**Fig. 1**).

Stage 1: Awareness

This is when someone first becomes aware of your company, product, or service. They may hear about you or your practice from a friend, drive by and see your sign, see a flyer in a local pet store, visit your website, and see an ad on the Internet. The goal with awareness, apart from the obvious, is to intrigue the consumer enough so that they learn about what you offer, even if they do not have a need just yet. The idea is to help them see that you have a solution to a problem they may not have now but may in the future. If they have a clear understanding of what you offer and

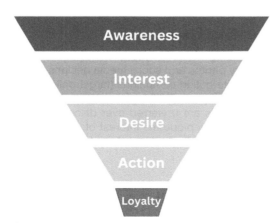

Fig. 1. Five stages of a sales funnel.

how it could potentially help them, they will be more apt to recognize the next exposure as a positive one. If possible, this is an ideal time to provide greater access to your practice via an email sign up, encouragement to follow you on social media, or even visit your website. With the right enticement, you may be able to capture an email address in exchange for helpful health information for their pet. At the same time, this first step in engagement allows the practice to gather information on respondents and analyze who your message is appealing to, furthering your ability to target subsequent ad messages.

Strategies for the awareness stage include.

- Develop a clear brand position or message—think differentiators; mission statement; core values; how you wish to be perceived
- Define your ideal customer with specifics—age, interests, relationship to their pets, and income
- Be very explicit as to what problem your practice or product solves and how choosing you will benefit them

Tactics to consider building awareness of your practice

Website, search engine optimization, Google Ads, social media, paid social media ads, email marketing, videos, affiliate marketing (co-promote your practice with a related business, ie, doggy day care, groomer, and pet friendly hotel), signage, community events.

Stage 2: Interest

After the initial awareness stage, you want to nurture the consumer's interest in your practice and learn about what you offer. Positive exposure to your brand over time helps to build credibility and trust. Consistently reaching out to consumers via social media, offers to subscribe to receive information, and even encouraging a question-and-answer exchange can all lead to an awakening of how you may benefit them. When this stage succeeds, the consumer will typically begin seeking information on how you can help them.

Strategies for the interest stage include.

- Adjustments/refinement to key words and search terms prospects are using when looking online
- Social media posts that drive traffic to your website
- Blog posts that educate, inform, entertain
- Demonstrate "how" you solve problems with success stories and content that addresses your ideal customer's needs

Tactics to consider building interest in your practice:

Use professional quality photos and social media designs that mirror your website and other brand assets, retargeting campaigns (target online ads to those who have already visited your site), quality content (blogs, social media posts), email campaigns, and special offers (value adds are preferred over discounts) and focus on creating quality content that will not only pique the interest of your target audience but more importantly, develop trust. After all, you want them to follow along and take the next step in the journey to client hood.

Stage 3: Desire

This is the stage where the consumer begins to actively seek the solution to their needs within their budget (think value for services). It is necessary to highlight your practice's differentiators here so that your practice stands out. But remember, not every pet owner is an ideal client of your practice so do not be swayed to try to solve everyone's problem. Stay focused on your ideal client and attract those who are most likely to choose and appreciate you. To assist the consumer in this stage of the sales journey, or the middle of the funnel, communicating how you help others through stories, testimonials, and reviews will show your value and allow pet parents to visualize themselves as your client. It is also time for a bit more transparency including pricing, or what goes into the price for a particular service. This is particularly important for those pet parents who may be "shopping" for a particular service where you need to explain why you do what you do and how those steps benefit their pet.

Strategies for the desire stage include.

- Relevant educational materials in exchange for email addresses or to be entered into a contest offering, surveys and polls (do not forget to publish the results)
- How-to videos
- Checklists
- Social media contests with prizes awarded and showcased on multiple platforms

Tactics to consider building desire for your practice:

Create and share educational videos using veterinarians, technicians, and client service representatives. Let potential clients get to know you and see how you approach caring for patients. Use social media and online ads to drive traffic to a landing page where you list the differentiators and benefits your practice offers, without having to name the competition. This will help the pet owner identify and relate to what you provide that is important to them. The competition may also offer it but if they have neglected to point it out, you win. If a member of your team has built a personal brand online, consider leveraging their network with mentions of your practice, use of links and hashtags that all support your brand. The goal with this stage is to persuade the potential client that they not only need quality pet care but also need it from your practice.

Stage 4: Action

This stage moves a potential client to a purchaser, completing the sales journey, but it is not the last step, because you must deliver on the brand promise. In other words, you must provide an experience that is expected based on the messaging that brought the client to you, or better. In essence, meet, or better yet, exceed expectations. To accomplish this, personalize the visit as much as possible, ask questions that elicit information about the client's relationship with their pet, gauge their understanding of general preventive topics, and listen to their concerns. *Strategies* for the action stage include.

- Keep building the relationship through regular communication that includes relevant information for their pet (think feline-specific info for cat owners)
- Express gratitude for choosing your practice and follow-up with a thank you and give the pet owner an opportunity to answer ask questions that might have arisen since the visit
- Stay top-of-mind by encouraging the client to download your practice app, inform them of your pharmacy, provide links to your social media, and offer up a subscription to your newsletter

Tactics to consider compelling action for your practice

Consider offering something special for the new client (a bundle of services, a wellness plan, a new client gift bag, and preferential scheduling for a follow-up visit). Then, survey their experience through a brief, online questionnaire to see how you performed and where there are opportunities for improvement. Show you are listening and you care.

Stage 5: Loyalty

Now that you have landed a new client, you want to do everything you can to keep them. Retention is far less expensive than attracting a new client. Furthermore, if your new client is enjoying your services, they are more likely to spread their positive views by word-of-mouth, leave an online review, and even share your social media platforms for even broader reach. Stage 5 is all about deepening the relationship with your new client.

Strategies for the loyalty stage include.

- Promote your loyalty program
- Engage with the client at regular intervals in their preferred form of communication (email, text, and direct mail)
- Continue the education between the visits and keep sharing all the services you offer. They may come in for one service but not be aware that you also offer boarding, grooming, training, and so forth.

Tactics to consider earning loyalty for your practice

If you have a loyalty program, send regular updates as to their status and how much they need to earn for the next freebie or value add, send a service specific video to lay the groundwork for a new offering (a before and after dental campaign, a rehab survival story, a weight loss success), highlight their pet in your newsletter, and acknowledge any client who refers another client. Last, if, or should I say, when there are any issues, address them quickly and kindly with the goal of listening first, then resolving. You cannot please everyone, but most people simply want to be heard.

INTEGRATING DIGITAL AND TRADITIONAL

The whole point of this article is that before you do any marketing, it is essential to understand who you are as a practice, who you want to serve, and what type of experience you want your clients to have when they interact with you. This then gives you a framework to build an effective marketing plan. Based on the brand positioning you have chosen, you can now develop the necessary strategies to achieve your goals, which will include both traditional and digital. *Hint*: This is where the four P's come in or in this case, six.

A final point: The practices that do this most effectively fully engage their team. After all, your team spends more time with the clients than veterinarians typically and they deliver on your messaging every day. For them to be practice ambassadors, they need to believe in your brand, be enthusiastic communicators of your brand messaging, and then be trained to deliver on your promises. When this is done well, clients are satisfied, team members are fulfilled, and practices thrive.

We are fortunate to have many tools in our marketing toolbox. Although traditional marketing is not dead, it is facing a great deal of competition from the seemingly instant gratification of digital tactics. However, integrating digital and traditional methods has been proven to reap more benefits than a one-dimensional approach. A qualified agency can work with you to define your brand, create compelling designs, identify your ideal client, and implement both traditional and digital campaigns aimed at reaching and motivating an intended segment of the pet-owning population. By setting realistic goals and strategically crafting and executing a marketing plan that is consistently deployed, you can achieve desired ambitions cost-effectively and with a high degree of success.

Finally, everyone wants to know, "what should all this cost"? Of course, the answer is, it depends. Although there are some very rough ballpark figures for how much a practice should spend on marketing, it really depends on your goals. If you are launching a new practice, or introducing a new service, or moving to a new facility, your goals will be different than if you are a mature practice that wants to maintain good contact with your clients in between appointments, have a steady stream of new clients, and put forth an inspiring opportunity to attract new team members. Once you have established clear, specific goals, then you can work backwards and determine the cost to achieve them. In general terms, we see practices spend anywhere from 1% to 8% of revenue or more on marketing, all based on their stage of business and goals. It is also important to classify marketing expenditures appropriately. In fact, you may want to have one line item on your profit and loss statement (P&L) for marketing, or you may want to break it down into traditional marketing, digital marketing, recruitment marketing, and so forth, especially if you are trying to understand the true ROI.

DISCLOSURE

The author has nothing to disclose.

REFERENCES

1. Burstein D, Marketing Chart: Which advertising channels consumers trust most and least when making purchases. Available at: https://www.marketingsherpa.com/article/chart/channels-customers-trust-most-when-purchasing.
2. An M, Why People Block Ads (And What It Means for Marketers and Advertisers). Available at: https://blog.hubspot.com/marketing/why-people-block-ads-and-what-it-means-for-marketers-and-advertisers.
3. The CMO Survey. Available at: https://cmosurvey.org/results/.
4. Burstein D, Marketing Charts: Why the value chain matters to the marketer. Available at: https://www.marketingsherpa.com/article/chart/customer-channel-preferences.
5. Social media influencers come under fire amidst widespread distrust. Available at: https://whatsnewinpublishing.com/social-media-influencers-come-under-fire-amidst-widespread-distrust/.
6. SuperListeners 2020. Available at: https://www.edisonresearch.com/wp-content/uploads/2020/12/Super-Listeners-2020.pdf.
7. Basic Marketing: A Managerial approach. Available at: https://babel.hathitrust.org/cgi/pt?id=inu.30000041584743&view=1up&seq=1.

Social Media and Digital Marketing for Veterinary Practices

Caitlin DeWilde, DVM

KEYWORDS

- Digital marketing • Veterinary medicine • Veterinary marketing
- Veterinary social media • Veterinary reputation

KEY POINTS

- Understand the fundamentals of digital marketing in veterinary medicine to enhance your practice's online presence.
- Develop a strategic multimodal marketing strategy by identifying your purpose and target audience.
- Decide which of the social media platforms are right for your practice, while leveraging email marketing, texting, online review platforms, Web sites, and search engine optimization.
- Learn how to create compelling content that converts and track relevant metrics to measure the success of your digital marketing efforts.

INTRODUCTION

In today's rapidly evolving veterinary landscape, success is no longer solely dependent on exemplary bedside manner and medical expertise. Veterinary practices need a solid online presence and strategic digital outreach to connect with pet owners, foster trust, build loyalty, and provide accurate pet health information that supersedes the flood of misleading online sources. Our professional commitment to leverage scientific knowledge for the benefit of society now extends beyond the confines of the examination room to the vast online arena.

To achieve these objectives, veterinary practices must embrace the power of digital marketing across multiple platforms and avenues to amplify their visibility, demonstrate expertise, and showcase their value. It is imperative to harness emerging technologies to connect with pet owners on their preferred platforms and within social communities. As technology and platforms continually evolve and expand, so do the opportunities for practices to establish enduring bonds and achieve business success.

Veterinary practices now have a wide array of marketing avenues at their disposal, ranging from traditional approaches like Web site and email marketing to social media

The Social DVM, LLC, 2200 South Vandeventer Avenue, St Louis, MO 63110, USA
E-mail address: cdewilde@thesocialdvm.com

Vet Clin Small Anim 54 (2024) 381–394
https://doi.org/10.1016/j.cvsm.2023.10.006
0195-5616/24/© 2023 Elsevier Inc. All rights reserved.

vetsmall.theclinics.com

platforms. With the advent of text messaging, custom practice apps, and beyond, practices have access to novel opportunities for engagement. Although there may be associated costs in terms of staff time and advertising expenditure, the unprecedented advantage lies in the ability to precisely target the ideal customer (existing or potential) at a relatively low cost. Today's social media and Web advertisements can effectively reach a specific audience for as little as a few dollars per day with no minimum spending required. Such campaigns yield instant results that can be analyzed and adjusted in real-time, providing unparalleled nimbleness and potential for success when coupled with the right messaging and imagery.

Over the past decade, pet owners have increasingly viewed a veterinarian's ability to effectively market their practice and leverage digital opportunities as a marker of trust and success. The significance of the Internet in seeking pet health information has also been firmly established.

The 2011 and 2014 Bayer Veterinary Care Usage studies showed, respectively, 39%[1] and 48%[2] of pet owner reliance on the Internet as the first option when a pet is sick, whereas more recent studies have data that suggest a reliance as high as 78%.[3]

Today, pet owners continue to rely on various online resources, including blogs, social media, Web sites, and online communities, either before consulting a veterinarian or alongside seeking veterinary advice. Encouragingly, recent research indicates that pet owners viewed their veterinarians as their most trusted source of pet health information[4] (but also prefer supplemental online information access).

The veterinary industry demonstrated the significance of online advertising and marketing in the wake of the 2009 recession. The 2011 Veterinary Care Usage study[5] identified just 4 key attributes for practices that had increased patient visits during the preceding 2 years, and the following 2 were related to marketing:

1. Active use of social media, such as Facebook
2. A belief that marketing and advertising were important to practice success

Nearly a decade later, adoption of social media and digital tools is still increasing, and a recent survey[6] found the following practice benefits:

- Increased communication with clients: 35%
- Positive client feedback: 23%
- Stronger client bonding: 16%
- New client acquisition: 7%
- Improved compliance: 7%
- Increased patient visits: 3%
- Boosted revenue: 2%
- Positive staff feedback: 2%

Another recent economic survey[7] of several successful practices demonstrated that they were continuing to expand social media and digital tools (**Fig. 1**).

By embracing social media and digital marketing, veterinary practices can seize opportunities to connect, engage, and thrive in the digital age. This article aims to provide valuable insights, practical guidance, and evidence-based strategies to assist veterinarians in effectively using social media and digital marketing tools for the growth and prosperity of their practices.

WHAT IS DIGITAL MARKETING: BEYOND SOCIAL MEDIA

It is not just about posting cute pictures on the practice's Instagram page or sharing a helpful article on its Facebook page. Digital marketing involves every representation

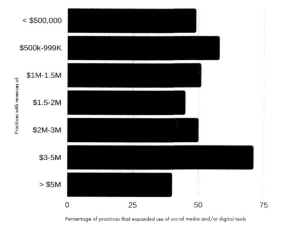

Fig. 1. Percentage of veterinary practices that expanded with digital or social tools versus their revenue. (*Data* sourced from the article "Decision Data: Adding digital tools, social media?" (https://www.dvm360.com/view/decision-data-adding-digital-tools-social-media))

and communication that is sent or received by a practice using an electronic medium. A practice's Web site, online review platforms, email communications, texting service, paid digital ads, podcast, practice app, and even digital reminders all combine to create a multimodal digital marketing presence.

However, the availability of multiple avenues does not mandate that a practice must use each one of them.

Just as practitioners weave medications, therapies, nutrition, and environmental changes together to help patients, veterinary teams need to collectively look at the social media, Web site, email, digital communication, and advertising their clinics are using. Used in concert and with a cohesive plan for creating and measuring their success, practices can better market themselves to new clients and build strong bonds with existing clientele.

DEVELOPING A MULTIMODAL MARKETING STRATEGY

When it comes to digital marketing, managing and excelling on multiple platforms and marketing messaging can be a daunting task, especially for short-staffed practices. Adopt a progress over perfection mindset and make the most of the practice's social media with these tips.

Know Your "Why"

One of the best strategies to use when narrowing a practice's marketing focus is to simply ask: "Why?" Why is the practice marketing at all? What is the practice hoping to accomplish? If the answer is not clear, then it is time to invest some serious thought and energy into defining your objective. For some practices, their "why" might be to increase new clients or booked appointments. For others, it is to improve existing client loyalty or to earn more 5-star reviews. When the "why" is clearly defined, it becomes much easier to think about what content will help the practice achieve that goal.

Know Your "Who"

When it comes to the pay-to-play environment of social media, it is important to have a clear idea of WHO a practice's clients are so that advertising dollars are not wasted marketing to people who are not or are unlikely to become clients. More importantly, it is important to market to the RIGHT clients whenever possible. Knowing their names, emails, or even general demographic information can help social media content get seen by more of the clients a practice is hoping to market to. Furthermore, knowing the ideal "who" can help refine the types of content the practice uses—and what platforms to invest more time and energy into.

Practices Do Not Have to Be Everywhere...Quality > Quantity

As the number of platforms increases, practitioners may feel tempted to attempt posting content on every new platform and maintain a strong presence across all of them. However, it should be acknowledged that most successfully marketed practices use a multimodal platform strategy rather than an all-encompassing approach.

Practitioners are advised to select the platforms that their clients and team members have identified as significant (conducting a survey can be helpful in this regard) and concentrate on developing a robust content strategy specifically for those platforms. In case there are concerns about potentially missing out on the next prominent platform, practitioners can create an account on it but clarify in their bio or pinned post where followers can access more up-to-date content.

Get Hyperlocal

Even the most viral #puppiesofinstagram post is unlikely to generate additional clients or bring a practice closer to their marketing goal. It is crucial to focus on what matters to the clients and the community served. Use community-specific hashtags, share photographs showcasing involvement in the local area, share content from other nearby businesses, and take pride in the community. Such content will strongly resonate with followers and clientele, ultimately fostering loyalty and enhancing overall satisfaction.

Listen and Engage

Last, but not least, it is important for veterinary teams to listen to what their followers are saying online—in comments, messages, and reviews. This crucial step and opportunity to engage in conversation with clients, whom they usually only see once or twice a year, are often overlooked by many practices. Although negative reviews can sometimes be frustrating, most reviews tend to be positive. Showing gratitude and responding to these reviews can further strengthen the relationship between the practice and the client. In addition, sharing positive reviews can serve as a way to express appreciation to the teams involved. Practices should make a regular effort to check mentions, tags, messages, and reviews. It is essential to recognize and acknowledge those who act as online ambassadors for the practice. Responding to reviews and messages, as well as expressing gratitude to those recognized as "Top Fans" in the Facebook Page's community section, helps in building relationships. Listening and actively engaging with social media content can provide valuable feedback and insights from clients, benefiting the practice.

MARKETING PLATFORMS
Social Media

Social media present the ultimate opportunity for veterinarians to literally and figuratively engage with their clientele on a daily basis, instead of the once or twice yearly in-person visits. In addition to sharing social media–friendly pet articles and photographs, practices have the opportunity to share trusted resources, client education materials, and more personalized content that differentiate the practice from its competition and allow clients to become more bonded to the staff of the practice. In addition, based on the practice's staff resources and online offerings, social media can present yet another opportunity for online booking, online pharmacy and refill requests, highly targeted yet low expense advertising, and online messaging (**Fig. 2**).

Facebook
Facebook is the most commonly used social media platform, both for general users and for the veterinary industry. Boasting 3 billion daily active users,[8] the platform is used by more than 80% of veterinary practices.[9] Photographs, videos, stories, and Web links can be shared easily, and Facebook offers specific business page features, including call-to-action buttons, targeted advertising, reviews and recommendations, user insights, and client messaging.

Instagram
Instagram is rapidly growing among users in the general population and in the veterinary community. There are more than 2 billion users[10] sharing photographs and videos via traditional posts, quick Instagram "stories" that are visible for just 24 hours, or long-form video reels. Ninety percent of the platform's users follow business pages,[11] so despite a more "informal" vibe, businesses and brands have significant opportunities to connect with their clients.

Instagram also presents a unique opportunity for the practice's business profile to connect directly with and tag an individual account—particularly pet accounts (manned by an estimated 25% of adults who have set up an account for their pet[12]).

Veterinary practices can take advantage of specific business account features, including call-to-action buttons, targeted advertising, user insights, scheduling posts, and client messaging. Instagram and Facebook tools, content, and management can be accessed together in Meta Business Suite.

Other social media platforms
Based on client and team demographics, marketing goals, and content availability, veterinary practices may also use other social media platforms like LinkedIn (Company Pages), TikTok, Snapchat, Pinterest, and Twitter. However, there are currently limited data to support their successful widespread usage within the industry and/or conversion to new veterinary business or increased marketing hires (two of anecdotally used

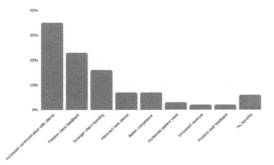

Fig. 2. Distribution of practices' primary reasons for expanding the use of digital tools and/ or social media in veterinary practices. X axis, primary reasons for expansion of digital tool usage; Y axis, percentage of respondents. (*Data* sourced from the article "Decision Data: Adding digital tools, social media?" (https://www.dvm360.com/view/decision-data-adding-digital-tools-social-media))

practice motivations for using these tools). Practices interested in using these platforms would be best served to survey their clients and teams to assess if these platforms would be effective given their practice's specifics.

General Social Media Best Practices: Hashtags and Tagging

Hashtags

Hashtags, classified by the "#" symbol, are words used by users on Instagram (and other social media platforms) to classify their data. This type of tagging allows users to easily search for content relevant to a specific word. For instance, a user posting a photograph of this journal may consider tagging the photograph with #veterinary-textbook, #veterinary, or #vetmed. Hashtags give content the benefit of being discoverable by not only followers but also people searching for content on a specific topic, like #vetmed. This way, practice accounts can reach new followers because many Instagram users *follow hashtags* just as they would accounts.

Instagram allows up to 30 hashtags in a post, either within the caption or as a comment. Recommendations vary on the number a user should use without appearing overly spammy, but on average, 10 hashtags has been a popular number.

Tagging

Tagging identifies someone else in a photograph or video, either by clicking "tag people" when a post is made or by typing the "@" symbol before their username in the posted caption. Tagging the user means that they will receive a notification that they have been tagged, and depending on their profile's settings, it may also appear in their "tagged photos" section. Unlike Facebook, Instagram will allow a business account to tag an individual in a photograph or video. As the number of pet Instagram accounts grows, you may be able to tag your patients in photographs you share of them!

Email Marketing

Email marketing can encompass mass email messaging sent from the practice (eg, client newsletters), emailed care reminders, and individual back-and-forth emailing with the practice's client service team.

Email may present additional, yet still affordable, methods of client engagement when a less-immediate approach is preferred, including the following:

- Appointment reminders and confirmations
- Postvisit surveys and online review links
- Promotion of new services and product
- Sharing relevant health topic information, -for example, emailing owners a specific list of resources on a particular disease topic

One recent study found that 98% of pet owners would like to receive pet health information via email from their veterinarian.[13] That same study also found that 94% of pet owners have, or would, open an email their veterinarian sent them and that 41% of pet owners have never received an email from their veterinarian.[14]

Answering client emails can also help create a dialogue preferred by many pet owners, as nearly 24% of millennial pet owners currently email questions to veterinary practices.[15]

Texting

Texting clients can be an economical and efficient way to engage with clients. Texting is widely adopted by today's population with some studies showing use as high as

97% of Americans. In addition, text messages are often read and responded to within 3 minutes, compared with 90 minutes for an email messaging.[16]

Among younger veterinary clients, texting is a preferred medium for contact. More than half of a large pet owner survey found that clients prefer to receive appointment reminders via text,[17] whereas younger clients preferred texts even more for a variety of reasons, including appointment reminders (86%), checkup reminders (58%), and refill reminders (48%).[18]

Furthermore, nearly 40% of pet owners said they preferred their veterinary clinic to update them on their hospitalized pet via text instead of phone.[19] Although perhaps best suited as a customer service avenue, texting with pet owners can present marketing opportunities as well. For instance, if a pet owner texts a question, the practice can respond with an answer, plus the link to book an appointment or visit a specific page on the Web site for more information.

Veterinary practices can use texting for a variety of client interactions, including the following:

- Appointment reminders and confirmations
- Hospitalized patient updates
- Boarding patient updates and photographs
- Dosing/medication reminders
- Routine diagnostic test results
- Health alerts/area outbreaks
- Emergency practice closings

Note that use as a client-initiated customer support channel is different from mass promotional texting, which requires clients to opt-in to remain in compliance with the Federal Communications Commission. This strategy, too, can be effective, but practices must first

- Obtain consent or opt-in from the customer
- Keep a record of all communication
- Give customers an option to opt-out (eg, "STOP") of text messages
- Only text during business hours

However, if clients do opt in, this is a chance for practices to market just as they would with any other channel—offering discounts, specials, lead magnets, and digital resources, and, of course, call to action to book an appointment.

Online Review Platforms

Although online review platforms like Google and Yelp collect online reviews, they also create a highly visual and easily accessible representation of a practice—complete with clickable practice contact information, hours, and call-to-action buttons (like Book Now and Send a Message). Bolstered by photographs from the practice and clients alike, online reviews, and connection to social media channels, online review platforms are an essential part of a veterinary marketing strategy.

An estimated 90% of consumers read reviews for small businesses.[20] They not only bolster the credibility of a practice and foster trust among clients but also serve as a catalyst for attracting new clients. Furthermore, these reviews provide invaluable feedback, offering insights into the aspects of our services that resonate with pet owners.

Online reviews are typically cultivated in 4 platforms: Facebook, Google Business, Yelp, and Nextdoor. Even without active participation, profiles for a practice may be created and populated with client reviews and information sourced from various online channels. Failure to claim these profiles relinquishes a practice's control over how their practice is perceived. Teams lose the ability to respond to reviews and remain unaware of their existence unless diligently monitoring review sites on a daily basis.

Practices are best served by claiming the business owner account for each platform, populating it with the correct and most up-to-date information, and adding photographs that paint the practice in a positive light: heartwarming photographs of team members caring for clients, highlights of services and the practice's behind-the-scenes facilities that will help set it apart from the competition.

Review numbers (both score and amount) are trending upward for veterinary practices, with an average Google rating of 4.6, Facebook rating of 4.7, and Yelp rating of 4 of 5 stars.[21] Most practices have adopted Google Business and Facebook, but a lesser number have claimed their Yelp account (which integrates with Apple devices on search and maps) and Nextdoor listing.

Once established, online review platforms need little maintenance. Practices can respond to good and bad reviews as needed and update only when something changes at the practice (such as hours, contact information, new photographs, and so forth).

Based on the platform, additional marketing capabilities may be available. For instance, Google Business and Yelp provide (optional) messaging functionalities that facilitate more direct engagement with clients. Nextdoor and Yelp offer targeted ads. Most of the platforms will allow reviews to be shared directly onto Facebook pages, and Google offers a custom social media graphic creation and videos using content from a practice's reviews with its marketing kit tools. Finally, both Nextdoor and Google offer the ability to share social media-esque posts onto platform feeds, increasing client engagement and driving business with call-to-action buttons.

Web Sites and Search Engine Optimization

Many practices have an existing Web site but may not be using it to its fullest potential. A practice Web site is an essential online representation of the business. At minimum, having a Web site gives pet owners information about the practice and allows them to communicate with the business. A Web site also serves as a source of "social proof" and credibility. Nearly 70% of consumers expect a business to have a Web site, even if they are a small business.[22] Practice Web sites can range from simple to robust, offering everything from basic information to full-service sites featuring pet owner portals, telemedicine, and online stores.

In addition to the need for basic information about the practice, practice Web sites can meet many other needs for both potential and existing clients alike. Practices have the ability to use their site not only to educate pet owners but also to provide access to key convenience offerings (pet portals, online pharmacies, ship-to-home food delivery), differentiate themselves from the competition, highlight the practice's personality, link to social media and online review sites, and facilitate appointments with online bookings.

Search engine optimization (SEO) relates to how well the practice's Web site performs in search engine rankings and how well it can match the search queries typed by clients. A higher search engine ranking means the practice will be found more readily, and in some cases, deemed more credible by appearing earlier in the search results. Mastering SEO could be an entire textbook in and of itself, written by a dedicated SEO specialist and Webmaster. However, some basic tips follow:

- Use keywords when appropriate: include topics, services, and the community(ies) the practice serves.
- Ensure the Web site is mobile-friendly and loads quickly.

- Claim and fully complete the Google Business Page for the practice and work on eliciting positive reviews. This will help link your Web site to Google's local search results.
- Regularly add new content to the site like blogs, using solid titles and descriptions.
- Ensure the practice is using *Google Analytics* and *Google Search Console* (formerly Webmaster Tools) to stay up-to-date with the latest from Google.
- Consider working with a *certified Google Partner* to regularly analyze and update the practice's Web site and keywords.

PAID DIGITAL ADVERTISING

Digital advertising can be one of the most effective and affordable methods of reaching clientele, particularly via Google, Facebook, and Instagram. Never before in the history of marketing could mere cents be spent to reach a highly targeted demographic–down to the age, education level, and home ownership status and within a particular mileage of an exact destination. In today's competitive and increasingly digital environment, veterinary practices need to use some degree of paid advertising in order to be found by new clientele and to build engagement and loyalty with existing clientele alike. Multiple opportunities for paid digital advertising exist within online search engine platforms, social media channels, and review sites.

Unfortunately, significant information and data on paid digital advertising in the veterinary industry are scarce. According to the 9th edition of the *AAHA Financial and Productivity Pulsepoints*,[23] practices spent an average of 1.4% of total income on advertising. However, American Animal Hospital Association's own definitions of advertising and promotion expenses include ads, newsletters, brochures, direct mail and promotional items, but do not include Web site or social media expenses. The equation used in the 9th edition of the *AAHA Financial and Productivity Pulsepoints* is advertising and promotion expenses/total income = % of advertising budget.

Similarly, the 2019 edition of the Well Managed Practices Benchmark Study[24(p75)] found practices spent 0.5% of fixed expenses on advertising and promotion. Anecdotally, practices spend anywhere from 0.8% to 3% of total revenue on advertising, but this large definition makes it hard to determine a benchmark specifically for digital advertising.

That said, although benchmarks are helpful, the reality is that each practice's budget is different, based on their needs, objectives, and cash flow. New practices or practices in highly competitive areas may need to spend closer to 3% of their revenue on advertising, whereas established practices or low-competition areas may enjoy a lower-cost advertising budget. Whatever the budget is, it should be paired with a marketing strategy and an effort to assess return on investment (ROI), to ensure whatever is spent is spent well.

CONTENT

More than 70% of veterinary clients report using the Internet to search for pet health information,[25] but 41% of veterinary practices provide no educational resources online.[26] Similarly, this need echoes the findings of the Bayer Veterinary Care Usage Study, in which 65% of cat owners reported that their veterinary team could provide better educational material to help them understand their pet's health needs.[27]

Social media and all marketing channels present an opportunity for veterinarians to provide educational content in a medium where pet owners are already spending a large amount of their time. Veterinary practices can present educational information via links, photographs, infographics, or, for the highest engagement, video. In addition to educational material, practices can create marketing content that promotes the practice, drives business and revenue, and creates bonds with clientele.

Traditional social media marketing best practices recommend following a rule of thirds when it comes to diversifying content: one-third shared content, one-third promotional content, and one-third personalized content. The latter may be even more important in the veterinary industry, where connection with the veterinary team and facility can reassure pet owners, create stronger bonds, and differentiate the practice from local competition.

Similarly, content should be varied in type: photographs, videos, graphics, blogs, articles, and so forth. Practices can create their own photograph and graphic content for social platforms using graphic creation tools like Canva or Adobe Illustrator; write blogs for Web site, email, and social content; and share media created by veterinary industry groups, clinical associations, and product manufacturers.

Video content gives your clientele a look at the "real people" behind the medicine and patient care at your practice—something no one else can replicate. Every social media platform's algorithm gives preferential treatment to video content. Better yet, memory and understanding are increased, with viewers retaining 95% of a message after watching it through video, as opposed to just 10% when reading the same message in text form.[28]

In veterinary practice, creating video gives team members the chance to share interesting, engaging content with clients and lets them get to know the team and facility. In addition to creating another digital touchpoint form of educational content, video also presents a content medium that can easily be repurposed and reused. For instance, when a video is recorded, the file can be submitted for transcription, creating a text file that can be repurposed into a blog post.

TRACKING THE METRICS THAT MATTER

When it comes to tracking marketing ROI, veterinary teams should gather data both online and within their practice. The abundance of data provided by digital advertising platforms and practice management systems can be overwhelming, with pages of information being exported for a single boosted Facebook post; for example, to navigate this sea of data, it is important to keep the marketing objective in mind and use it as a guide to narrow down the relevant data points.

Although online marketing tools like Facebook Ads Manager or Google Analytics offer valuable insights, it is essential to correlate these data points with the ones that are specifically relevant to the practice. For instance, if the goal of a particular Facebook campaign is to increase appointment bookings, the Facebook ad may show metrics, such as a cost of $0.89 per click, 72 clicks, 500 post reach, and 36 reactions. By incorporating Google Analytics, the landing page associated with the Facebook ad may show 72 appointment booking page visits, and/or 15 booking conversions. However, the ultimate measure that truly matters is the number of people who actually booked and showed up for the appointment. Practices can gather more helpful information by asking clients to mention a specific ad, use a particular code at booking, or click on a designated tracking link.

Regardless of the level of depth a practice wants to pursue in assessing ROI, it is crucial to track both costs and rewards. This includes not only advertising expenditure but also the "cost" associated with content creation and staff time required for marketing activities. To enhance overall marketing efforts, veterinarians should use SMART goals and leverage the front desk and practice management system to support conversions and quantify data. Instead of getting overwhelmed by numerous metrics, it is advisable to start with one or 2 key metrics that align with the practice's objectives and identify the data and metrics associated with the SMART goals to refine the focus. Using a central tool to track and measure the data in one place allows practices to quickly assess the success of their marketing efforts.

MAKING MARKETING MORE EFFICIENT

As practices are stretched to an unprecedented level of thinness, marketing may be one of the last things team members want to spend time on. That said, marketing allows us to reach our clients with information they need (meaning fewer calls), facilitate online or asynchronous action like booking appointments and processing online pharmacy requests (fewer ringing phones), and best of all, reach a TARGETED audience— so those calendars are full of the appointments the practice actually wants and clients who are the best fit.

- Schedule time to plan: Allocate at least 30 minutes to plan a month of content in advance.
- Use a content calendar: Strategically place content by filling in holidays, closures, and health awareness events. Develop weekly posts that align with practice goals, including team member spotlights, reminders, and convenience offerings.
- Schedule time to create and deploy: Block off one to 2 hours per month to create, assemble, and schedule content across social media and marketing platforms.
- Use marketing tools: Use recommended marketing tools to save time during content search, creation, and posting.
- Do not reinvent the wheel: Repurpose successful content, such as holiday graphics and evergreen posts, while adding a unique touch.
- Outsource when needed: Seek assistance from freelance marketers, veterinary marketing companies, or online platforms for tasks beyond the practice's expertise, such as video editing or graphic design.
- Use a style guide: Maintain consistency in font, color scheme, logo, and messaging by following a brand style guide. Compile commonly used assets in a cloud-based folder for easy access.

SUMMARY

Veterinary practices can enhance their digital presence and reach a wider audience through strategic digital marketing. Investing in a solid understanding of a practice's why and ideal clientele, followed by a survey of the practice's clients and team, can help narrow which platforms and content will be most effective for a specific practice's needs and goals. In general, a multimodal strategy that includes social media, email, a web presence, and online review listings will serve as a solid foundation. Based on a practice's goals, time and financial budgets, and specific demographics, paid advertising and an expansion into marketing avenues may be indicated.

CLINICS CARE POINTS

1. Here are some common "Whys," but remember that some practices may have multiple, and that they may change over time:
   - Increased appointments
   - Increased revenue
   - Increased service utilization (eg, online booking, app downloads, and so forth)

- Client education
- Loyalty
- Increased/improved ratings and reviews
- Staff time saved
- Convenience offering

2. Consider building a VIP list of favorite clients—those whose pets are up-to-date on all recommendations, the ones who leave unprompted 5-star reviews, and the clients that treat staff with respect and are fun to work with. Reach out to them to ask them what content and platforms are important to them. The results will help teams create content more likely to resonate with the best clients and those who share their interests and values.

3. Listen and engage with your clients
   - *Respond to reviews and messages.*
   - *Make a note of positive reviewers in practice management system and thank them in person on their next visit.*
   - *Visit the practice's Facebook Page community section to recognize and thank "Top Fans."*

4. Some additional tips for hashtag usage include the following:
   - Scan local profiles and influences: Find out what hashtags are popular in your local community and favored by relevant groups (for instance, a local dog training group or rescue, as well as other local businesses)
   - Get specific: Be sure to use hashtags relevant to your niche and location. Although using the hashtag #dogsofinstagram may earn your photograph more likes, it is unlikely that an internationally popular hashtag will net you any new local clients. It would be better to use a hashtag like #dogsofspringfield for appearing in the searches of dog owners in Springfield.

5. Example marketing text messages:
   - A discount on product or service (eg, 20% off geriatric examinations this month)
   - An alert to give a particular regular dosing product (eg, monthly preventative) with a link to refill if out
   - A message that the pet is due soon for preventative care with a booking link
   - Notification of a last-minute appointment opening
   - An alert to refill a prescription
   - A text with a link to download a new e-book from the practice
   - A notification of a new service offering (eg, telemedicine, online pharmacy, cat-only hours) and link to the service on the practice's Web site

6. Whenever possible, videos should be captioned. Facebook provides a free automatic caption generator when uploading files to the platform, although the punctuation and spelling can be inaccurate. Submitting the file to an online service is very affordable and more effective, often generating the required SubRip (srt) file type cost-effectively and within a few hours. Up to 85% of video on social media is watched without sound,[29,30] so adding captions (which will automatically appear if sound is not turned on) will increase both watch time and comprehension of the material.

7. Depending on the objective, experience, and interest levels, the following tools present a range of options when it comes to obtaining more data to help quantify marketing return on investment.
   - Meta Business Suite/Facebook Ads Manager
   - Facebook Pixel
   - Google Analytics
   - Practice Management System

8. How can a practice know if a client found them on Facebook or Yelp if they are not asking? Most practices use some type of initial client registration form, and this is a perfect tool to determine how the client learned about the practice. Whenever possible, be specific. Rather than including a "How did you hear about us?" followed by a blank line, create boxes for each possible source (eg, word of mouth, Google search, Facebook, Instagram, Yelp, Nextdoor, other online source _____).

When the client returns the form, use the practice management software's referral tracking in the new client setup. For instance, if a client indicated that they found the practice on Nextdoor, select "Nextdoor" from the drop-down menu of referral sources.

DISCLOSURE

The author has nothing to disclose.

REFERENCES

1. Executive summary of the Bayer veterinary care usage study in." https://avmajournals.avma.org/view/journals/javma/238/10/javma.238.10.1275.xml. Accessed 14 June. 2023.
2. Executive summary of phase 3 of the Bayer veterinary care usage " https://pubmed.ncbi.nlm.nih.gov/24649990/. Accessed 14 June. 2023.
3. UK pet owners' use of the internet for online pet health information." https://bvajournals.onlinelibrary.wiley.com/doi/abs/10.1136/vr.104716. Accessed 14 June. 2023.
4. Pet owners' online information searches and the perceived effects " 8 Jan. 2021, https://veterinaryevidence.org/index.php/ve/article/view/345. Accessed 14 June. 2023.
5. Executive summary of the Bayer veterinary care usage study in." https://avmajournals.avma.org/view/journals/javma/238/10/javma.238.10.1275.xml. Accessed 14 June. 2023.
6. Decision Data: Adding digital tools, social media? - DVM360." 26 Nov. 2019, https://www.dvm360.com/view/decision-data-adding-digital-tools-social-media. Accessed 14 June. 2023.
7. Decision Data: Adding digital tools, social media? - DVM360." 26 Nov. 2019, https://www.dvm360.com/view/decision-data-adding-digital-tools-social-media. Accessed 14 June. 2023.
8. Pride, representation, and inclusion in vet med - DVM360." 7 June. 2023, https://www.dvm360.com/view/pride-representation-and-inclusion-in-vet-med. Accessed 15 June. 2023.
9. Meta Reports First Quarter 2023 Results - Meta Investor Relations." 26 Apr. 2023, https://investor.fb.com/investor-news/press-release-details/2023/Meta-Reports-First-Quarter-2023-Results/default.aspx. Accessed 14 June. 2023.
10. 2022 Veterinary Marketing Benchmark Report Presented by iVET360." https://ivet360.com/veterinary-marketing-benchmarks/. Accessed 14 June. 2023.
11. Global social networks ranked by number of users 2023 - Statista." 14 Feb. 2023, https://www.statista.com/statistics/272014/global-social-networks-ranked-by-number-of-users/. Accessed 14 June. 2023.
12. "Instagram for Business: Marketing on Instagram | Instagram for " https://business.instagram.com/. Accessed 14 June. 2023.
13. One in four pet owners have created social media accounts for their ." 30 Mar. 2022, https://swnsdigital.com/uk/2022/03/one-in-four-pet-owners-have-created-social-media-accounts-for-their-furry-friends-with-many-having-more-followers-than-their-own-page/. Accessed 14 Jun. 2023.
14. Pet Owner Research - Vetsource." https://vetsource.com/pet-owner-research/. Accessed 14 June. 2023.
15. Pet Owner Research - Vetsource." https://vetsource.com/pet-owner-research/. Accessed 14 June. 2023.

16. 2023-2024 APPA National Pet Owners Survey." https://www.americanpetproducts. org/pubs_survey.asp. Accessed 14 June. 2023.

17. 10 Stats that Will 100% Convince You to Start Texting Your Clients." https://www. pattersonvet.com/vet/blog/10-stats-that-will-100-convince-you-to-start-texting-your-clients. Accessed 14 June. 2023.

18. Updates and appointment reminders? Text, please! - DVM360." 7 May. 2019, https://www.dvm360.com/view/updates-and-appointment-reminders-text-please. Accessed 14 June. 2023.

19. Finding the right channels to reach pet owners - MWI Animal Health." 7 Apr. 2022, https://www.mwiah.com/our-insights/finding-the-right-channels-to-reach-pet-owners. Accessed 14 June. 2023.

20. Medical Updates and Appointment Confirmations: Pet Owners " 25 Feb. 2019, https://www.frontiersin.org/articles/10.3389/fvets.2019.00080/full. Accessed 14 June. 2023.

21. Do Online Reviews Matter? - ThriveHive." 13 Feb. 2018, https://thrivehive.com/do-online-reviews-matter/. Accessed 14 June. 2023.

22. 2022 Veterinary Marketing Benchmark Report Presented by iVET360." https:// ivet360.com/veterinary-marketing-benchmarks/. Accessed 14 June. 2023.

23. A Guide to Build Your Online Presence - Google for Small Business." https:// smallbusiness.withgoogle.com/digital-essentials-guide/. Accessed 14 June. 2023.

24. Financial and Productivity Pulsepoints, Tenth Edition - AAHA." https://ams.aaha.org/ eweb/DynamicPage.aspx?site=store&webcode=prodredirect&code=FPPU10. Accessed 14 June. 2023.

25. 2019 Well-Managed Practice® Benchmarks Study (WMPB ." 9 Mar. 2021, https:// wellmp.com/2019-well-managed-practice-benchmarks-study-wmpb-provides-insights-to-the-top-veterinary-practices-in-the-country/. Accessed 14 Jun. 2023.

26. Perceptions and Behaviors of Pet Owners and Veterinarians." https://ispub.com/ IJVM/8/1/12921. Accessed 14 June. 2023.

27. Up Your Website Game | Merck Pet Owner Paths | MERCK." https:// merckpetownerpaths.com/action-steps/step-10/.

28. Executive summary of the Bayer veterinary care usage study in." https:// avmajournals.avma.org/view/journals/javma/238/10/javma.238.10.1275.xml. Accessed 14 June. 2023.

29. Report: Marketing in Software, SaaS, & Technology - Insivia." https://www.insivia. com/2023-saas-marketing-report/. Accessed 14 June. 2023.

30. The Ultimate Roundup of Compelling Closed Captions Statistics - Rev." 19 May. 2021, https://www.rev.com/blog/caption-blog/ultimate-roundup-closed-captions-statistics. Accessed 14 June. 2023.

Veterinary Practice Profitability
You Have to Measure It to Manage It

Karen E. Felsted, CPA, MS, DVM, CVPM, CVA*

KEYWORDS

- Profit • Profitability • Financial • Cash flow • EBITDA • No-Lo practice • Expenses
- Revenue

KEY POINTS

- The gold standard measure of a practice's financial success is the operating profit, which ultimately drives cash flow and practice value.
- Typical veterinary financial reports do not include a profit calculation; therefore, most practice owners/managers do not know how profitable the practice is.
- A lack of profitability comes from revenues that are too low, expenses that are too high, or a combination of the two.
- There are many changes a practice can make, some easy and others more time-consuming, to increase the profits.

INTRODUCTION

The gold standard measure of a practice's financial success is the operating profit. Profits are, essentially, the amount left over after deducting all the normal and necessary expenses of the practice (paid at fair market value rates) from the revenue.

Unfortunately, most practices do not really know how profitable they are. Because profitability drives current cash flow as well as the sales value of a practice, an understanding of how it is calculated and what drives it is essential to making good operating decisions. Before delving down into where profits come from, it is first necessary to discuss why this concept is so important and how to calculate the overall profit margin of the practice.

In addition to the obvious impact on current cash flow, profitability is also a critical determinant of practice value. Historically, practice owners have assumed that when they decided to sell their practices there would be buyers ready to purchase them and willing to pay a good price. In other words, they have assumed there was value in

PantheraT Veterinary Management Consulting, Richardson, TX, USA
* 412 Lawndale Drive, Richardson, TX 75080.
E-mail address: Karen@pantherat.com

Vet Clin Small Anim 54 (2024) 395–407
https://doi.org/10.1016/j.cvsm.2023.10.003
0195-5616/24/© 2023 Elsevier Inc. All rights reserved.

these businesses that could be transferred to someone else. Of course, there have always been a few practices for which this assumption did not hold true. A buyer could not be found or what buyers wanted to pay was not remotely what the seller thought the practice was worth. Typically, these practices have been easy to identify and had several traits in common. They tended to be smaller practices with owners who had not focused much on the business side of things. Often the facility and equipment were old, and the doctors had not kept up with the changes in medicine as much as they should have. These practices had little profit in them, and because the bulk of practice value is determined by profitability, the practices had little value. Fortunately, there were not too many of these practices.

Years ago, practices tended to be very similar in how they operated and in their levels of profitability. Over time, however, the profitability of practices started to vary greatly and the number of practices with no or little value increased—to the point where the VetPartners Valuation Council coined the term "No-Lo^{SM} practice" to describe these practices. More and more practices, when appraised, did not have the value that would normally have been expected or was desired by the practice owner. Moreover, in almost all cases, the owners of these practices were totally unaware of the problem. Some of these practices had traits in common with the practices that have historically had little or no value. They were small practices that did not keep up with changing client demands regarding service, quality of medicine, advanced technology, and improved facilities. The other practices with no or less value, however, were a surprising group. On the surface, these practices would seem to be doing very well. They are located in very attractive facilities, practice good medicine, have all the latest equipment and a large support staff, offer comparatively high compensation and benefits to their employees and, in the owners' eyes, cash flow is strong. However, practice value is largely based on profits, and the very factors that make these practices look attractive on the surface are those that are reducing profitability.

TERMINOLOGY

As noted above, a simple definition of profitability is the amount left over after deducting all the normal and necessary expenses of the practice (paid at fair market value rates) from the revenue.

None of the standard financial or management reports a practice usually gets includes a true profitability number, and therefore, many practice owners are unaware of the true profitability of their practice. Neither the taxable income from the tax return, the net income from the profit and loss statement or practice cash flow from a cash flow report represents true profitability. Using those numbers as an estimate of profitability can result in some serious miscalculations in value expectations and in management decision-making.

Most privately held veterinary practices are small businesses and their accounting systems are often not very sophisticated. Some common differences between profitability and net income/taxable income/cash flow result from the following:

- Accounting errors such as in how payroll or the principle portion of debt payments are calculated and entered in the various reports
- Owner personal expenses may be incorrectly included in practice financial statements, cash flow reports, or tax returns
- Nonoperating items such as interest/dividend income or interest expense are often (appropriately) included in a profit and loss statement, cash flow report, or tax return but would not be part of a profit calculation

- Expenses are often not stated at a fair market value; common examples of this include owner compensation and rent expense (when the practice real estate is also owned by the practice owner)
- Differences in tax law that exist for different kinds of entities—the bottom line "taxable income" number can vary greatly just because of the entity structure used by the practice (eg, S corporation vs sole proprietorship)
- Corporate groups will often provide profit and loss statements to each practice in their group but these may not accurately include the costs for services paid for by the parent company

All of these problems and others result in information that is not accurate from a profitability calculation perspective although the reports may be accurately prepared for their intended purpose.

A term that has become more common in veterinary medicine is EBITDA, which stands for Earnings before Interest, Taxes, Depreciation, and Amortization. This is similar to a profitability calculation; however, a profitability calculation often includes an estimate of the amount typically spent by the practice each year on equipment purchases, whereas an EBITDA calculation will not.

With both EBITDA and profit calculations, adjustments *must* be made to correct the types of errors and other issues outlined above in order to come to a figure that truly estimates profitability; that is, what is left over after all the normal and necessary expenses of the practice are paid at fair market value rates.

CALCULATION OF PROFITABILITY

The operating profit is the difference between the operating revenues and expenses of a practice. Operating revenue and expenses include only items normally and necessarily seen in the day-to-day operations of the practice such as fees for professional services and drugs and medical supplies expense. These items should be stated at fair market value rates. For ease of comparison with other practices, the profit margin is generally stated as a percentage—this is calculated as practice profits divided by gross revenue. Some of the items that must be calculated differently to determine operating profit include the following: practice owner payments, debt payments, facility rent if the real estate is owned by the practice owner and leased to the practice, services provided by family members to the practice, depreciation, interest income, and expense and personal expenses (perks) paid by the practice on behalf of the owner.

So how is operating profit calculated? The following steps are generally those needed to get to this figure although there can be some variations in individual practices. Taxable income per the practice's tax return or net income per the practice's profit and loss statement is usually the starting point (**Fig. 1**). Various adjustments are made from there.

- Add back: depreciation, amortization, and equipment lease payments treated as an expense in the tax return.
- Deduct the estimated average amount spent on equipment per year—depreciation as determined by tax law is not the best estimate. A reasonable estimate in many companion animal practices is 1% to 1.5% of gross revenue. This expense is usually higher in emergency and specialty hospitals.
- Determine how much the owner was paid in compensation and rent (if the practice owner owns the practice facility as well) during the year.
- Adjust owner compensation to represent a fair amount that should be paid for the owner's medical/surgical work—20% to 22% of personal production is often used in a small animal practice. Owner compensation for medical/surgical

	P&L	2022 Adjustment	Adjusted P&L		Explanation
REVENUE					
Fees for Professional Services	$2,016,452		$2,016,452	100.0%	
Total Revenue	$2,016,452	$0	$2,016,452	100.0%	
EXPENSES					
COST OF PROFESSIONAL SERVICES					
Drugs & Medical Supplies	$302,111	($3,600)	$298,511	14.8%	Remove personal expense
Laboratory Services	$134,789		$134,789	6.7%	
Animal Disposal/Mortuary Costs	$14,002		$14,002	0.7%	
Dietary Products	$11,596		$11,596	0.6%	
Outside Veterinary Services	$4,516		$4,516	0.2%	
Total Cost of Professional Services	$467,014	($3,600)	$463,414	23.0%	
COMPENSATION AND BENEFITS EXPENSE					
Owner Veterinarian Compensation	$70,000	$139,740	$209,740	10.4%	Adjust owner compensation to FMV
Associate Veterinarian Compensation	$227,662		$227,662	11.3%	
Contract Labor (Relief Veterinarians)	$1,250		$1,250	0.1%	
Staff Compensation	$493,530	($12,000)	$481,530	23.9%	Remove non-FMV family compensation
Payroll Taxes	$63,295	$5,746	$69,041	3.4%	Adjust taxes to FMV
Employee Benefits	$14,019		$14,019	0.7%	
Meals & Entertainment	$1,508		$1,508	0.1%	
Total Compensation and Benefits Expense	$871,264	$133,486	$1,004,750	49.8%	
FACILITY & EQUIPMENT EXPENSE					
Rent on Practice Real Estate	$50,000	$40,000	$90,000	4.5%	Adjust rent to FMV
Repairs and Maintenance, inc. Service Contracts	$28,126	($5,214)	$22,912	1.1%	Remove fixed assets
Housekeeping & Janitorial	$6,061		$6,061	0.3%	
Utilities and Telephone	$59,961		$59,961	3.0%	
Insurance	$6,608		$6,608	0.3%	
Depreciation Expense	$27,140	($27,140)	$0	0.0%	Remove non-cash expense
Reinvestment in Equipment	$0	$30,247	$30,247	1.5%	Adjust to average annual equip purchase
Real Estate Tax	$33,784		$33,784	1.7%	
Practice Vehicle	$3,989	($3,989)	$0	0.0%	Remove personal expense
Total Facility Expense	$215,669	$33,904	$249,573	12.4%	
ADMINISTRATIVE EXPENSE					
Office and Computer Supplies	$18,941		$18,941	0.9%	
Postage	$398		$398	0.0%	
Printing	$1,457		$1,457	0.1%	
Bank Charges	$1,372		$1,372	0.1%	
Advertising and Promotion	$43,957		$43,957	2.2%	
Payroll Services and Employee Benefits Administratic	$1,069		$1,069	0.1%	
Accounting & Bookkeeping Services	$6,216		$6,216	0.3%	
Credit Card Merchant Service Fees	$55,246		$55,246	2.7%	
Charitable Contributions	$11,855		$11,855	0.6%	
Total Administrative Expense	$140,511	$0	$140,511	7.0%	
OTHER EXPENSE					
Interest Expense	$21,255	($21,255)	$0	0.0%	Remove non-operating expense
Amortization Expense	$4,970	($4,970)	$0	0.0%	Remove non-cash expense
Total Other Income	$26,225	($26,225)	$0	0.0%	
NET INCOME/ADJUSTED PROFITS	$295,769	($137,564)	$158,204	7.8%	

Fig. 1. Example of an adjusted profit and loss statement.

work should be calculated similarly to how other veterinarians in the practice or community with similar experience and skills would be paid.

- Adjust owner compensation for management work—if the hospital has a practice or office manager, the owner should get less than if there is no such manager in place. About 1.0% to 1.5% of gross revenue is often used to represent owner management compensation when the practice has a manager.
- Adjust rent expense to fair market value if currently paid to the owner at a rate greater or lesser than fair market value.
- Determine the dollar amount of personal expenses (perks) paid by the practice and remove this expense—perks are items not necessary to the operation of the

practice but paid by the practice generally to gain a tax advantage for the owner (examples include nonbusiness meals and entertainment, nonbusiness auto costs, swimming pool payments, personal furniture purchases, trips to Tahiti, and so forth).
- Deduct the cost associated with free services provided to the practice; for example, family members may provide bookkeeping or other services to the practice at no charge. If the practice had to hire someone to do this work, there would be a cost involved and this should be included as an expense.
- Add back any compensation and benefits paid to family members that are above what would normally be paid for these services. This includes payments to family members who do *no* work in the practice.
- Remove any true nonrecurring income or expenses such as one-time insurance proceeds, expenses related to a natural disaster or the paycheck protection program (PPP) loans seen during the COVID-19 pandemic. These kinds of nonrecurring items are not commonly seen in practices.
- Add back interest expense.
- Subtract interest and dividend income.
- Recalculate the earnings figure.
- Divide the new profit number by gross revenue in order to see the profit figure as a percentage of revenue.

This resulting percentage can be compared with other practices. Although there are no exact figures available and opinions vary on the exact ranges, the following chart (**Table 1**) indicates how profit percentages are often interpreted for a small animal general practice.

"The No-Lo Practice" booklet available free from: https://www.vetpartners.org/practice-valuation-resources/includes a worksheet to guide you through the calculation process. Remember that every practice may have some unique items that need to be adjusted in order to get to the true profit number. The VetPartners guide and the information above are excellent starting points but working with a financial consultant who works specifically with veterinary practices can also be helpful in calculating *your* practice's specific profit margin. A directory of such consultants can be found at www.VetPartners.org.

PROFITS BY DEPARTMENT

Once the overall profit margin of the practice has been determined, a further analysis can be done to determine which areas of the practice contribute the most to profitability. This is most commonly done when a large amount of revenue is generated from multiple departments. Both revenue and expenses must be allocated to each department or division of the hospital. Departments can be determined in several different ways; in a general practice, they would usually include outpatient, pharmacy, surgery, dentistry, hospitalization, boarding, and grooming. A mixed animal practice might first look at

Table 1 Interpretation of profit percentages	
Percentage Range	
≥20%	Superior
14%–19%	Above average
12%–13%	Average
7%–11%	Below average
<7%	Poor

profits by species, for example, by equine, dairy cow, companion animal, and the other species seen in the practice. A specialty hospital will generally calculate profits by service—internal medicine, surgery, dermatology, and so forth.

These departments generally have different cost structures and different levels of profitability, and unless the departments are reviewed as independent businesses within the larger entity, it will not be possible to manage them most effectively.

It is generally easy to categorize revenue separately for each of these departments but expense allocation is harder to do and most practices do not even try. The goal, however, is to create a profit and loss statement for each department. For example, total staff costs may look a little high when they are reviewed in total for a general practice with a large and elaborate boarding component. After costs are allocated between the 3 entities (medical practice, boarding, and grooming), however, it may become apparent that staff is used efficiently in the medical practice but costs are very high in the boarding/grooming departments in comparison to the revenue brought in.

Setting up systems to accurately allocate expenses is a little time-consuming in the beginning but will pay big dividends in the end: Ways of allocating some common expenses are discussed below.

- Drugs and medical supplies—set up the inventory system to track usage by department; for example, all drugs and supplies may be received into central supply and subsequently issued to each department
- Outside laboratory test costs should be assigned individually to the department to which the patient's revenue was allocated
- Usage of internal laboratory or imaging facilities/equipment—the number of tests used by each department must be captured and total costs for the equipment (including related personnel, supplies, and an allocation of the original purchase price) is allocated to each department based on usage
- Compensation—amounts related to doctors or staff assigned solely to one department should be assigned to that department. Costs related to floating or shared staff need to be allocated monthly by usage. For example, receptionists' compensation may be allocated based on the percent of transactions for each department. Benefits may be assigned individually (often done for doctors) or allocated using payroll percents (more commonly done for staff)
- Facility rent—assign costs based on the square footage used by each department. Shared space can be allocated based on the number of transactions per department
- Other facility costs (janitorial, utilities, property taxes, and so forth) are often allocated based on the same percentages used to allocate rent
- Marketing—individual marketing programs can be assigned to the department involved; joint marketing can be allocated based on the number of transactions per service
- Credit card fees should be allocated based on the percentage of total or credit card revenue per department

There needs to be a balance between the complexity of the allocation methodology and the usefulness of the information obtained. In general, a reasonably based allocation system (even if not perfect) is better than none.

The same adjustments that were included in calculating the overall profitability of the practice also need to be considered at this level of analysis. For example, if the owner doctors' salary was adjusted to fair market value in the first calculation, this adjusted number is the one that should be used when allocating his/her salary by department.

WHERE TO GO NEXT?

If the practice's profits are not at the desired level, what can be done about it? A lack of profitability comes from revenues that are too low, expenses that are too high, or a combination of the two. Understanding not only the profitability of the practice but also the kinds of factors that lead to this state is critical. Until the practice has an idea of the root causes of the problem, it is difficult to determine what the correct solution is. Discussed below are some of the most critical revenue and expense areas that should be reviewed regularly. The practices that are most successful in increasing revenue and profitability are those that have a strong sense of who they are and the kinds of clients they want to attract. If the practice has not identified its vision and mission as well as a value proposition, this is the place to start.

REVENUE AND REVENUE DRIVERS

Shown below is a chart outlining some of the key drivers of revenue followed by a discussion of the metrics that provide information about these drivers (**Fig. 2**). Not all revenue metrics are included here but it is a good starting point. Just reviewing total revenue for a month, quarter or year is not enough to determine if the practice is doing well financially; more detail is needed to fully use this information to improve practice operations. Revenue by itself is not sufficient to monitor a practice's financial health; a practice must monitor expenses as well as practice profitability.

It is possible to have a practice with a very high level of revenue and an impressive revenue growth rate and still have a low level of profitability.

Total Practice Revenue

A review of total practice revenue for a particular period compared with a prior period is useful in that it measures the overall growth or decline of the practice and can be compared with published benchmarks in order to understand how this practice is doing compared with others. A more in-depth analysis of the factors driving revenue is necessary, however, to determine *why* a practice is growing or declining and what management changes are needed to correct problems in this area.

Transactions (Invoices)

Total revenue can be derived by multiplying the number of transactions by the average transaction charge (ATC). (Note that the terms invoice and transaction are often used

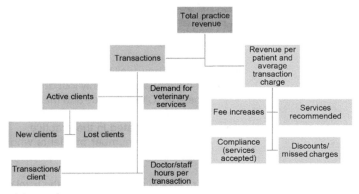

Fig. 2. Key drivers of revenue.

interchangeably.) A transaction is any invoice whether for a single bag of dog food or a high-dollar surgery.

Similar to revenue analysis, the analysis of total practice transactions for a particular period compared with a prior period is useful in that it measures the overall activity growth or decline of activity in the practice and can be compared with published benchmarks in order to understand how this practice is doing compared with others. A deeper analysis is again needed to determine why the practice is growing or declining and what management changes are needed.

Examples of important areas to investigate in order to improve transaction numbers include the following:

- Changes in the number of new clients/patients, active clients/patients, and transactions per clients/patients
- Client retention/lost clients
- Competition and the perceived value of other practices compared with the subject practice
- Practice standards of care
- Changes in the economy
- Staff and doctor efficiency in seeing clients
- Client compliance with key recommendations by doctors and staff
- Time management skills of each team member
- Practice workflow
- Appropriate appointment, procedure, and staff scheduling
- Effective delegation skills by all team members

Client Analysis

Obviously one of the key drivers of transactions and revenue is the number of clients and patients seen by the practice. Client-related key performance indicators include the following:

- Number of active clients and patients
- Number of new clients and patients
- Number of lost clients and patients
- Number of transactions or visits per clients and patients

The calculation of active clients and patients per full-time-equivalent (FTE) veterinarian is a measure of the overall productivity of the practice. A low number of active clients per FTE doctor may indicate a practice that has too many doctors compared with the number of clients or it may indicate a practice that is in the early stages of its growth cycle. Some boutique practices may have fewer clients than an average practice but generate much more revenue per client for the specialized services they provide.

The number of new clients is an indication of how well the practice is doing in generating real growth and in replacing the clients that are invariably lost due to the death of a pet or clients who move from the service area. Client service and marketing generally drive new clients into the practice, and these are the areas that should be focused on if these figures are declining or are lower than anticipated in the practice.

Lost clients represent, as the name implies, the number of clients who leave the practice. Knowing how many leave is not enough; however. The practice needs to ascertain why these clients are leaving.

The number of transactions (visits) per client is an indication of the level of care clients provide to their pets and is dependent on the quality of the workups done by the doctors and recommendations made as well as the quality of the communication in making these recommendations.

Doctor/Staff Hours per Transaction

One particularly helpful efficiency metric is the average number of staff and doctor hours per transaction.

Average staff hours per transaction is calculated as follows:

$$\frac{Total\ number\ of\ hours\ worked\ by\ all\ support\ staff}{Total\ transactions}$$

Average doctor hours per transaction is calculated similarly as follows:

$$\frac{Total\ number\ of\ hours\ worked\ by\ all\ doctors}{Total\ transactions}$$

And then, of course, average *total* hours per transaction is calculated as follows:

$$\frac{Total\ number\ of\ hours\ worked\ by\ all\ doctors/staff}{Total\ transactions}$$

There are not any published benchmarks for the hours per transaction metric but this number is often between 2 and 3 hours per transaction. The best practices are at 1.5 hours/transaction; very occasionally, a practice will have a slightly lower number but the medical care and service quality can suffer when this number gets too low. The goal is to reduce the total number of hours per transaction and shift hours from doctors to nondoctors.

Revenue per Patient and Average Transaction Charge

Another driver of revenue is the amount spent by each client in a transaction or in a particular period. Most practices look at the ATC figure but both are useful and give the practice different kinds of information. These are blended numbers. The revenue per patient figure includes all spending at the practice during a particular period. ATC is an average of both medical and nonmedical transactions ranging from a US$20 bag of food to a US$3,000 surgery.

Areas to be investigated if these figures are low include the following: the fee schedule in the practice, the extent of pet care recommendations made to and accepted by the pet owner, and the amount of missed charges or discounts in the practice.

Fee Increases

Fee increases are obviously a key driver of client spending and, ultimately, total revenue. Pricing strategies are generally not sophisticated in veterinary medicine and most practices simply price their services similarly to others and increase them by some arbitrary percentage each year with limited focus on increasing value at the same time.

It has become clear that practices need to be more strategic in their fee setting and fee increases.

Implementing a pricing strategy is not just about deciding what percentage to use to increase fees every 6 to 12 months. Pricing is a marketing issue and just one component of the traditional 4 "P's" of the marketing mix: place, promotion, product, and price, all of which must be considered in price determination in addition to value, reference prices, the business's value proposition and price execution.

A detailed analysis of pricing strategies is outside the scope of this article but a practice must have a process in place to continually review both product and service fees. Many pricing resources are available from the Veterinary Hospital Managers Association at www.VHMA.org.

Revenue/Transactions/Average Transaction Charge per Full-Time-Equivalent Veterinarian

Two revenue drivers in the figure above include "services recommended" and "compliance (services accepted)"—these are both components of doctor productivity. Metrics used to understand doctor productivity include revenue per FTE veterinarian, transactions per FTE veterinarian, and ATC. These can be calculated in various ways. The example calculations shown below are done using revenue but similar calculations can also be done for transactions.

The first calculation is to determine the overall productivity of the practice as a whole.

$$\frac{\text{Total practice revenue}}{\text{Number of FTE DVMs}}$$

The second way is to analyze the productivity of the doctor-only work in the practice.

$$\frac{\text{Total medical revenue}}{\text{Number of FTE DVMs}}$$

The difference between the 2 calculations above is that nondoctor revenue from boarding, grooming, over-the-counter (OTC) product sales and other similar nonmedical services is not included in the second calculation. Although there are variations among practices about what is included in medical revenue, it generally comprises about 85% to 90% of total revenue in a companion animal practice.

The above calculations provide information about *average* productivity per doctor. The last component of this doctor productivity analysis is to review actual revenue per *each individual* doctor in the practice from their production reports.

Total practice transactions and ATC, medical transactions and ATC, and individual doctor transactions and ATC should also be reviewed.

Once these top-level calculations have been done, the practice should drill down further into areas that may need improvement. Even if doctors are not paid on a production basis, it is critical that the practice know how much their doctors produce and how it correlates with their salaries. Some areas to investigate include the following:

- Number of hours worked each week by the doctors
- Number of appointments, surgeries, and dentals done by each doctor during this time frame
- Support staff help used by each doctor
- Number of key procedures (eg, CBCs, chemistry panels, and x-rays) performed by each doctor in relation to the number of transactions they generate
- Measurement of client compliance with key recommendations by doctors and staff
- Dollar amount of discounts and missed charges per doctor

Remember that doctor productivity either in total or for a specific doctor is not all about how that doctor performs; it is also very dependent on the overall management of the practice. For example, productivity may suffer because the practice simply does not have enough patients coming in the door, a poor level of client service, fees that are too low, poor support staff help, or other reasons.

Discounts and Missed Charges

The establishment of an appropriate fee schedule is obviously a critical driver of the ATC and revenue in total but it is equally important that the services are captured on the invoice and paid for by the clients.

Discounts are a reduction in fees deliberately given to a client by doctors or staff. Missed charges represent products or services given to the client that are accidently not charged for. Discounts and missed charges have a similar impact on the finances of a practice and can have a dramatic effect on the profitability. It is important for practice owners and managers to understand what this impact is when making decisions about how much to discount and the changes that are needed to reduce missed charges.

Discount reports available in the practice's practice information management system (PIMS) generally only include a fraction of the total amounts discounted or given away and, obviously, none of the missed charges. A manual audit comparing medical records to client invoices is often necessary to identify the magnitude of discounts and missed charges.

Discounts come in many different forms—employee, senior citizen, multiple pets, marketing, or for bundled services. Discounts are not always "bad" as long as they are accomplishing the goals set by the practice when the discount was put into place.

As noted above, the metrics discussed here do not include all of the important metrics a practice should review regularly. Additionally, other more detailed metrics should be used to dive further into the areas discussed above. For example, if the practice chooses to focus on improving doctor productivity, some additional metrics to be analyzed include the following: the number of appointments, surgeries and dentals done by each doctor, and the number of FTE technicians and veterinary assistants per FTE doctor. Which metrics to use will depend on which area the practice is hoping to understand better or improve.

EXPENSES AND EXPENSE DRIVERS

Because profitability is determined by subtracting expenses from revenue, expenses must also be controlled in order to maintain high levels of profits. The most critical (ie, the largest) expense areas to review are as follows:

- Inventory costs—drugs, supplies, and food
- Doctor compensation/productivity
- Staff (nondoctor) compensation/productivity

All costs can get out of control, and therefore, all expenses should be reviewed in detail at least annually but more time and effort should be spent on the larger ones because control of those expenses will have the most impact on profitability.

Inventory Costs

This is one of the largest expenses in every practice and controlling inventory can significantly improve the practice's bottom line. Most practices have some kind of inventory system in place but many systems need improvement. Most practices look at the cost of the various inventory item categories as a percentage of gross revenue as a starting point in understanding if these costs are too high. The most common expense categories used are drugs and medical supplies expense, dietary product expense, and OTC product expense although some practices will have more categories and/or more detailed subcategories.

Inventory costs may look high simply because the practice is using a cash basis of accounting rather than an accrual basis, which means the amount of inventory expense on the profit and loss statement represents items purchased rather than used. In order to assess inventory costs accurately, an estimate of the dollar amount of the products sold or used in-house is essential. Changes needed to improve the efficiency of the inventory system are not hard to make but require time and an attention to detail. Areas to focus on in order to improve profitability include regular counts of key items, improved ordering, physical control, and the addition of various checks and balances to make sure inventory related data is captured accurately.

Doctor Compensation

This is another very large expense item in every practice and is best analyzed by correlating it with doctor production. In general, compensation should be 20% to 22% of the doctor's production for a small animal general practice but there can be variations depending on the specific circumstances of the practice. This percentage range represents W2 compensation only, not including benefits, payroll taxes, or other employee costs. See the section above "Revenue/Transactions/Average Transaction Charge per Full-Time-Equivalent Veterinarian" for more information on doctor production.

Staff Compensation

The amount of staff compensation is influenced by the following:

- Number of team members
- Number of hours worked by each team member
- Compensation paid to team members
- Overtime
- Team member skills and knowledge
- Workflow efficiency
- Scheduling

Team numbers and scheduling must correlate with doctor scheduling and production and review of the above items can help determine where problems lie if costs are high.

Other tips for reviewing and controlling expenses include the following:

1. Review the detailed list of transactions in any account that seems to be high (or low)—sometimes there are expenses recorded in that account in error, which should be included elsewhere.

2. Set up easy to access electronic or paper files containing all the bills, receipts, packing slips, contracts, or other backup documentation related to the expenses. When analyzing costs, it may be necessary to review this type of documentation, and if it has been thrown out or is too hard to access, good quality analysis may not be possible.

3. It is not enough to know whether the practice's expenses fall within accepted norms when compared with the veterinary benchmarking studies publicly available. For example, the average amount of drugs and medical supplies expense (excluding laboratory and dietary products) may range from 15% to 20% depending on the study reviewed. Assuming all other expenditures are equal, if a practice's drugs and medical supplies expense increases from 15% to 20%, the profitability will be significantly eroded even though the expense seems to

be "normal." This does not mean that the studies are "bad" but they represent an average of the group surveyed, and average may not be good enough in a particular practice situation if the owners want the highest level of profitability. Comparing a practice's expenses to outside studies is a useful component of the financial analysis process but the calculation of profitability and internal trend tracking is also important.

4. Do not assume that just because the practice is locked into a certain dollar expenditure that there is nothing that can be done to better control it. For example, the practice may contractually be obligated to pay US$10,000 per month in rent. The practice cannot change the dollars paid but it can make sure the space is used as efficiently and productively as possible.

WHERE TO GET HELP?

There are many outstanding management resources available to practitioners from organizations such as VetPartners (www.vetpartners.org), the Veterinary Hospital Managers Association (www.VHMA.org), the AVMA (www.avma.org), AAHA (www.aaha.org), AAFP (www.catvets.com), as well as conferences and webinars, publications, and other industry groups. Working with a financial advisor or practice consultant may help in not only gaining a greater understanding of the issues affecting profitability but in identifying and implementing solutions. VetPartners (www.vetpartners.org) can help in locating an appropriate individual. Joining a study group such as those offered by Veterinary Management Groups, WTA Veterinary Consultants, and others can also be an excellent way to improve a practice.

SUMMARY

There are many actions a practice can take to improve its profitability but the management team must first *know* what the profitability of the practice actually is. Fortunately, there are multiple resources available to practice owners and managers to get this information. If the practice's profits are not at the desired level, it is because the revenue is too low, the expenses are too high, or both. Understanding not only the profitability of the practice but also the kinds of factors that lead to this state is critical. Until the practice has an idea of the root causes of the problem, it is difficult to determine what the correct solution is. Fortunately, there are also many resources available to help a practice change and improve.

DISCLOSURE

The authors have nothing to disclose.

FURTHER READINGS

The No-Lo Practice: Avoiding a Practice Worth Less by the VetPartners Valuation Council (https://www.vetpartners.org/practice-valuation-resources/).

Valuation Essentials for Veterinarians: Measuring Value Over the Life of Your Practice by the VetPartners Valuation Council (https://www.vetpartners.org/practice-valuation-resources/).

Karen E. Felsted, Leslie A. Mamalis, David F. McCormick, "The Profitable Vet: Strategies for Financial Success in Veterinary Practice" with authors Dick Goebel.

Building Value for Veterinary Practice Sale

Leslie A. Mamalis, CVA (Emeritus)

KEYWORDS

- Practice value • Valuation • Value • Goodwill

KEY POINTS

- The purpose of the valuation drives the value itself. Be certain that the expert valuing the business has a clear understanding of why it is being done.
- To maximize value, the business must be profitable, generate consistent levels of earnings year after year, and operate well in the absence of the owner.
- No reliable "rules of thumb" exist for valuing veterinary practices. Rules of thumb are merely observational statistics, not predictive of business value.
- The 2 most reliable methods for maximizing a veterinary practice's value are through optimizing profits and minimizing the risk of owning the business.

WHAT IS VALUE?

Like Plato's definition of beauty, value is in the eye of the beholder. What holds great value to one person may have little or no value to another. For example, a filet mignon may be highly valued by a diner who enjoys red meat but entirely unpalatable to a vegetarian.

Travelers expect all hotel rooms to be reasonably clean with beds, a television, and bathroom. With choices from economy to luxury, how does a guest select the room with the best value? It may depend on whether the guest plans to spend a brief overnight or a lengthy stay, the size of their party, whether they want a pool to entertain children, or an onsite restaurant to make meals convenient. A family of 4 spending one night as part of a long road trip will have different definitions of value than a business traveler in town for a week.

Business value is less relative than the examples above. For a veterinary hospital, value is driven by financial earnings but other factors, some difficult to quantify, also influence value. For example, a highly profitable practice in a rural area without access to emergency veterinary clinics to handle caseloads on nights, weekends, and holidays, will be less attractive to many buyers than a somewhat less profitable hospital

Summit Veterinary Advisors, 2250 South Ellis Court, Lakewood, CO 80228, USA
E-mail address: Leslie.Mamalis@gmail.com

Vet Clin Small Anim 54 (2024) 409–421
https://doi.org/10.1016/j.cvsm.2023.10.013
0195-5616/24/ **vetsmall.theclinics.com**

in a suburban area where emergency hospitals are present. In this case, individual work–life balance priorities are in play.

At any point in time, a business may have several different values, depending on what is being valued and why. The purpose of the valuation has an impact on the methodology used and will affect the result. This underscores the need for the client and the valuation analyst to determine many facts at the onset of the valuation engagement.

REASONS FOR A VALUATION

For veterinary practices, the most common reason for a valuation is for the sale of all or a portion of the business. However, there are other reasons for a valuation, including the following:

1. Mergers with other veterinary practices or hospitals
2. Updates to buy/sell agreements or life insurance policies
3. Strategic planning
4. Tax planning, including estate and gift tax planning
5. Litigation, most commonly in cases of divorce or partner disputes

Even when a sale is not anticipated, it is critical for veterinary hospital owners to have the hospital undergo a periodic examination so they know how much money a sale potentially would bring to them. Practice value is critical information for retirement planning, including developing a plan for sheltering sales proceeds from income taxes. Most valuation analysts recommend that practice owners have their practice valued every 3 to 5 years. By doing this, the owners have an opportunity to respond to any unexpected trends.

DIFFERENT DEFINITIONS

Many consultants who establish selling prices for their clients use the term "valuation" but there is a significant difference between a true business valuation and establishing an asking price. Many professionals act as advocates for the practice owner and arrive at a price that emphasizes their clients' best interests. Similarly, buyers may work with consultants who advise them regarding an appropriate purchase price. Neither consultant determines a true business value. Instead, they are establishing a price, either the highest price supportable when working for the seller or the lowest reasonable price when working for the buyer for the purpose of negotiation. By definition, a business valuation must be an unbiased, professional determination of business value. According to the Professional Standards for the National Association of Certified Valuators and Analysts,[1] the valuator may not act as an advocate for any side of a potential transaction and must verify they have no conflicts of interest before accepting the valuation engagement. The professional fees paid for a valuation may not influence the value in any way.

Readers of valuation reports should look for language that describes what type of report was prepared. Does it state that the report follows the standards for an official business appraisal organization? If not, the conclusion of value may not reflect an unbiased point of view.

VALUATION CREDENTIALS

Several different valuation credentials are recognized in the industry, including the Certified Valuation Analyst through the National Association of Certified Valuator and Analysts (NACVA),[2] the Accredited Member, and Accredited Senior Appraiser through the American Society of Appraisers,[3] and the Accredited in Business Valuation through the American Institute of Certified Public Accountants.[4] The Certified Business Appraiser (CBA) designation was offered by the Institute of Business Appraisers until it was acquired by NACVA in 2008. NACVA continued to offer credentialing to new candidates until 2016. Although the designation is no longer available, NACVA allows valuation professionals to maintain their CBA credential if they comply with recertification requirements.

The credentialing process typically includes preparatory coursework, a rigorous examination, and a peer-reviewed written case study. With all the work that goes into becoming a credentialed business appraiser, one can understand why the business valuations they produce are so highly valued in financial, legal, and insurance circles.

Although the credentialing process provides an understanding of appraisal methodology, a credential alone does not signify that the professional understands veterinary practices. The credential demonstrates that the individual received education specific to valuation and meets continuing education requirements. Years of experience in the veterinary industry is also important. Members of the VetPartners Valuation Council, many of whom hold a valuation credential, have experience specifically working with and valuing veterinary practices. This specialization means that members understand the unique nature of veterinary medicine and valuation of closely held businesses. (The Internal Revenue Service [IRS] defines a closely held business as one where 50% or more of the stock is owned by one to 5 owners.[5])

RULES OF THUMB

The International Glossary of Business Valuation Terms[6] defines a "rule of thumb" as "a mathematical formula developed from the relationship between price and certain variables based on experience, observation, hearsay, or a combination of these; usually industry specific." In the veterinary industry, a rule of thumb may be derived from actual practices sales, along with a healthy dose of hearsay, an average of one or more variables and comparing that average to the sales price. In other words, a rule of thumb would apply to an "average" practice.

Rules of thumb are problematic, particularly in a profession where most practice sales are private, meaning access to data regarding those sales is difficult to obtain. Instead, many people rely on values recounted "through the grapevine" to develop these rules. The inability to compare similar practices in veterinary medicine makes the rule-of-thumb approach an unreliable method of valuing veterinary practices. Even more problematic, if the rule of thumb relies on a multiple of earnings, there is no consensus regarding how earnings are quantified, what they include and do not include, or even whether owner compensation is subtracted from earnings, or is added back into them.

The value of any business is based on the specific characteristics of that business. In the valuation world, rules of thumb are sometimes used as sanity checks but never as a primary valuation method. The tremendous changes in veterinary medicine during the past 15 to 20 years must not be overlooked. Old formulas and multipliers of revenue are not and likely never were reliable methods of determining value.

The disadvantages of relying on a rule-of-thumb valuation are many. The most serious concerns relate to establishing a selling price that is much lower than the true fair market value of the practice. There are instances of sellers losing hundreds of thousands of dollars in sales price because they or their advisors did not take the time to get a formal appraisal. On the other side of the transaction, if a buyer overpays for a practice, it could result in a situation where the buyer cannot afford to make the payments. If the seller is financing all or part of the sale and the buyer defaults on the loan, then that seller may never receive full payment. In a worse scenario, the retired owner may be forced to take back the practice, which may be generating a fraction of the original presale revenue. Finally, no rule of thumb can encompass the wide variation of practices, modalities, facilities, specialties, geographic locations, economic situations, equipment availability and condition, staff training, and all the other intricacies of veterinary medicine.

Rules of thumb are observational statistics that report on averages of sales transactions that have already occurred. They are not predictors of future sales. Business value is affected by many different variables unrelated to revenue or EBITDA (Earnings Before Interest, Taxes, Depreciation, and Amortization), including financing terms, whether it is an asset sale or an equity sale, how long the seller will remain with the practice and how they will be compensated. Other factors that influence practice value are whether payment contracts with laboratory and imaging equipment will be assumed by the buyer, facility lease terms, staff turnover, and many other factors too numerous to mention.

Unfortunately, there are no shortcuts. Using shortcuts or rules of thumb are fraught with errors, misunderstandings, and a false belief in what may be inflated values. Determining a business' true value is complex and time consuming. The process can be overwhelming but relying on a rule of thumb to avoid due diligence is dangerous. Although rules of thumb are easy to apply, they should not be relied on for such a significant investment.

STANDARD OF VALUE

The purpose of the valuation also dictates the standard of value used. The standard of value reflects the type of valuation needed and for whom. These are as follows:

- Fair market value (FMV): The IRS defines the FMV as "the price at which the property would change hands between a willing buyer and a willing seller, when neither is under any compulsion to buy or to sell, and both having reasonable knowledge of relevant facts." Under the FMV standard, the value is based on a typical buyer or a typical seller in the market, rather than the investment needs of a specific buyer or seller. This value is often applicable to private transactions between a practice owner selling to a private buyer with conventional financing. This value often assumes that the buyer will be able to replicate the success of the practice as was experienced by the previous owner.
- Investment value: The primary difference between the FMV standard and the investment value standard is that the valuation reflects the needs of a specific buyer or seller. If either the buyer or seller were motivated to act based on criteria unique to them, the appropriate value would be investment value. For example, if the seller were moving out of state in 60 days, there might be urgency on their part to sell, and a lower price might be acceptable if the timeline was met. In another example, a buyer may be willing to pay more for a specific practice if it is in an area where they wish to live and have been searching for a practice to buy for an extended period.
- Strategic control value: The veterinary market contains many "atypical" buyers, specifically corporate consolidators. These buyers value veterinary practices according to their internal *investment value* standards and not the FMV standard. Furthermore, the amounts that corporate consolidators will pay include a

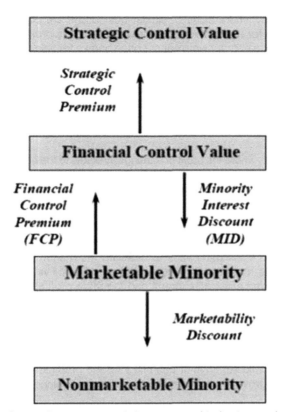

Fig. 1. Flowchart of control premiums and discounts used in business valuation.[7]

premium that reflects a "strategic control value"[7] rather than the typical financial control value for a private owner of a veterinary practice (**Fig. 1**).

The difference in the standard of value leads to much higher prices when corporate consolidators are the buyers. These values are not accurate representations of the FMV appropriate for a private veterinarian. Individuals do not have access to the same capital markets that the consolidators use and do not benefit from economies of scale that allow consolidators to dramatically reduce the cost of goods or the cost of employee benefits.

APPROACHES TO VALUE

The 3 approaches to value are as follows:

1. *Asset approach*, where the value of each physical asset is assessed, and the numbers added together. Because it does not consider intangible assets such as goodwill, the asset approach is rarely used as the primary valuation approach for veterinary practices. However, valuators may use it to establish a minimum value or use the results as a "sniff test" when assessing the value determined through a different approach. This approach can also be used when a practice is iquidating by selling the assets and not transferring goodwill.

2. *Market approach*, where sales of similar businesses are compared and used to develop a value for a given veterinary practice. This approach uses the principle of substitution, the primary way realtors price homes for sale. Realtors maintain databases of home sales information. By searching for recent sales prices of homes of the same size and condition with similar features in comparable neighborhoods, realtors assess what the target home is worth.

The market approach is more difficult to use with veterinary practices because sales information is private. At least 2 large veterinary practice brokers have proprietary sales databases but those are not normally available to valuators outside those brokerages.

3. *Income approach*, where the profit or earnings available to the buyer are quantified and capitalized (divided by a percentage that represents ownership risk). This is the most common approach used for businesses that generate most of their money through professional services as opposed to manufacturing or merchandise sales. Depending on the consistency of earnings, 2 different methods may be used, the capitalization of earnings/cash flow method, or the discounted earnings/cash flow method.

Because the asset approach does not include intangibles and few valuators have access to large sales databases to use with the market approach, the income approach is the most common approach to value for veterinary practices. The practice is viewed as an investment and the more profitable the investment, the higher the business value. Although medical and computer equipment can be costly, goodwill is often the most valuable business asset.

Under the income approach, the valuation analyst must make astute decisions concerning the following:

- The appropriate *capitalization rate* or *multiple* (see later discussion)
- The true economic earnings or cash flow for the practice
- The expected growth in the practice's economic earnings or cash flow

If any of these does not reflect the true nature of the business, the resulting value could be materially affected.

The income approach includes several different methods. The most common for veterinary practices are the single period capitalization method and the discounted cash flow method. Some valuators use the excess earnings method, which combines features from both the asset and income approaches. A discussion of each appears as follows:

Discounted cash flow (DCF): The DCF method values a business based on projections of how much money that investment will generate in the future. Those projections are then "discounted" to reflect the time value of money (TVM). The TVM concept holds that money today is worth more than the same amount of money in the future. There are several reasons for this. First, if invested, the money would earn interest. Second, inflation increases the price of goods and services over time, reducing purchasing power. For example, a US$100 gas card in January 2009, when gasoline was US$1.74 per gallon, would have been worth more than in June 2022 when the national average for a gallon of gas was US$5.00.[8] In 2009, the gas card would have purchased 57.5 gallons compared to 20 gallons in 2022.

The DCF method uses projections for a discrete time frame, usually 3 to 10 years, plus a "terminal value," a number that represents profits in perpetuity. Those figures are discounted and added together to determine the current business value. The largest concern when using DCF is the reasonableness of the financial forecasts. Ideally, the practice owner and their financial advisors and accountants develop forecasts for the valuator to use.

Single period capitalization (SPC): The SPC method determines business value by capitalizing profits generated by the entire pool of assets present in the business. The analyst adjusts historical results for 3 to 5 years and identifies which year or years offer the best representation of the future. Although the name "single period capitalization" suggests that only one period is included, the valuator may select 1 year or several years as proxies for the future.

SPC is essentially a simplified version of DCF where future earnings grow at a constant rate. Therefore, the SPC method is most appropriate for established veterinary practices with stable earning histories. When less history is available, such as for a start-up clinic, or where historical earnings do not represent the future, as with a move to a new location or the addition or loss of clinicians, the SPC method will not return a reasonable value. Instead, the DCF method is used.

Excess earnings: This model was developed in the 1920s to appraise closely held businesses where intangible assets represent a major component of the business value. The excess earnings method "artificially divides a company's earnings into two separate earnings streams: one for tangible assets and one for intangible assets. The problem is that these assets do not generate earnings by themselves. Rather, a company's earnings are derived from a combination of tangible and intangible assets working together."[9]

Two major shortcomings of the excess earnings method are as follows:

1. The method is highly dependent on accurate values for the tangible assets. The most accurate way to obtain these values is through hiring an equipment appraiser, which can add thousands of dollars in cost. Instead, the owners, their accountant, or the appraiser estimates value based on rules of thumb, depreciation schedules, or balance sheets. These are mere approximations of value that may or may not have much validity, and using such approximations can result in a significant misstatement of practice value.
2. There is neither an agreed upon capitalization rate for intangible assets alone nor is there an agreed upon method for determining that rate.

Until the late 1990s, excess earnings was the most common method used in veterinary practice valuations. Because the profession of business valuation has evolved and modernized, excess earnings is used much less frequently.

CALCULATING ADJUSTED EARNINGS

When the asset approach is the only method used, the valuation assessment is complete once the assets have been individually appraised. Under the income and market approaches, the valuator determines the most likely earnings available to a buyer.

When calculating earnings, the valuator must review the financial statements and federal income tax returns and make informed decisions about whether those reports reflect the future of the business. Tax preparers are educated about how to legally report the lowest income for the individuals and businesses they serve. The goal in tax preparation is to show the lowest possible income and thus reduce the income tax burden for their clients. A valuator must "normalize" the financial statements, removing the tax planning reflected in the financial statements and the owner's discretionary spending, to show the true profits of the veterinary hospital. Those profits are 50% of the valuation equation, so it is imperative that each adjustment made is appropriate to the individual practice.

Common adjustments include the following:

- Adding back depreciation and amortization expense and subtracting an allowance for equipment and facility reinvestment. The US tax laws provide businesses with the option to accelerate depreciation and "write off" equipment purchases long before the equipment becomes outdated or unusable. For valuation purposes, tax depreciation is replaced with an economic depreciation factor, which more accurately reflects a veterinary hospital's regular consumption and replacement of equipment and furnishings. This adjustment is most often a percentage of gross fees and reflects the nature and modality of the practice. A dermatology specialist, for example, requires less equipment than an orthopedic surgery specialty practice.

- Normalizing owner compensation: An owner may pay themselves however they wish. Ideally, their tax professional makes recommendations that reflect both business and personal tax planning. For a valuation, owner compensation will be adjusted to reflect what one or more third parties would be paid to carry out the same duties the owner performs. For example, for owner veterinarians, the valuator will determine what an unrelated veterinarian would be paid for the same position. When associates work in the practice, the owner's veterinary compensation is adjusted to what those associates are paid relative to the revenue they produce. Often this compensation is based on a percentage of the clinical production the owner generates.

Owners are also involved in the management of the business. Even when highly competent managers are in place, some responsibilities remain with the owners, such as performance reviews for employed doctors, strategic decisions related to the facility and equipment, or determining the manager's compensation and benefits package. For this management oversight, valuators often use a percentage of annual gross fees, from as little as one-fourth of 1% to as much as 4%. The owners should be paid the equivalent of what someone else would earn when performing the same duties.

- Facility rent: When the practice owner also owns the real estate on which the practice sits, facility rent will be set to an amount that provides the greatest tax benefit to both the veterinary hospital and the property-owning company. This rent may have little to no relation to fair market rent. If a decision has been made regarding what the rent will be in the future, the valuator will substitute that amount for rent. If not, the appraiser will estimate a fair market level of rent expense. This estimate is made easily if the property has been recently appraised. The annual fair market rent is within the range of 8% to 12% of the value of the building and property.
- Nonrecurring income/expense: These represent one-time events, such as money from the Paycheck Protection Plan (PPP) loans or economic impact disaster loans that were part of the US government's coronavirus taxpayer relief . An example of a nonrecurring expense might be either the accounting fees related to PPP loan forgiveness or the cost of the valuation itself. Nonrecurring income is subtracted, and nonrecurring expenses are added to earnings.
- Nonoperating income/expense: Again on advice from their tax preparer, some owners run expenses for their personal automobiles through the business. Although equine ambulatory, mixed animal, and house call practices require one or more vehicles to provide veterinary services, companion animal practices have no business reason for owning or maintaining vehicles. For the companion animal practices, vehicle expenses are added back to earnings.

This category of adjustments also includes business interest income and expenses if those will not continue after a sale.

- Discretionary expenses: Particularly in small businesses such as veterinary practices, the line between personal and business is easily crossed. Cell phone plans
for the hospital may include the owner's family members. Travel and meal expenses, office supplies, cable/Internet service, and repairs and maintenance accounts should be reviewed, and any personal expenses identified and adjusted.
Included in this category are health insurance premiums for the owner's family
members.

Care must be taken to adjust *only those things that will change after the valuation*. If
facility rent has been higher than the local market rate but will not be lowered in the
future, the expense should not be adjusted. The following example demonstrates
the difference between adjustments made for a 100% sale compared with those
made for a 20% associate buy-in (**Table 1**).

The only appropriate time to adjust COGS (Cost of Goods Sold) in a valuation is
when the owner has recorded personal expenses here. Even then, such expenses
must be clearly identified and easily quantified. It is never acceptable to adjust
COGS to levels seen in other veterinary hospitals, or to figures published by industry
sources. This type of adjustment results in overvaluing the business.

There are 2 ways to maximize practice value: maximizing profit and minimizing the
risk of owning the business. Most practice management consultants, owners, and
managers focus on maximizing profits through managing expenses. Other articles
address doing so in detail. One must understand that while expense management
is key, there is a limit to the degree to which expenses can be reduced before patient
care and client service are affected.

ESTIMATING RISK

Practice value is the interrelationship of profit and risk. A person buying a business is
purchasing the stream of future earnings the business will generate. Those earnings
will cover payments on the acquisition loan for the business itself and provide a return
to the owners beyond fair compensation for the work they perform in the business.
However, these earnings are never guaranteed.

Before making a commitment, investors evaluate the expected return on a potential
investment vehicle. Informed investors will require a higher potential rate of return for a
risky investment than they would require for a safer investment. Similarly, a buyer of a
veterinary hospital will be willing to pay a higher price for a stable business with less
risk than they would for an unstable or poorly performing business with more substantial risk.

Although the assessment of risk is more subjective than the adjustment of earnings,
there has been extensive research in the veterinary market to help guide valuators
when establishing capitalization rates. The Valuation Council of VetPartners has spent
more than 15 years studying, quantifying, and developing internal and external factors
that contribute to the risk of owning a veterinary practice.[10] Internal factors relate to
the situation within the practice, all of which are largely controllable by the owner.
External factors are those related to the environment within which the practice oper-
ates. Business owners cannot control these risks but can mitigate them to some
extent.

Internal Risk Factors

1. *Volatility of adjusted profitability*: When earnings are steady or increasing, there is
less risk to a buyer than when earnings are high in 1 year and low in the next. Unless
the volatility is easily explained and expected to level off, the buyer has no way to

Table 1
Controlling and noncontrolling adjustments to earnings

Adjustment	100% Asset Sale	20% Equity Sale
Depreciation/Amortization	Added	Added
Owner's compensation	Adjust to market rate	Must reflect how all owners will be paid after the buy-in
Associate compensation	No change	No change
Rent	Adjust to postsale amount	Adjust to postsale amount
Interest expense	Added *unless* the buyer is assuming a liability, like an equipment lease	No change. Interest continues because the liabilities remain with the practice
Discretionary travel	Added	Only if neither owner will charge personal travel to the business
Family cell phone plans	Added	Usually increased to include the new owner's family
Cost of goods sold	No change	No change

know what the following year holds. Will it be a year with average earnings? Will earnings fall to a low point? A practice with a consistent level of low earnings scores better on this factor than a hospital with higher earnings that fluctuate from year to year.

2. *Ability to effectively transfer goodwill*: This factor measures the risk related to the ability to continue operations after a sale. The practice's goodwill can be attached to the clinic as a whole or to specific individuals within the clinic. With large, multi-doctor clinics, the goodwill is much less likely to be tied to a particular owner and is less likely to be at risk when an owner departs. In contrast, the goodwill in a single-doctor practice is often directly tied to the owner and can create significant risk to the buyer when the owner is no longer at the hospital.

The less the clients care about the sale of the practice, the better it is for the buyer. The best scenario is when the seller has gradually reduced their schedule and the other doctors in the practice, including the buyer, have become well known to clients. If clients are concerned about who will be running the business after a sale, they are more likely to switch to another practice that might be closer to them. Solo doctors selling to someone outside the practice can use several methods to reassure both the clients and the buyer.

- Sellers should plan to remain with the practice for several months after the sale. Sellers can reduce their schedules but should remain visible for a while.
- Introduce the buyer to clients through a letter or email. Express appreciation for the trust pet owners have placed in the seller and the practice and clearly convey confidence that their pets will be well cared for.
- Tell the staff the same thing. They will be watching for signs that the buyer should not be trusted.

3. *Revenue growth*: On average, primary care practices grow 5% annually, through a combination of fee increases and gaining new clients. If revenue has not been growing, owners and managers should monitor whether the hospital is gaining more clients than it loses in a year, and ensure that the fee schedule is keeping up with the increasing costs of running the business. Are reductions in gross

income temporary and easily explained? For example, was a highly productive doctor out of the hospital for several months on parental leave or for a temporary disability?

4. *Quality of doctors and staff*: The number of credentialed veterinary nurses as well as if the manager is a Certified Veterinary Practice Manager[11] are indications of the quality of the employees working in the hospital. Are any of the doctors boarded? Do they have certifications for acupuncture or rehabilitation? Staff longevity also comes into play. In a hospital with high staff turnover, the clients may not develop strong connections to the practice. In contrast, practices where the employees demonstrate palpable pride in their employers are less likely to lose key employees in an ownership transition, provided the culture is not changed dramatically.

5. *Equipment and instrumentation* in the hospital, and its current condition. Some hospital owners who plan to retire in a year or two may stop investing in equipment to make the business seem more profitable. This decision will backfire if the buyer must replace or repair critical medical equipment or resurface the parking lot. Every dollar the buyer must invest in necessary equipment and maintenance is a dollar that cannot be spent on practice value.

External Risk Factors

1. *Local demographics*: The American Veterinary Medical Association (AVMA) publishes the AVMA Pet Ownership and Demographic Sourcebook with statistics that indicate which demographic factors influence pet and horse ownership as well as data on the number of pet owners needed to support a full-time veterinarian. (The most recent edition was published in May 2022.)

   There is little a business owner can do about the demographics of the area surrounding the veterinary hospital but management can ensure the practice reflects the ethnicity of the neighborhood. Do the doctors or staff speak a second language? Does the practice participate in local community and cultural events?

2. *Veterinary competitive environment*: This factor addresses the risk associated with the loss of clients to current or potential competing veterinary practices. Compare the services offered as well as the quality of medicine and client service to other practices in the area. The more the practice demonstrates its strengths to clients, through both actions and words, the more bonded clients will be to the practice.

3. *Facility lease terms*: Part of the value of the practice lies in the affordability of the facility lease. When the building is leased from an unrelated third party, the lease must be assignable to the new owner under the current or similar terms. Ideally, the lease has several renewal options remaining, and annual increases are within reason.

   If the practice owners also own the real estate and plan to keep it for rental income for a period, include a right of first refusal to the buyer. They want assurance that the property will not be sold to another buyer who may force the hospital to move.

4. *Marketability/desirability of practice type*: The most easily sold veterinary practice is a companion animal practice in an urban/suburban area. It is harder to find buyers for specialty, equine, or production practices because fewer veterinarians are trained and interested in that work. The location of the practice comes into play here, as well. Urban and suburban practices usually have plenty of interested buyers, whereas rural practices and those in up and coming or revitalized neighborhoods may take longer to sell.

Each of these factors influences the risk of owning a given veterinary practice. For veterinary hospital valuators, the most critical factors that come into consideration are the first 3 internal factors: volatility of earnings, ability to transfer goodwill to a buyer, and revenue growth. All of these are largely within the business' control. By monitoring and addressing changes in these factors in the years before a sale, the owners can maximize the sales price of their practice.

SUMMARY

A veterinary practice often represents the most valuable asset in a veterinarian's investment portfolio. This asset requires constant attention to grow into an asset that not only supports its owner and employees but also represents a highly valuable business the owner can sell. Practice owners must learn how to manage a profitable business and maintain that profitability throughout their ownership. However, profitability alone does not ensure a valuable business. Understand the factors that represent risk to a future buyer and take steps to mitigate them where possible. Practice owners should not wait until they wish to retire to determine the value of their investment. The hospital should be valued by a credentialed valuation professional every 3 to 5 years, more often as the owners approach retirement. If the value is not where the owners want or need it to be, there will be time to make improvements before a sale.

CLINICS CARE POINTS

- At some point, the business will not be able to further reduce expenses without sacrificing patient care or client service. The business must increase revenue to drive profits.
- The assumptions used in the valuation can significantly affect the results.
- A practice with a low level of consistent year-to-year earnings carries less risk than a practice with alternating levels of high and low earnings.

DISCLOSURE

The author has nothing to disclose.

REFERENCES

1. NACVA Professonal Standards. Available at: https://www.nacva.com/Files/NACVA_Professional_Standards_Effective_06-01-23.pdf.
2. NACVA- National Association of Certified Valuators and Analysts. Available at: https://www.nacva.com/.
3. ASA- American Society of Appraisers. Available at: https://www.appraisers.org/.
4. AICPA- American Institute of Certified Professional Accountants. Available at: https://www.aicpa-cima.com/.
5. IRS- Internal Revenue Service. Available at: https://www.irs.gov/faqs/small-business-self-employed-other-business/entities/entities-5.
6. International Glossary of Business Valuation Terms. Available at: http://web.nacva.com/TL-Website/PDF/Glossary.pdf.
7. Christopher Mercer Z, Harms Travis W. Business valuation: an integrated theory. 3rd Edition. Wiley Finance Series; 2021. pg. 37.
8. Gas Prices December 2022: Latest Winners And Losers From Recent Gas Price Trends. Available at: https://www.forbes.com/sites/qai/2022/12/02/gas-prices-december-2022-latest-winners-and-losers-from-recent-gas-price-trends/?sh=5dc3fd5c76ad.

9. The excess earnings method: When is it appropriate? Available at: https://www.cshco.com/articles/the-excess-earnings-method-when-is-it-appropriate/#:~:text=The%20excess%20earnings%20method%20artificially,t%20generate%20earnings%20by%20themselves.
10. VetPartners. Available at: https://www.vetpartners.org/Practice-Valuation-Resources/.
11. The Certified Veterinary Practice Manager (CVPM) credential by Veterinary Hospital Managers Association (VHMA). Available at https://www.vhma.org/home.

FURTHER READINGS

Valuation Essentials for Veterinarians. Available at: https://www.vetpartners.org/wp-content/uploads/2018/10/Val-Essntl-for-Vets-2017-version-10.pdf.

AVMA Pet Ownership and Demographic Sourcebook https://ebusiness.avma.org/ProductCatalog/product.aspx?ID=2050.

Caruso GR. The art of business valuation, accurately valuing a small business. Hoboken (NJ): John Wiley & Sons, Inc; 2020.

Top Veterinary Practice Issues that Negatively Affect Culture, Retention, and Performance

Jeffrey R. Sanford, MBA[a],*, Richard M. DeBowes, DVM, MS, DACVS[b]

KEYWORDS

- Leadership • Community • Attracting • Talent • Discounting • Change • Inflation
- Inventory

KEY POINTS

- The absence of leadership is the greatest problem in practice destroying culture, employee retention, patient care, value, and growth.
- Across the country, practices are experiencing a drop in patients and invoices due mostly to the patient shift from wellness to urgent care.
- Price inelasticity was also overestimated as fees increased significantly across the country with no correlation in value.
- Attracting and retaining talent is dependent on creating a great work environment including fostering a sense of community and friendships at work.
- Discounting and expansive inventories cut a practice's ability to maintain earnings while payroll increased.

PROBLEM: THE NEED FOR LEADERSHIP
Explanation

General Patton once said, "An army is like spaghetti. You can't push a piece of spaghetti, you got to pull it." Deficits in directional leadership do exist in most practices. Most of the following issues are evidence of weak leadership. With full medical curriculums, veterinarians are generally not exposed to leadership training as part of their medical education. In practice, few recognize anything beyond positional leadership as the default for being the owner, veterinarian, practice manager, or lead technician. Working too much "in" their practice instead of "on" their practice, few with essential

[a] University of Georgia College of Veterinary Medicine, Office of Academic Affairs, 501 D.W. Brooks Drive, Athens, GA 30602, USA; [b] Clinical Communication, Leadership and Practice Management, Washington State College of Veterinary Medicine, PO Box 647010, Pullman, WA 99164-7010, USA
* Corresponding author.
E-mail address: jsanford@uga.edu

Vet Clin Small Anim 54 (2024) 423–440
https://doi.org/10.1016/j.cvsm.2023.10.014
0195-5616/24/© 2023 Elsevier Inc. All rights reserved.

management responsibilities realize the importance of leadership in providing their people daily and even longer more strategic direction. Additionally, many practice "leaders" are blind to their own leadership styles, depending on context, can inspire or demoralize their people.

We recently visited a practice that had a hard time keeping staff and did not grow during the pandemic. Oblivious to the owner but obvious to the staff was the owner's controlling behavior and her habit of yelling at staff when problems arose. Despite the owner stating she deeply cared about her people, her lead registered veterinary technician said they had to walk on eggshells around the owner. If a practice is not growing, and doctors and staff are stressed and "burned-out," or staff are just quitting, leadership is generally the issue. This void of leadership is being compounded by the corporate accumulators where previous owners have left the practice or have become disengaged. Instead of determining what is proper and right for each practice, I hear many in corporate leadership focus too much on increasing production and assessing elasticities with price increases. Having little regard to the vision and purpose of a practice in providing direction, many of these practices are producing subpar, losing people, revenues, invoices, and patients.

How to Change This

Many have said leaders are "born" and not made. The authors disagree. To lead, one must be able to connect with people, motivate them with common beliefs, and inspire a sense of ownership.[1] The authors believe leadership building in the profession starts with veterinary schools: (1) recruiting students with past leadership experience; (2) providing leadership mentorship at the colleges; (3) provide scholarships/awards for those that volunteer for leadership positions; (4) integrate leadership elements though out new required curriculums; and (5) provide outside leadership experiences that encourages self-awareness, critical thinking, communication, and team building.

Too often traits for leadership are confused with the traits of those that do great technical work. This fallacy is described in Michael Gerber's and Peter Weinsteins' book, *The E-Myth Veterinarian*. A great veterinarian or a great technician might be great at what they do but typically lack the training, skill sets and tools needed to be a great manager and leader. Considering the importance of leadership to a practice, leadership education must become just as important in practices as updates on new pharmaceuticals or training in new therapeutic techniques.

True leadership is the foundation for practice success as it provides a vison and direction for the entire team, supports proactive behaviors, and determines and celebrates success. We believe true mentoring for leadership must begin with 1 root question, "What can we do to make sure this employee and possible future leader is a success in this practice?" A proactive approach to mentoring and training every teammate with the tools required for leadership is essential to practice culture and the attainment of optimal medical, professional, and financial outcomes by the practice.

PROBLEM: THE NEED FOR BETTER CULTURE
Explanation

According to the 2020 Census of Veterinarians[2] and 2022 American Veterinary Medical Association Report of the Economic State of the Veterinary Profession,[3] poor work culture is 1 of the key reasons for veterinarians wanting to leave the profession. Of those thinking of leaving, 47% gave poor work culture as the reason. Over the years, college surveys of alumnae show 30% of new graduates change employers within their first year of working. Based on calls we receive from them; poor culture is a core reason for leaving an employer.

The organizational culture of any practice is the collective mindset of its team members, typically centered on what values the owner and practice believe are important; what evidence clients see of the practice team caring for their pets and for them; and the overall "secret sauce" for maintaining a healthy work environment and its competitive advantage. The pandemic has shifted the culture for many practices, from a more organized, wellness-oriented practice toward the more spontaneous nature of urgent care. This urgent care mindset has changed the nature and closeness of relationships between the client and the healthcare team. Most practices saw their urgent care cases double and even triple in the past 3 years. Regular, routine healthcare appointments were canceled or postponed in deference to only handling cases that 'needed' to be seen. This was exacerbated with general practices (GPs) scheduling 20 to 30-min appointments. Team members saw themselves as overworked and variably demoralized by the backup of surgical and procedural waiting lists. This workload shift, combined with a lack of leadership and an inadequate investment in culture, created the perfect storm for poor cultures in many practices. Because of this patient compliance, client retention, successful recruitment and onboarding, and overall practice wellness suffers in a practice.

How to Change This

To manage culture, it is essential for leadership to understand that the motivation, inclination, and performance of their team is a direct result of their level of engagement and commitment to a shared raison d'etre; a "Why" statement. That galvanizing 'Why' is the main reason employees choose to work where they work. It is important for employees to believe that they make valuable contributions at work, that they feel needed and make a difference at their practice. When we visit practices, too often we hear what is wrong with employees including their mistakes, their bad attitudes or poor work ethic. We don't hear enough of what people are doing right. To move this mindset, leadership has to guide behavior using a set of core values, collaboratively developed, agreed by all, and illustrated by good work and reviews. These behavior guardrails should be reaffirmed at the beginning of every meeting and illustrated by recent examples of great behaviors and successes displayed by veterinarians and staff. "Shout outs" for great work and behavior are critical for practice culture and wellness. Supporting and illustrating values allows teammate to be able to see, feel, and embrace that culture which sets their behavior and contributes to their individual and collective sense of fulfillment.

In a practice where the culture has developed organically and without intentionality, the relationships, the level of engagement, and the work product outcome vary considerably, often as the result of who is working on any given day. Culture is NOT a moving target! As the collective mindset of the group, it is how people work together in a practice to meet the various challenges of the day while honoring our agreement as to how we would work together in pursuit of our 'Why'. For a practice or any service group to be successful they must set time aside to focus on what they do and how they see their work. With core values serving as the principle cornerstone of the practice, they set behaviors that become obvious to any client who observes their actions, behaviors, and communications.

PROBLEM

A lack of a 'cohesive community' in the veterinary workplace is adversely affecting the completeness of medical care and the client experience, while negatively impacting employee retention and recruitment.

Explanation

Community building in the workplace is getting more attention with the current labor shortage. Current research found that 65% of people didn't feel any sense of community at their place of work.[4] Scott Galloways, *Adrift: America in 100 Charts*, illustrates a steady decline in a person's sense of community leading to a problem of rising isolation and loneliness. He demonstrates this with a decrease in church attendance, participation in Boy Scouts and Girl Scouts as well as the change from movie theaters to Netflix, shopping malls to Amazon, playing outside to playing computer games.[5] Cigna reports 52% of Americans are lonely. Veterinarians are no exception. Due to these trends, we believe many employees don't want their workplace to be just a place to earn a paycheck; instead, they are seeking a sense of belonging, a sense of community where they work. This is evidenced by Gallup's recent findings around friendships at work.[6] The importance of having a friend at work has grown greatly over the past decade. Furthermore, data show that when employees have a close friend at work, they are less likely to leave their employers.

Furthermore, Gallup engagement data suggest that employee engagement in the workplace is dropping at noteworthy rates. Engagement dropped from 2020 levels of 36% to 34% in 2021 and down to 32% in 2022. At the same time, actively disengaged employees increased from their 2020 levels of 14% to 16% in 2021 and 17% in 2022.[7] The consequences of team member disengagement to a veterinary practice are considerable and few practices seem to be aware of the risks they face. Beyond the difficulty and costs of finding, recruiting, and retaining team members; patient care, compliance, medical outcomes, and revenue generation are all at peril as fewer numbers of people are actively engaged. If the healthcare team exists merely as a work group and not as a team whose hallmarks are a commitment to a shared goal, guided by shared values and whose primary strength is the synergy they demonstrate through their collaboration, their value to the practice will be markedly limited.

How to Change This

When people had a sense of community at work, 58% reported thriving at work, 55% were more engaged, and 66% were more likely to stay with their organization.[4] Overall, they were experiencing less stress and were far more likely to reach a better work/life balance. How does a veterinary practice build a sense of community? First, we believe this process begins by having a good culture with common beliefs and values as before described. Second, we believe a practice must work on building open communications within your team by really giving each employee their "voice" within a practice. This can be accomplished using several different approaches including one-on-one check-ins to find out how an employee is doing, what they want to accomplish and what leadership can change or provide support; daily rounds where employees can give their input on tackling the day's schedule; weekly meetings to praise successes, set direction and tasks, and ensure meaningful connections with people are made.

If used properly, communications and a sense of community can be greatly enhanced using technologies such as Slack or BlueNote. Here is a short string over 15 minutes at 1 practice.

5:15pm- Savannah and Ellie killed it today as far as handling appointments and schedule with no complaints. I appreciate you guys.

5:45pm Thank you AT for helping me get a cysto on 1 dog and attempting rad on another -crazy cat.

5:20pm. No complaints—well done!

5:54 Way to go KP for doing her first blocked cat just before closing!!!!
5:55 Yep, I witnessed it.

Third, practice leadership should be creating mutual learning experiences. Naturally, many would be thinking of medical learning. While good and necessary, we want to think outside the veterinary box. Bond Vet, a DeNovo chain in the Northeast, often holds cooking classes for employees and new recruits. We think another fun approach would be to find expertise within your practice and have employees teach their skill. We have heard of sewing classes, drink making, and wrapping presents perfectly. Beyond learning experiences, we also believe practices should encourage shared activities outside of work. We have seen employees take on these activities such as book clubs, baseball games, kickball with their significant others, yoga, escape rooms, massages, etc. Shared memories from past positive activities and events can help enhance culture, build a sense of community, and sustain morale. *"Nostalgia can help counteract anxiety and loneliness, encourage people to act more generously toward one another, and increase resilience."*[4]

Dr. John Younker, owner of Common Companion Vet Co-a high growth DeNovo practice in Atlanta, stated, *"It was not until my people really knew that I cared about them that my problems with recruiting and retaining doctors and staff virtually disappeared."* This reminds me of the quote made famous by Theodore Roosevelt, "People don't care how much you know until they know how much you care."[8] Dr. Younker hired 7 doctors and even more staff in the past 2 years with little posting or advertising for positions. Common Companion has a great buzz for being a great place to work. In fact, employees are driving most recruitment now, wanting to work with those they know that have the same values and beliefs. Additionally, Dr. Younker uses engagement surveys and one-on-one sessions to get valuable feedback from his people. Most important is addressing the issues and suggestions provided by employees. Leadership can ruin trust quickly if employee issues are not addressed quickly. For example, Dr. Younker received feedback that his employees were tired of going home late, well after closing. After meeting with doctors and staff to discuss the issue, the practice collectively decided to stop urgent care at 4:00 PM and wellness at 5:00 PM so that everyone can finish their tasks, discharge their patients, and leave the practice by 6. Not only did he support a sense of community in determining the right course of action, but he also claimed this 1 step improved morale, culture, and overall wellness of the practice.

A word of caution, mature practices with older veterinarians and staff might have to work especially hard to be relevant to new grads and younger employees. Regardless of how great a practice is with their culture, communications, and sense of community, we have worked with several older practices with older doctors and staff that had difficulty retaining younger veterinarians and technicians. Think about it. If you were 25 and a new veterinarian, would you want to work in a practice where everyone was at least 20 to 30 years your senior? The long game for these older practices and a caution for younger practices is to keep relevant not with just the medicine but also by the age of employees.

PROBLEM

It may be that owners and medical directors are expecting too much from high-salaried, newly hired associates.

Explanation

Recently, I spoke to an owner who wanted to tell me how awful her new associate hire was. "She has no resilience, no grit, and runs away from conflict," she stated and went on to complain that she was overpaying this new graduate with $110,000 and benefits. I asked the owner to describe how the new doctor was on-boarded their first day. The owner stated that this person was scheduled for 14 appointments. The owner also made herself available to answer any questions throughout the day. I asked, "Over the past 10 months how many hours have you spent developing medical competence and confidence with this new hire." She stated, "about 10 to 15 hours." I further asked, "How many hours has the new hire been trained on leadership, teambuilding, communications, and resiliency? She stated none. "Did you give her your best technician to work with her the first couple of weeks so she could figure out what was expected?" "No," she responded quickly, "she is my technician!" After hearing this, I told her a saying my father was quite fond of, "Grass is greenest where it is watered—you need to get watering." While this is an extreme example, we hear owners and medical directors voicing similar complaints about the high base pay and high signing bonuses even for the inexperienced newer graduates.

Market pressures have rightly increased associate starting pay. Personal experience with new graduate employment agreements suggests that many new graduates have total compensation packages more than $150,000. In a recruitment frenzy, some are offering 6 figure signing/commitment bonuses. Students coming out of school are under considerable pressure to generate revenue or face a reduction in their base compensation. Few new graduates have the clinical experience and the communication competence to meet these expectations. Many practices are discovering that they need to develop individualized intense, focused, on-boarding, and mentoring programs to make up for this lack of key experiences that are essential for professional and financial success in private practice. When the pressure gets to be overwhelming and/or the production becomes difficult or impossible, students find that they need to seek employment in a different environment.

How to Change This

First thing! Ditch your narration of, "when I took my first job 10, 20, 30, 40 years ago...." Talking about how great and resourceful you were when you started despite no real mentoring will get you no closer to understanding the needs of your new graduate hire. Begin your understanding by objectively looking at the typical experience of most new graduates. In their efforts to get accepted into appropriate colleges and veterinary schools, most worked hard focusing on grades rather than meaningful work experiences. National labor statistics show 16 to 19-year-olds employment has dropped from 50% in 1990 to 25% in 2010.[9] While technically competent, preparation for GP/urgent work is often deficient at most veterinary colleges working their 4th year under specialists, residents, and interns. Many graduating with only having done half of a spay unless they were fortunate to have a rotation at a spay-neuter clinic. So, after 4 years of high school, 4 years of college, and 4 years of vet school, many graduates have little recent work experience and most graduate with incomplete understanding of GP/ER care. With this in mind, leadership should really reframe their onboarding, literally considering their new hire's 4th year GP/urgent care education as their first year working in the practice.

One of the major problems we have with employment contracts is their limitations in scope with mostly informing a new hire what they are required to do and what activities they are restricted from doing. In these contracts, where are the practice's promises in supporting the new hire and assuring their path in achieving success? New graduates come to an employing practice filled with knowledge, potential and enthusiasm. They too are often overwhelmed, and most have fears of fitting in and overcoming their imposter syndrome. It is essential that they feel looked after and cared for as a valued team member. We believe the practice's "promise" for the success of the new hire should be understood by everyone in the practice. Acceptance and legitimate validation can help build confidence and ultimately resilience, a key attribute amongst successful clinicians.

We believe mentoring is an overused word and a misunderstood concept. Some veterinarians believe mentoring refers negatively as employee "hand-holding" while others believe passively the availability of experienced veterinarians to answer questions. Mentoring often fails in practice because there is a lack of leadership support, a lack of staff willingness to work with new hires, no clear plan with understood objectives and goals, no budget for DVM time and production flexibility, and poor organization with weak communication of a mentoring plan.[10] Overall, new hires do not want hand holding and they also don't want to feel as if they are inconveniencing veterinarians with questions. Overall, what they want is a plan! A plan for onboarding with dedicated time and support; a plan determined by both the new hire and the practice to build competence and confidence with exams, diagnostics, treatment, and surgery. They want guidance in understanding practice values and expected behavior as well as joining your special practice community.

Overall, a new employee's value to a practice will be dependent on successful onboarding. Not to be confused with orientation, onboarding encompasses everything required to acclimate a new team member to a workplace community. Research shows 69% of employees are more likely to stay with a company for 3 years if they experienced successful onboarding. Those with a consistent onboarding process experienced 50% greater new-hire productivity.[11]

Fundamental to successful onboarding is selecting the right candidate for your practice to begin with. Through behavioral interviewing techniques, determine if a candidate is a solid match for the practice's mission and value beliefs as well as fitting in with your practice community. Though we understand the need to fill positions, we strongly recommend working interviews lasting more than just a day or 2 to evaluate a potential candidate. If you are unsure of what behaviors that need to be identified, we recommend reading Patrick Lencioni's book, *The Ideal Team Player*. Lencioni identifies 3 behavior traits that identify "an ideal team player": (1) They are *humble*; demonstrate by putting the needs of the team above themselves; (2) They are *hungry*; demonstrated by a strong work ethic and a need to grow; (3) They are *people smart*; demonstrated by emotional intelligence in understanding people and how words and actions to bring out the best in others.[12]

PROBLEMS: PRACTICES CAN'T FIND OR ATTRACT GOOD TALENT
Explanation

Though some believe there are enough veterinarians graduating from veterinary colleges, most practices are having trouble attracting and retaining talent. Rural areas have an even harder challenge. Currently, well over 13,000 job postings for veterinarians are listed on the site Indeed. Probably many more are posted on association and college sites. Mental health, work/life balance and practice culture were key reasons for veterinarians wanting to leave the profession. According to recent research, job postings have around a 14% success rate in attracting professional talent.[13]

How to Change This

For those that have great success in attracting and retaining talent, we found the following.

A. Priority #1. Make sure the practice is a great place to work. See the 4 points mentioned earlier! Set practice and individual boundaries. Pay attention to doctor and staff stress. Research suggests that burnout is directly due to poor work environment and excessive production expectations.

B. "Your Network Is Your Net Worth;" very true today. Ten years ago, every available DVM job had 5 to 10+ veterinary candidates applying: today new graduates mostly limit their options to 3 to 5+ practices. According to the research mentioned before, acquaintances make up 75% of all professional job placements. Much like the 6° of separation from Kevin Bacon, networks have become the critical driver for finding talent. The challenge for most is that personal networks typically get smaller over time. Imperative for network health is to get out there! Get visible! Meet new people by joining organizations, going to meetings, getting active with veterinary colleges and technician schools, etc.

Also expand your network with social media. We recently saw a fantastic example of this when I took 8 students and the owners of a successful practice out for dinner. During dinner 1 of the owners was taking fun pictures while the other was asking if the students would like to join their Instagram. After dinner, everyone received gift bags with a thank you note and lots of practice swag including a sweatshirt and mug filled with energy bars, The pictures of the dinner went out that night and 62 veterinary students saw the post the next day. Remember 80% of new grads join practices that they know. The practice had a buzz on campus.

C. Optics are important. Make sure your website has been updated. Your site will likely be the first place a job seeker will go to check out a practice. Update your website with professionally taken photos and videos; keep away from stock puppy and kitten photos. Also hire a professional to update content including a career page where you can promote positions and externships. If you plan to post, hire a professional that knows how to differentiate you on job posting boards. Remember, it is not about the practice; most job seekers do not care how many medical toys the practice has. They want to know if they could "fit in" and what path is available for their success. With loneliness a real concern, many are also thinking how they would fit in with your practice, where would they live and what quality of life activities could they do outside the practice. On your website and job postings, provide job seekers a narration making it easy to see them working at your practice.

D. Externships are fantastic opportunities to recruit. This could be a challenge; most schools have no system to match students with practices. Often, externships are based on word of mouth with those who had a great experience. Third year students often investigate by asking 4th years. In 2022, 15 students at University of Georgia College of Veterinary Medicine participated in veterinary emergency group externships. Based on their exceptional experience, all wanted to become a "veggie" but only 11 were offered employment. Including the learning goals of the student, make an experience that would create a great experience, meet the recruiting goals for you and generates a buzz back on their campus. As Bonnie Rait sings, "Let's give them something to talk about."

PROBLEM

Over the course of the pandemic, practices have shifted their focus from 1 of family practice and wellness to 1 of urgent care or emergency medicine.

Explanation

According to VetWatch, revenues are up collectively for practices across the country; however, invoices are down, and client/patients are down.[14] A review of practice visited by us over the past 2 years shows a decrease in yearly/wellness visits from 70%-80% of all visits to 40%-50% of all visits. While practices experienced higher ACTs and revenues with more urgent care; on the other hand, most experienced drops in revenues for wellness services including fecals, heartworm test (HWT), vaccines, dentals, prevention and diets. This year we witnessed 3 practices where rabies coverage dropped to less than 30% of patients. Stacking urgent cases back-to-back, especially with GP scheduling with 20 and 30 minute appointments, puts a lot of pressure on veterinarians and staff. With employees stressed and overworked, the industry experienced a great resignation and shortage.

We believe many practices experienced a change in practice behavior in what we call the "ER effect." Starting with curbside services, practices found efficiency examining and treating animals in the treatment area or in examination rooms without the owner present. With this efficiency, some practices achieved levels of medical revenues far exceeding their examination room capacities. At the same time, most practices experienced increased urgent care invoices as a response to the pandemic. Anecdotally, many say they experienced a puppy explosion in their practices while at the same time they noticed clients, staying home due to the pandemic, were much more sensitive to pet changes. During the pandemic, most practices prioritized urgent care cases as they: (1) split staff into 2 or more shifts to protect and to assure the practice remained open. (2) experienced greater volume of patients, as other practices stop accepting new patients, had excessive waiting periods, or were closed due to the pandemic. In fact, many "open" practices had clients driving great distances over 2 hours not wanting to wait to be seen. And (3) experienced veterinarian and staffing shortages.

So, when practices reach a level of urgent care more than 40%-50% of all examinations, we believe a shift happens in practice behavior where doctors and staff maintain an urgent care rhythm or a reactive way of doing care throughout the day. While blood laboratories and pharmaceuticals improved in most practices, intentional recommendations for wellness services suffered. While the "one and done" of urgent care can be appealing for veterinarians, we worry about the long-term implications for many GP practices, especially with so many competing resources having entered the market such as Chewy, Walmart, Vetster, Pawp, and Dutch-most offering convenient telemedicine options.

This "ER affect" also adversely impacts client bonding and client retention to the practice. First, we have witnessed clients with wellness appointments being inconvenienced with long waits when doctors and staff prioritize urgent care visits over their appointments. Second, we have witnessed many doctors still wanting their patients to be examined in treatment, only performing the request of clients collected by the technician. Even if care is performed in examination rooms, the "ER affect" creates a pattern where efficiency is still prioritized over effectiveness. Recommendations become suggestions with little client education or client understanding. Additionally, forward scheduling is less of a priority. With wellness not a primary focus, forward scheduling was frequently dismissed, and reminder systems failed. Client retention falls with many clients not given a reason to return. Before the pandemic, we saw client and patient retention between 80%-90%. Today, many of those same practices are seeing only 50%-60% of their clients and patients returning. While some practices may see the drop in invoices and patients as a needed break, the concern for the near future is the sustainability of future revenues with the higher urgent care mix, the diminished experience by wellness appointments, and the elasticity of higher fees.

How to Change This

Going forward, veterinary business models are unlikely to look like they did just 5 years ago. Urgent care facilities have sprung up and thrived during the COVID pandemic. Many presenting complaints that were handled routinely pre-Covid by general practices were referred to specialty practices, emergency rooms, or urgent care facilities. Furthermore, providers offering 24/7 access to a veterinarian such as Chewy and other telemedicine companies are filling in for wellness where GP practices are failing. This redirection of clients to other providers, particularly established clients, weakens the relationship between the historical provider and their established clients.

To protect practice health, we believe most practices should start becoming much more intentional with the type of medicine offered rather than the current reactional way of practicing, many trying to be all things to all people. This process begins by determining a practice's identity, basically who they are and who they want to be (get pumped about this and listen to Roger Daltrey belting out "Who are you!") Before determining its position, a practice may want to objectively assess the practice and its competitive environment using a strengths, weaknesses, opportunities, and threats analysis—strengths and weaknesses being internal conditions within your control and opportunities and threats relating to external conditions from which a practice must position. Additionally, a practice must take a hard look at how the practice conducts itself with clients and patients. Over the past 3 years, many new workflow and communication habits and behaviors were formed which may counter efforts in creating a universally accepted identity. According to researchers, a person can develop a new habit between 18–254 days, and it takes an average of 66 days for a new behavior to become automatic.[15] Know that if a practice wants to be something different in the future, it must achieve acceptance, provide training, monitor progress, and celebrate results.

If a practice decides to get back to basics and grow back wellness care instead of rolling the dice that urgent care will replace increasing lapsed patients ever year, we recommend becoming more intentional and taking control of wellness. This begins with generating and monitoring 3 basic reports, (1) a compliance report which evaluates wellness coverage for the total number of patients; (2) monthly tracking of the quantity of wellness services (HWT, fecal, dental, rabies, etc.) compared to wellness visits; (3) Client/Patient retention report. Compliance with total patients will be low if retention is low. This may also be indicative that the culture and practice behavior has not changed to the targeted practice identity. We actually had a client increase her practice 7 figures in 18 months when the practice became more intentional toward wellness care by generating these reports. The key to these reports is to set practice goals and to raise awareness for doctors and staff. Have you ever noticed that most high growth DeNovo practices focus greatly on wellness?

Once you define who you are and become more intentional with your medicine, the next step is to refine the client experience to fit your practice's identity and to make sure appointments are geared for intended results. This overall process is what we call Appointment Mapping. Typically facilitated by a trained moderator, the session starts with each team member writing down what tasks are required for an ideal appointment and which team member is responsible for getting those tasks done-reception, technician, and veterinarian. When everyone shares their "map" of an appointment, we typically see differences in what tasks are required, when tasks should be done, and often see conflicts on who is responsible—many assuming others were handling a task. Once we identify gaps in perception, it is imperative to really map out an appointment as a team. We recommend writing out individual tasks on individual sheets and tape them to a wall or large surface. Collectively, the team agreed to what should be done and who is responsible. We recommend mapping different types of appointments—puppy, wellness, sick/urgent, emergency, etc. This process can also be used to introduce new services or pharmaceuticals into the practice.

The next step is to create another layer on the appointment map(s) adding what needs to be said or asked and by whom. Important to this process is to bring in expertise that can guide with examples of what works at other practices or other resources that can. Once everyone agrees with the map, it is time to get busy putting words into action. It is often said that repetition is the mother of all learning. Expect some inefficiencies while learning to be more effective with your appointments. As you repeat the ideal over and over, efficiency will follow.

Working on the aforementioned will set in motion efforts to support the practice's vision and values creating a path for the future of your practice. Typically, practices that know who they are, are directed by a common belief and values system, and have a great culture and sense of community, tend to be more consistent, attract the right type of clients for their practice, become a magnet for the best talent, and perform financially at a much high level.

PROBLEM

Practices have increased fees considerably without increasing value.

Explanation

Remember the outrage over an $8 carton of eggs? Inflation, especially with gas, groceries, clothing, and travel hit people hard across this country and all over the world. For veterinary practices, operational cost generally increased; however, labor costs rose the greatest, especially with the shortage of veterinarians and technicians. Practices that had combined or total labor cost around 35% of revenues saw these cost increase in excess of 40% in less than a year. In response to the rising operational costs over the past 18 months and to also increase the profitability, we witnessed practices generally raising prices from 10% to 30%. Some chose to raise fees over time and others did it all at once.

One must think about the elasticity of demand for veterinary services, especially considering revenues are up for most practices but most practices also have dropping invoices, particularly with wellness care. I saw a meme on Facebook, it read, "I don't often brag of my expensive trips, but I just returned home from the vet." Like $8 eggs, many are looking for the change in the value proposition when fees increased. With so many practices putting their energies to be more efficient rather being more effective, I wonder if clientele are confused by the optics or the total lack of appropriate messaging?

This is very true when many veterinarians seemed all too happy to avoid direct interaction with the client and instead, focus on their happy spot—the patient. Despite the end social distancing for most, we still see some veterinarians still engaged in curbside service and many more who became accustomed to working at a distance from their clients, performing physical examinations in their treatment areas and essentially performing services on patients away from the pet owner. This trend greatly diminishes the value of the veterinarian and the client experience by eliminating the opportunity to educate clients by contemporaneously sharing with the client, the results of the physical examination. With 20%-30% increases in fees (like $8 eggs), clients are wondering what they are paying for. With a lack of understanding, a client's perception is that vet med has seemingly become 'all about the money', especially with high invoices and a lack of clear direction from their doctor as to what would be in the best interest of their pet.

How to Change This

The 2 most common pricing models in veterinary medicine is market pricing and cost-based pricing. Market pricing typically involves getting a staff member on the phone to call competitive or similar practices and find commonly paid fees for a specific service. Some vendors and private services can also provide this service. Basing fees on this assumes that all practices are comparable and undifferentiated. Mostly used with pharmaceuticals, cost-based pricing determines the fee by adding the cost of a pharmaceutical or service and adding an appropriate profit margin. Easy to do for pharmaceuticals, much more difficult for veterinary services when trying to determine total cost including labor, facility, supply, equipment, and overhead.

With increased competition from Chewy and Walmart and their efforts to commoditize veterinary services putting downward price pressure on pharmaceuticals and veterinary services, in the face of the shortage of veterinary and technician talent drive up costs for veterinary services. It is no wonder why mass merchandisers and large corporations want a midlevel veterinary position. Overall, we don't think competing with Chewy on price will be a rewarding strategy. Instead, a practice may want to adopt an alternative pricing model to reflect the specific approach the practice uses to build and capture value for its service. Points to remember in determining value pricing: (1) What is the probability the practice can consistently deliver the expected experience or benefit for the charges? The lower the likelihood, the lower the price. (2) What is the emotional impact of the service the team provides? Higher impact, higher charge. (3) What is the client's ability to pay what the practice is charging? This requires understanding the area demographics and the target clientele. Special note: Some clients, no matter what their ability to pay is, will not accept value pricing.

Overall, the client expectations and experience are paramount to the value proposition tied to practice charges. Think of the practice experience as a series of touchpoints. Evaluating touchpoints involves not only what people see and hear but also what they smell and feel. Reviewing these touchpoints, what do you want clients/patients to think, feel and do? Really watch and evaluate the client experience. Based on this, does the experience fully justify the rise in fees and the full charge on an invoice? To justify fees, every team member should have an understanding of the cost to perform services and also understand the value proposition to support the profit margins. Team members will sabotage charges by either not making recommendations and discounting, or dropping charges when value is misunderstood. A training investment would be critical if this is likely.

For many owners, wellness care beyond vaccines has become fairly expensive. Yearly examinations, laboratories, prevention, vaccines, dentals, and diets can be well over $1,000. This can be challenging for many pet owners. For the future, we think it will become more imperative to equip the practice with financial options to ease the financial burden for clients including insurance, financing, and wellness plans. Ideally, a practice would have a "finance" person who was well versed with options and would help clients with which option was best for them.

PROBLEM

Discounting fees in practices is seemingly commonplace.

Explanation

Discounting, both intentional as well as unintentional, has always been a challenge in veterinary medicine. Healthcare team members enjoy their role as caring care providers, but many find the fee for service paradigm to be stressful and often undesirable. In their effort to be liked by them or at least avoid upsetting them, many look for ways to keep the medical invoice as affordable as possible. The most popular ways to lower charges are to discount, drop the charge, or find a lower cost fee option. In our experience, veterinarians and staff will discount invoices over a year totaling 3% to 5% of revenues. We know of 1 practice that gave away over $600,000.00 in 1 year by regularly downgrading to the lower cost examinations and allowing any staff member to adjust charges. At this practice we noticed 1 invoice was discounted 3 times from discharge to check out, from $260 to $95.

Recently, we were at a practice with 3 older male doctor owners that all discounted, each doctor had an average ACT around $140. They brought in a new graduate associate whose average transaction was over $220 within her first year. Being seen as the expensive doctor, the associate asked if she could discount like the other doctors. They denied her this request and she quit soon after. We visited another practice where a practice owner discounted a $1,500 dental and mass removal invoice by $600. This was done in the examination room in front of a technician who was only making $100 more a week than what was discounted. Even worse, this discount was given to a successful cardiologist in the area. This technician quit the following week. From these 2 examples, it is easy to see why discounting at a practice can be so problematic.

As mentioned, discounting is common in practice and too often has negative effects including: (1) Discounts can be very disruptive to the culture of a practice. Too often, inconsistent values form when doctors charge differently in a practice. This also can get the entire team in a mindset on keeping the invoice cost low, disregarding good care and patient results. (2) There are no reliable data showing that discounts in a practice grow clientele and repeatable business. Since dropped charges, intentional discounts, and bundled discounts are not itemized on an invoice, clients often are unaware of the benefit (3) Discounts are very unfair to those clients who did not receive the benefit. (4) Discounts directly rob your practice of earned profit. The practice has already performed the work; discounts take dollar for dollar away from your bottom line. Along those lines, why raise prices if you plan to discount to a comfortable ACT? (5) Discounts rob the practice of pay raises, better benefits, new equipment, continuing education, etc. Discounting only hurts your business, your team, and ultimately your ability to care for clients.

How to Change This

How does a practice know if veterinarians and staff are 'addicted' to discounts. First, ask doctors how much they discount. Most practice management software can monitor changed charges on invoices by DVM. Many have period totals of discounts. Compare with doctor's estimate. If the amount is large overall or much larger than estimated, the practice more than likely has a systemic discounting problem. If the Cost of Goods Sold as a percentage of revenues is excessive, above 28%, more than likely a discounting problem exists. A great method to check discounting is by finding the average fee charged for a service item and comparing it to the set fee (total revenues of item divided by the quantity of the item is compared to listed fee). If the difference is greater than 2% to 3% with several of your fees, the practice likely has a discounting problem.

Once a problem of discounting has been found, how does a practice change? First, the entire team needs to be aware of discounting behaviors, the magnitude of the problem at the practice and why the use of discounting must change. Second, we believe the practice should start with how the practice uses its software. All charges should be reviewed; any duplicates should be removed, and unclear descriptors should be changed; and blocks on changing the values of fees should be set except by approval. We were in 1 practice where cleaning and polishing for dentals was given a 10% discount. When we reviewed invoices of dentals, we noticed 10% was given off the entire invoice including other procedures and products.

We think it very important for doctors and head technicians to review fees at least twice per year for clarity on the charges and the appropriateness of the fee. Once a set fee list has been determined, everyone in the practice should review and understand. If discounting and dropped charges are a problem with a couple of people, make sure the veterinarian and technician look over the final invoice together to assure everything was captured and without discounts. If CSR's are giving discounts, dropping charges, or as we saw in many practices, cutting the quantity of products at check out, we recommend technicians check out clients in the examination room using credit card readers or quick response codes. Clients can leave with products given to them in the examination room. Again, when changing behavior with discounting, start with awareness of the problem, build desire to change (higher incomes, better equipment, better care, etc.), build systems that make it very inconvenient to discount, and monitor.

Some practices do appropriately discount. For any good purposes, we recommend keeping discounting under 5% of the charge and not cumulative. Exceptions include.

- Wanting client to accept additional care. Eg, agreeing to schedule a dental appointment today.
- Correcting a wrong. Eg, an unnecessarily long wait. Instead of discounting though, a more meaningful alternative to this example would be to give a gift certificate for coffee or ice cream. You still charge the same, showing no flexibility with your fees, but the client is rewarded for their inconvenience.
- Rewarding military or service providers. Only give 1 discount and not cumulative for having different qualifiers (eg, 15% off for veteran (5%), police (5%), over 60 (5%).

PROBLEM

Many practices fail to effectively control their inventory.

Explanation

With the increase in labor costs, many practices are looking for other opportunities to maintain their profit. One of those opportunity areas is with the cost of goods sold (COGS). For financial reporting, COGS is primarily the inventory cost of pharmaceuticals, vaccines, medical supplies, and diets as well as the cost of laboratories and cremation. Important is the relationship of COGS to practice total revenues, reported as a percentage of revenues. Healthy GP practices can get this value below 22% of revenues (practices with large boarding revenues can drive COGS much lower). Practices with COGS in excess of 25% typically have counterproductive behaviors creating a higher percentage. These include behaviors that suppress revenues such as discounting, dropped charges, low fees, and embezzlement. Many practices have too much inventory, too high and too deep! Too many options and too many of each option.

There are several behaviors that cause this including: (1) Bulk buying to cut down the number of times to order, often disguised as achieving a discount from a vendor. (2) Allowing doctors to order whatever pharmaceuticals or supplies they want regardless of cost or duplication. (3) Allowing clients to dictate what they want a practice to carry. (4) Wanting to be liked by the sales representative and ordering whatever they think appropriate (opposite of discounts given clients). (5) No management of inventory of turns, often holding past expiration date.

For most GP practices, 20%-40% of revenues are pharmaceuticals, vaccines, and diets. This is significant and needs to be managed and protected! We too often hear defeatism doctors and staff with prevention and pharmaceutical revenues being a lost cause because a practice can't compete with Chewy or Walmart. In my opinion, this is like saying the Ritz Carlton can't beat Best Western, because they both sell the same product, both have 4 walls, bathroom, bed, and television. What about the value a practice and a veterinarian add to the experience and care for the pet. We find bonded clients, wanting what is best for their pets, buying pharmaceuticals from the practice or the practice's online store.

Additionally, alternative pharmacy providers such as Chewy are starting to provide mail order laboratories (fecals and cytology). Most are getting very active in telemedicine, providing 24/7 access to veterinarians. These providers will script pharmaceuticals often without a Veterinary Client Patient Relationship (VCPR). Additionally, these companies can further mine clientele for prevention, pharmaceuticals, and service. While many believe practices and their patients are protected by the VCPR, we believe this may be short lived. First, most pet owners have no awareness of a VCPR. They follow ads on Facebook, LinkedIn, and Instagram. If a pet owner is technically savvy or under the age of 35 and did not realize a full value for price at the last veterinary appointment, telemedicine may provide a more convenient and personal experience even though examination, diagnosis, and treatment is subpar.

How to Change This

Serving as the source of medications and diets for your patients bonds clients to your practice. A practice should be seen as the 'go to' resource for products and services for their pet and having complete information on pet's care and their pet's Rx scripts is imperative in providing the best care. The more clients are in touch with your practice, either in person or via a client support portal, the stronger your relationship grows with those clients. However, when a practice has too many pharmaceutical options for patients such as with preventatives, doctors get confused, staff get confused and the client definitely gets confused with weak or no real recommendation except with what may be cheapest.

To deliver the best care and to cut down pharmacy options, we believe doctors should review all pharmaceuticals and decide what the practice should carry. First, determine if an Rx has purpose and common use, agree that no 2 Rx treat the patient the same way. Why do we have 2 Ivermectin products? (May want pill, liquid, injectable options). A new Rx must meet a unique need, be an improvement, or something not currently offered. This reminds me of my girls when they were younger. My wife was frustrated with the quantity of stuffed animals they collected each year, too many for my children to manage decently on their beds. She told both they could have 20 stuffed animals on their bed. First, they had to determine what stuffed animals they loved the most to get the number down from about 75. The new rule was that if they received another stuffed toy, it could only be brought in if it replaced 1 of the 20. Either way, a stuffed toy was sent to charity for another family to love. Additionally, each inventory line item should be evaluated on what is best for the patient, what is best for the client, and what is best for the practice. While most products are outstanding for the patient, many fall short for the second and third qualifier.

Once the doctors determine what needs to be in inventory, the inventory manager/practice manager should be the one who determines how much. One of the big problems we see with inventory management is that most practices don't have a person whose only responsibility is inventory management. Too often we see inventory control take a second level of importance to other practice responsibilities. Let's say a practice does $4M in revenue; and has a COGS at 30% or $1.2 M. How much more profit would a practice earn if the COGS dropped to 23% or even 17% as some have done? Is inventory worth a manager's full attention? We think so.

So, what products the practice carries should be primarily set by the veterinarians. How much should be carried should be set by the inventory managers. How much should be based on the historical quantities sold, how fast product quantities turn (turnover), and the availability of products. They should also be aware of the margins for products. We see some practices making the mistake of setting margins in the software. If the product cost continually increases, this practice is fine but what if practice takes advantage of a presale product discount? The practice will have no real gain on profit due to the drop in price with all savings passed on the client.

Lastly, everyone in a practice should have a firm "stop" based on the following.

- Is this product still relevant? Is it old? Should we carry the newer or upgraded formula?
- Is it a low volume product with better alternatives? Should we outsource or special order instead of keeping on shelf?
- Is the product in a similar class or does it offer similar benefits as other products? Which more popular with your doctors and clients?
- Does the hospital need the product immediately in case of an emergency? Is it a product you must always have!
- Once you stop, get it off your computer as soon as possible. If you can't, watch for future revenues for a product that is no longer carried.

ALL OF THE AFOREMENTIONED
Explanation

It may be hard to fathom, but there are practices that have ALL 9 of the earlier mentioned problems, to 1° or another, at the same time. The best thing we can say in these situations is that they recognized the issues and sought outside help.

How to Change This

Practice owners, managers, and administrators, must be fully aware of what is going on with their practices at all times. Using data and discussion to diagnose issues should be performed routinely.

It is strongly suggested that most practices can benefit from an appraisal (not for sale but for business purposes) of their practice value every 5 years or so to determine their profitability and based upon those results dive deeper to find ways to be more successful OR in a best-case scenario continue to replicate what is done well.

The last few years may have been a blip on the veterinary radar screen. However, based on our experiences in the thousands of hospitals we have visited, the pandemic revealed the multitude of issues that practices have long ignored. The future of the profession truly will be determined by the ability to address the aforementioned issues and others that impact the enjoyment and profitability of those in the profession.

CLINICS CARE POINTS

- It is essential that practices collectively develop and affirm a WHY statement around which the entire team can rally. Support that WHY statement or mission with a unanimously supported set of core values that guide the thinking, communication and service behaviors of team members in their interactions with one another and their stakeholders.

- Develop a preferred pathway to care that will serve as the cornerstone of your practices medicine. Best care is evidence based and intentional. Without a thoughtful approach to provide the most common medical services uncommonly well, a practice will regress in the quality and consistency of care that it offers and the practice will cease to function as a team and instead, resemble a collection of seemingly independent 1 doctor practices, operating under the same roof.

- Recruiting good team members is important but keeping them is even more important. A well established, engaged, and supportive on-boarding program is central to supporting and retaining healthcare team members. On-boarding is not a 1 size fits all orientation program. Successful practices explore the unique needs of every new team member and provide support tailored to the needs of those colleagues in order to optimize their personal fulfillment and their value to the practice.

- Work with your team members to provide clients with a healthcare experience and not merely a veterinary appointment. Create a healthcare environment in your practice where 'Mayo level' medicine is infused with 'Disney level client care' to create a value-added healthcare experience focused both on client education and patient care', appropriate to create patient outcomes marked by happy, healthy, pain-free longevity.

DISCLOSURE

"The authors have nothing to disclose."

REFERENCES

1. Website: Valcour M. Anyone can learn to Be A better leader. Harvard Business Review Leadership Development; 2020. Available at: https://hbr.org/2020/11/anyone-can-learn-to-be-a-better-leader%20%20/. Accessed July 10, 2023.
2. U.S. veterinarians 2020, American Veterinary Medical Association (avma.org).
3. 2023 AVMA Economic State of the Veterinary Profession.
4. Website, Porath C, Sublett C. Rekindling a sense of community at work. Harvard Business Review Leadership Development; 2022. Available at: https://hbr.org/2022/08/rekindling-a-sense-of-community-at-work. Accessed July 1, 2023.
5. Galloway S. Adrift: America in 100 Charts. USA: Penguin Random House; 2022. p. 64–5.
6. Website, Patel A, Plowman S. The increasing importance of a best friend at work. Gallup: Workplace; 2022. Available at: https://www.gallup.com/workplace/397058/increasing-importance-best-friend-work.aspx. Accessed April 22, 2023.
7. Website, Harter JUS. Employee engagement needs a rebound in 2023. Gallup: Workplace; 2022. Available at: https://www.gallup.com/workplace/468233/employee-engagement-needs-rebound-2023.aspx. Accessed April 22, 2023.
8. Website: U.S. Office of Personnel Management. Theodore Roosevelt, In Our Mission, Role and History. No Date. Available at: https://www.opm.gov/about-us/our-mission-role-history/theodore-roosevelt/Accessed July 30, 2023.

9. Website: U.S. Bureau of Labor Statistics. Employment-population ratio 16-19 yrs. FRED Economic Research; 2023. Available at: https://fred.stlouisfed.org/series/LNS12300012. Accessed June 30, 2023.

10. Website: Winstanely G. Mentoring programs fail (and how you can avoid them). Mentorloop; 2023. Available at: https://mentorloop.com/blog/7-reasons-mentoring-programs-fail/. Accessed June 5, 2023.

11. Website: Hirsch A. Don't underestimate the importance of good onboarding. In SHRM: Talent Acquisition. 2017. Available at: https://www.shrm.org/resource-sandtools/hr-topics/talent-acquisition/pages/don't-underestimate-the-impor-tance-of-effective-onboarding.aspx. Accessed: November 2022.

12. Lencioni P. The ideal team player: how to recognize and cultivate the three essential virtues. New Jersey: Jossey-Bass; 2016. p. 155–62.

13. Granovetter M. Social networks and getting A job. YouTube; 2016. Available at. https://youtu.be/g3bBajcR5fE. Accessed January 16, 2023.

14. Website: VetWatch. Veterinary Trend Watch: Monthly Insight For U.S. Veterinary Market Trends. Rolling Date. Available at: https://www.vetwatch.com/Accessed July 23, 2023.

15. Website: Frothingham S. How long does it take for a new behavior to become automatic? (medically reviewed by Timothy J. Legg, PhD, PsyD). Healthline 2019. Available at: https://www.healthline.com/health/how-long-does-it-take-to-form-a-habit#takeaway. Accessed June 13, 2023.

Moving?

Make sure your subscription moves with you!

To notify us of your new address, find your **Clinics Account Number** (located on your mailing label above your name), and contact customer service at:

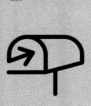

Email: journalscustomerservice-usa@elsevier.com

800-654-2452 (subscribers in the U.S. & Canada)
314-447-8871 (subscribers outside of the U.S. & Canada)

Fax number: 314-447-8029

Elsevier Health Sciences Division
Subscription Customer Service
3251 Riverport Lane
Maryland Heights, MO 63043

*To ensure uninterrupted delivery of your subscription, please notify us at least 4 weeks in advance of move.

9780443131455